Allergic Skin Diseases

Editors

PECK Y. ONG
PETER SCHMID-GRENDELMEIER

IMMUNOLOGY AND ALLERGY CLINICS OF NORTH AMERICA

www.immunology.theclinics.com

Consulting Editor
STEPHEN A. TILLES

February 2017 • Volume 37 • Number 1

ELSEVIER

1600 John F. Kennedy Boulevard • Suite 1800 • Philadelphia, Pennsylvania, 19103-2899

http://www.theclinics.com

IMMUNOLOGY AND ALLERGY CLINICS OF NORTH AMERICA Volume 37, Number 1

February 2017 ISSN 0889-8561, ISBN-13: 978-0-323-49651-3

Editor: Jessica McCool
Developmental Editor: Kristen Helm

Immunology and Allergy Clinics of North America (ISSN 0889–8561) is published quarterly by Elsevier Inc., 360 Park Avenue South, New York, NY 10010-1710. Months of issue are February, May, August, and November. Periodicals postage paid at New York, NY and additional mailing offices. Subscription prices are $320.00 per year for US individuals, $528.00 per year for US institutions, $100.00 per year for US students and residents, $395.00 per year for Canadian individuals, $220.00 per year for Canadian students, $670.00 per year for Canadian institutions, $445.00 per year for international individuals, $670.00 per year for international institutions, $220.00 per year for international students. To receive student/resident rate, orders must be accompanied by name of affiliated institution, date of term, and the *signature* of program/residency coordinator on institution letterhead. Orders will be billed at individual rate until proof of status is received. Foreign air speed delivery is included in all *Clinics* subscription prices. All prices are subject to change without notice. **POSTMASTER**: Send address changes to *Immunology and Allergy Clinics of North America*, Elsevier Health Sciences Division, Subscription Customer Service, 3251 Riverport Lane, Maryland Heights, MO 63043. **Customer Service: 1-800-654-2452 (U.S. and Canada); 314-447-8871 (outside U.S. and Canada). Fax: 314-447-8029. E-mail: journalscustomerservice-usa@elsevier.com (for print support); journalsonlinesupport-usa@elsevier.com (for online support).**

Reprints. For copies of 100 or more, of articles in this publication, please contact the Commercial Reprints Department, Elsevier Inc., 360 Park Avenue South, New York, New York 10010-1710. Tel. 212-633-3874, Fax: 212-633-3820, E-mail: reprints@elsevier.com.

Immunology and Allergy Clinics of North America is covered in MEDLINE/PubMed (Index Medicus), Current Contents/Life Sciences, Science Citation Index, ISI/BIOMED, Chemical Abstracts, and EMBASE/Excerpta Medica.

Contributors

CONSULTING EDITOR

STEPHEN A. TILLES, MD
Executive Director, ASTHMA Inc Clinical Research Center; Partner, Northwest Asthma
and Allergy Center; Clinical Professor of Medicine, University of Washington, Seattle,
Washington

EDITORS

PECK Y. ONG, MD
Division of Clinical Immunology and Allergy, Children's Hospital Los Angeles; Associate
Professor of Clinical Pediatrics, Department of Pediatrics, Keck School of Medicine,
University of Southern California, Los Angeles, California

PETER SCHMID-GRENDELMEIER, MD
Professor, Allergy Unit, Department of Dermatology, University and University Hospital of
Zurich; Christine-Kühne Center for Allergy Research and Education (CK-CARE), Zurich,
Switzerland

AUTHORS

SABINE ALTRICHTER, MD
Department of Dermatology and Allergy, Allergie-Centrum-Charité,
Charité – Universitätsmedizin Berlin, Berlin, Germany

FLORIAN ANZENGRUBER, MD
Department of Dermatology, University Hospital Zurich, Zurich, Switzerland

MEAGAN BARRETT, MD
Resident Physician, Department of Dermatology, Keck School of Medicine, University of
Southern California, Los Angeles, California

MURAT BAS, MD
Clinic of Otorhinolaryngology, Klinikum rechts der Isar, Technische Universität München,
Munich, Germany

MARK BOGUNIEWICZ, MD
Department of Pediatrics, National Jewish Health, University of Colorado School of
Medicine, Denver, Colorado

PHILIPP BOSSHARD, PhD
Mycology Laboratory, Department of Dermatology, University and University Hospital of
Zurich, Zurich, Switzerland

KNUT BROCKOW, MD
Department of Dermatology and Allergy Biederstein, Technische Universität München,
Munich, Germany

ADEEB BULKHI, MD
Fellow, Division of Allergy and Immunology, Department of Internal Medicine, University of South Florida, Tampa, Florida; Department of Internal Medicine, College of Medicine, Umm Al-Qura University, Makkah, Saudi Arabia

THOMAS B. CASALE, MD
Professor, Division of Allergy and Immunology, Department of Internal Medicine, University of South Florida, Tampa, Florida

ANDREW J. COOKE, MD
Fellow, Division of Allergy and Immunology, Department of Internal Medicine, University of South Florida, Tampa, Florida

MARJOLEIN S. DE BRUIN-WELLER, MD, PhD
Department of Dermatology & Allergology, University Medical Center Utrecht, Utrecht, The Netherlands

DAVID H. DREYFUS, MD, PhD
Associate Clinical Professor, Yale School of Medicine, Gesher LLC, Allergy, Asthma and Clinical Immunology, Waterbury, Connecticut

MASUTAKA FURUE, MD, PhD
Department of Dermatology, Kyushu University, Fukuoka, Japan

MARTIN ROBERT GAUDINSKI, MD
National Institute of Allergy and Infectious Diseases, NIH, Bethesda, Maryland

MARTIN GLATZ, MD
Allergy Unit, Department of Dermatology, University and University Hospital of Zurich; Christine-Kühne Center for Allergy Research and Education (CK-CARE), Zurich, Switzerland

CAROLINE GUILLOD, MD
Department of Dermatology, University Hospital Zurich, Zurich, Switzerland

TOMASZ HAWRO, MD
Department of Dermatology and Allergy, Allergie-Centrum-Charité, Charité – Universitätsmedizin Berlin, Berlin, Germany

DIRKJAN HIJNEN, MD, PhD
Department of Dermatology & Allergology, University Medical Center Utrecht, Utrecht, The Netherlands

MAKIKO KIDO-NAKAHARA, MD, PhD
Department of Dermatology, Kyushu University, Fukuoka, Japan

LISA KOSTNER, MD
Department of Dermatology, University Hospital Zurich, Zurich, Switzerland

MAREK L. KOWALSKI, MD, PhD
Professor and Chairman, Department of Immunology, Rheumatology and Allergy; Chair of Clinical Immunology and Microbiology, Medical University of Lodz, Lodz, Poland

MINNELLY LUU, MD
Assistant Professor of Clinical Dermatology, Department of Dermatology, Children's Hospital Los Angeles, Keck School of Medicine, University of Southern California, Los Angeles, California

MARCUS MAURER, MD
Department of Dermatology and Allergy, Allergie-Centrum-Charité,
Charité – Universitätsmedizin Berlin, Berlin, Germany

JOSHUA D. MILNER, MD
National Institute of Allergy and Infectious Diseases, NIH, Bethesda, Maryland

TAKESHI NAKAHARA, MD, PhD
Division of Skin Surface Sensing, Kyushu University, Fukuoka, Japan

ALEXANDER A. NAVARINI, MD, PhD
Department of Dermatology, University Hospital Zurich, Zurich, Switzerland

NOREEN HEER NICOL, PhD, RN, FNP
College of Nursing, University of Colorado, Aurora, Colorado

PECK Y. ONG, MD
Division of Clinical Immunology and Allergy, Children's Hospital Los Angeles; Associate
Professor of Clinical Pediatrics, Department of Pediatrics, Keck School of Medicine,
University of Southern California, Los Angeles, California

MIKE RECHER, MD
Immunodeficiency Clinic, Medical Outpatient Unit and Immunodeficiency Laboratory,
Department Biomedicine, University Hospital, Basel, Switzerland

PETER SCHMID-GRENDELMEIER, MD
Professor, Allergy Unit, Department of Dermatology, University and University Hospital of
Zurich; Christine-Kühne Center for Allergy Research and Education (CK-CARE), Zurich,
Switzerland

NICOLE SCHOEPKE, MD
Department of Dermatology and Allergy, Allergie-Centrum-Charité,
Charité – Universitätsmedizin Berlin, Berlin, Germany

ANNA SCHUCH, MD
Department of Dermatology and Allergy Biederstein, Technische Universität München,
Munich, Germany

FRANK SIEBENHAAR, MD
Department of Dermatology and Allergy, Allergie-Centrum-Charité,
Charité – Universitätsmedizin Berlin, Berlin, Germany

RADOSLAW SPIEWAK, MD, PhD
Department of Experimental Dermatology and Cosmetology, Faculty of Pharmacy,
Jagiellonian University Medical College, Krakow, Poland

DI SUN, MD, MPH
Department of Pediatrics, Keck School of Medicine, University of Southern California, Los
Angeles, California

JONATHAN S. TAM, MD
Assistant Professor, Division of Clinical Immunology and Allergy, Department of
Pediatrics, Children's Hospital Los Angeles, Los Angeles, California

JUDITH L. THIJS, MD
Department of Dermatology & Allergology, University Medical Center Utrecht, Utrecht,
The Netherlands

DUGARMAA ULZII, MD
Department of Dermatology, Kyushu University, Fukuoka, Japan

KARSTEN WELLER, MD
Department of Dermatology and Allergy, Allergie-Centrum-Charité,
Charité – Universitätsmedizin Berlin, Berlin, Germany

ANNA ZALEWSKA-JANOWSKA, MD, PhD
Department of Psychodermatology; Chair of Clinical Immunology and Microbiology,
Medical University of Lodz, Lodz, Poland

Contents

Atopic dermatitis and allergic urticaria are common conditions of the skin that can also be the presenting symptoms of uncommon diseases. Defects leading to immunodeficiency may be associated with atopic dermatitis or allergic urticaria. Unusually severe or otherwise atypical presentations of atopic dermatitis or allergic urticaria may lead to clinical suspicion of an underlying immunodeficiency.

Atopic dermatitis (AD) is a common inflammatory condition of the skin that is usually seen in childhood, but can onset or persist into adulthood. The characteristic distribution and morphology based on age, chronic relapsing course, and pruritus comprise the clinical criteria used in the diagnosis of AD. However, the numerous morphologies ranging from acute, weeping erythematous papules to chronic lichenified plaques, can be simulated by multiple other conditions, including inflammatory, infectious, neoplastic, and photo-dermatoses. Recognition of the distinguishing features and clinical mimickers of atopic dermatitis is vital for an accurate and timely diagnosis, and initiation of proper treatment regimens.

The use of standardized, valid, and reliable clinical measures is an important element in modern patient management, particularly in diseases that are not objectively assessable and are associated with a high disease burden. Chronic urticaria is such a disorder for which several new and well-developed clinical measures became available. These measures comprise tools to assess disease activity, disease control, and health-related quality-of-life impairment. This review provides an overview of the currently available clinical measures for chronic urticaria. In addition, it provides information on their strengths and limitations and how to best use them and evaluate their results.

Atopic dermatitis (AD) is a heterogeneous disease and many attempts have been made to define subsets of patients based on clinical character-istics. However, the current characterization of patients with AD might not adequately reflect the pathophysiologic diversity within patients with AD. This article reviews current biomarkers for AD and future perspectives. In the future, patients with AD will be stratified based on biomarker expres-sion levels in body fluids and tissue, genetic variants, or combined biomarker expression patterns. With new targeted therapies for AD currently investigated in clinical trials this will lead to better identification of patients that can benefit from these highly specific, but expensive new treatments.

There is little doubt that *Malassezia* spp plays a role in atopic dermatitis because it may interact with the local skin immune responses and barrier function, and sensitization against this skin-colonizing yeast can correlate with disease activity. Also, antifungal therapy shows beneficial effects in some patients. However, the pathogenetic mechanism and mutual inter-action between *Malassezia* spp and atopic dermatitis still remain partly un-clear and need further investigation.

Atopic dermatitis is characterized by the interplay of skin barrier defects with the immune system and skin microbiome that causes patients to be at risk for infectious complications. This article reviews the pathogenesis of atopic dermatitis and the mechanisms through which patients are at risk for infection from bacterial, viral, and fungal pathogens. Although these complications may be managed acutely, prevention of secondary in-fections depends on a multipronged approach in the maintenance of skin integrity, control of flares, and microbial pathogens.

Chronic urticaria (CU) is defined as wheals, angioedema, or both, that last more than 6 weeks. Second-generation antihistamines are considered the first-line therapy for CU. Unfortunately, many patients will fail antihista-mines and require alternative therapy, including immune response modi-fiers or biologics. Multiple biological agents have been evaluated for use in antihistamine-refractory CU, including omalizumab, rituximab, and intra-venous immunoglobulin; omalizumab is the most efficacious. Because of the success of omalizumab, multiple new biologics that are directed at the IgE pathway are under investigation. This review summarizes the rele-vant data regarding the efficacy of biologics in antihistamine-refractory CU.

Chronic itch in inflammatory skin diseases, such as atopic dermatitis, markedly diminishes the quality of life of affected individuals. Comprehensive progress has been made in understanding itch signaling and associated mediators in the skin, dorsal root ganglia, spinal cord, and central nervous system, which may amplify or suppress atopic itch. Conventional therapies for atopic dermatitis are capable of reducing atopic itch; however, most patients are not satisfied with the antipruritic capacity of conventional treatments. Exploring itch pathways and mechanisms may lead to novel therapeutic approaches for atopic itch.

National and international guidelines address stepwise atopic dermatitis (AD) management. Wet wrap therapy (WWT) is important as an acute therapeutic intervention for treatment of moderate to severe AD. Using clothing instead of bandages makes this intervention simpler, less time intensive, and less expensive. Education of patients and caregivers is critical to success; methodology must be standardized. Future studies must carefully describe all procedure components. Incorporation of validated outcomes tools would help with interpretation. WWT should be considered as a potential treatment option ahead of systemic immunosuppressive therapies for patients failing conventional therapy.

Allergic contact dermatitis (ACD) is a common skin disease caused by a T cell–mediated immune reaction to usually innocuous allergens. ACD can have grave medical and socioeconomic consequences. ACD and irritant contact dermatitis often occur together. A detailed history and clinical examination are crucial and guide patch testing, which is the gold standard to diagnose ACD. T-cell clones persisting in the skin may explain the tendency of ACD to relapse even after years of allergen avoidance. Traditional treatments for ACD are topical steroids, calcineurin inhibitors, phototherapy, retinoids (including the recent alitretinoin), and immunosuppressants. Targeted therapies are lacking.

This article updates current knowledge on epidemiology, risk factors, triggers, and management of anaphylaxis in patients with mastocytosis. Hyperactive mast cells and higher number of effector mast cells are speculated to facilitate anaphylaxis in this condition. In children, increased risk is limited to those with extensive skin involvement and high tryptase. In adults, manifestations of anaphylaxis are severe with high frequency of cardiovascular symptoms. Hymenoptera stings are the most common triggers for these reactions; however, idiopathic anaphylaxis and reactions to food or drugs occur. Patients with mastocytosis should be informed about risk of anaphylaxis and prescribing emergency self-medication and installing emergency preparedness before general anesthesia is considered.

Drug hypersensitivity reactions may manifest with either organ-specific or systemic symptoms, but cutaneous eruptions are the most common manifestations. Different medications may cause identical skin symptoms, whereas hypersensitivity to a single drug may manifest with various patterns of symptoms depending on the pathomechanism of hypersensitivity. Drug reactions should be also taken into account in the differential diagnosis of numerous skin rashes. Analysis of morphology of drug-induced lesions, about potential immunologic or nonimmunological mechanisms, is important for the final diagnosis. Thus, here the authors present a morphologic approach to the diagnosis of cutaneous drug-induced eruptions.

The angiotensin-converting-enzyme inhibitor induced angioedema (ACEi AE) is the most commen angioedema in the upper airway. The bradykinin B2 receptor antagonist icatibant is effective in ACEi AE. The drug is not approved officially for this indication and has to be administered in an emergency situation off-label. Corticosteroids or antihistamines do not seem to work in this condition. The effectiveness of C1-esterase-inhibitor in ACEi AE must be verified in a double-blind study.

Differential diagnosis of urticaria and angioedema has been based on the phenotype as either acute or chronic depending on the duration of more than 6 to 8 weeks, respectively. Additional subdivisions include poorly defined terms such as idiopathic, spontaneous, or autoimmune. In this article, the author suggests that an increased understanding of the acquired and innate immune system and data from novel proteomic technology have blurred the lines between these categories of diagnosis. Specific molecular pathways and response to specific medications should be incorporated in classification and diagnosis schemes.

Hypersensitivity reactions to foods can have diverse and highly variable manifestations. Cutaneous reactions, such as acute urticaria and angioedema, are among the most common manifestations of food allergy. However, cutaneous manifestations of food allergy encompass more than just IgE-mediated processes and include atopic dermatitis, contact dermatitis, and even dermatitis herpetiformis. These cutaneous manifestations provide an opportunity to better understand the diversity of adverse immunologic responses to food and the interconnected pathways that produce them.

IMMUNOLOGY AND ALLERGY CLINICS OF NORTH AMERICA

FORTHCOMING ISSUES

May 2017
Biologic Therapies of Immunologic Diseases
Bradley E. Chipps and Stephen P. Peters, *Editors*

August 2017
Angioedema
Marc Riedl, *Editor*

November 2017
Drug Hypersensitivity and Desensitizations
Mariana C. Castells, *Editor*

RECENT ISSUES

November 2016
Aspirin-Exacerbated Respiratory Disease
Andrew A. White, *Editor*

August 2016
Severe Asthma
Rohit K. Katial, *Editor*

May 2016
Rhinitis
Jonathan A. Bernstein, *Editor*

ISSUE OF RELATED INTEREST

Dermatologic Clinics, July 2015 (Vol. 33, No. 3)
Granulomatous Disorders of Adult Skin
Joseph C. English, *Editor*
Available at: http://www.derm.theclinics.com/

THE CLINICS ARE AVAILABLE ONLINE!
Access your subscription at:
www.theclinics.com

Foreword

Allergic Skin Disease and the Practicing Allergist: Growing Unmet Need, New Science, and New Treatments

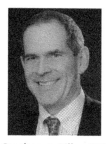

Stephen A. Tilles, MD
Consulting Editor

Historically, allergic skin diseases have taken a back seat to allergic respiratory diseases in the day-to-day practices of Allergy/Immunology specialists. For many decades, our clinics were fine tuned to primarily perform efficient consultations for allergic rhinitis and asthma, including same-day specific immunoglobulin E (IgE) testing to confirm which inhalant allergens were responsible for the patient's suffering. Back in the day, in the absence of effective and well-tolerated pharmaceutical treatments, we recommended immunotherapy for the majority of these patients, and its impressive efficacy has withstood the test of time. In the past three decades, with the advent of a plethora of safe and effective treatment strategies, including second-generation antihistamines, intranasal corticosteroids, and high-potency inhaled corticosteroids—combined with continued refinements in allergen immunotherapy strategies—we have seen the unmet needs in allergic rhinitis and asthma shrink drastically.

Diagnoses such as atopic dermatitis and chronic urticaria have always been on our "top 10" list, but until recently, these were relatively uncommon primary reasons for referral to an allergist. Well, times have changed. Together with IgE-mediated food allergy, allergic skin diseases have asserted themselves as major drivers of Allergy/Immunology referrals, and treatment paradigms for these diagnoses are also changing. In the case of atopic dermatitis, there has been tremendous progress in our understanding of its underlying pathophysiology, including the genetic and epigenetic factors responsible for challenging phenotypes. This knowledge has led to remarkably effective new treatments that are just now becoming available. Our clinical approach to chronic urticaria is also much different now than it was 10 years ago. We still do not understand its cause, but we do know that a thorough clinical history and Systems

Immunol Allergy Clin N Am 37 (2017) xiii–xiv
http://dx.doi.org/10.1016/j.iac.2016.10.002
immunology.theclinics.com

Review are more helpful than an elaborate diagnostic workup. In addition, the seren-dipitous realization that monoclonal anti-IgE works well for many of the most refractory chronic idiopathic urticarial cases has resulted in a significant upgrade in our treat-ment armamentarium.

This issue of *Immunology and Allergy Clinics of North America* contains a practical collection of articles geared to help clinicians who evaluate and treat chronic skin dis-eases. There is an overall emphasis on differential diagnosis, biomarker utility, and treatment strategies that will no doubt serve as a useful reference for both primary physicians and Allergy/Immunology specialists.

Stephen A. Tilles, MD
ASTHMA Inc. Clinical Research Center
Northwest Asthma and Allergy Center
University of Washington
9725 Third Avenue Northeast, Suite 500
Seattle, WA 98115, USA

E-mail address:
stilles@nwasthma.com

Preface

Allergic Skin Diseases

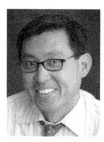 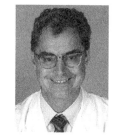

Peck Y. Ong, MD   Peter Schmid-Grendelmeier, MD
Editors

The current issue on Allergic Skin Diseases aims to provide a collection of practical tools for clinicians in their management of common allergic skin diseases, such as atopic dermatitis and urticaria. These tools include differential diagnosis, measurement of severity, evaluation of triggers, and treatments for severe cases and complications. Drs Gaudinski and Milner provided their insight on the pathogenesis and differential diagnosis of atopic dermatitis and urticaria based on a monogenetic approach of primary immunodeficiency conditions. A practical pictorial guide for the differential diagnosis of atopic dermatitis was delivered by Drs Barrett and Luu. Dr Weller and colleagues and Drs Thijs, de Bruin-Weller, and Hijnen contributed with updated reviews on the clinical measures and biomarkers for chronic urticaria and atopic dermatitis, respectively. Infectious triggers and complications of atopic dermatitis were discussed by Drs Glatz, Bosshard, and Schmid-Grendelmeier, and Drs Sun and Ong. Drs Bulkhi, Cooke, and Casale summarized the use of biologics in chronic urticaria, whereas Dr Kido-Nakahara and colleagues and Drs Nicol and Boguniewicz provided a concise review of potential anti-itch medications and a practical guide on wet wrap therapy for atopic dermatitis, respectively. In addition, this issue includes other allergic skin diseases and related conditions that are commonly encountered by primary physicians and allergists, including allergic contact dermatitis (Dr Kostner and colleagues), mastocytosis (Drs Schuch and Brockow), drug allergy (Drs Zalewska-Janowska, Spiewak, and Kowalski), angioedema (Drs Bas and Dreyfus), and food allergy (Dr Tam). These authors share their perspectives from Europe and

Immunol Allergy Clin N Am 37 (2017) xv–xvi
http://dx.doi.org/10.1016/j.iac.2016.10.001
0889-8561/17/© 2016 Published by Elsevier Inc.

immunology.theclinics.com

the United States on each topic. We hope that this issue will add to the clinicians' armamentarium in their day-to-day management of these diseases.

Peck Y. Ong, MD
Division of Clinical Immunology and Allergy
Children's Hospital Los Angeles
Department of Pediatrics
University of Southern California
Keck School of Medicine
4650 Sunset Boulevard, MS 75
Los Angeles, CA 90027, USA

Peter Schmid-Grendelmeier, MD
Allergy Unit, Department of Dermatology
University Hospital of Zurich
Christine-Kühne Center for Allergy Research
and Education (CK-CARE)
Gloriastrasse 31
8091 Zurich, Switzerland

E-mail addresses:
pyong@chla.usc.edu (P.Y. Ong)
peter.schmid@usz.ch (P. Schmid-Grendelmeier)

Atopic Dermatitis and Allergic Urticaria

Cutaneous Manifestations of Immunodeficiency

Martin Robert Gaudinski, MD, Joshua D. Milner, MD*

KEYWORDS

- Atopic dermatitis • Urticaria • Immunodeficiency

KEY POINTS

- Atopic dermatitis and allergic urticaria are common conditions of the skin that can also be the presenting symptoms of uncommon diseases.
- Defects leading to immunodeficiency may be associated with atopic dermatitis or allergic urticaria.
- Unusually severe or otherwise atypical presentations of atopic dermatitis or allergic urticaria may lead to clinical suspicion of an underlying immunodeficiency.

...for people who feel disgraced blush, and those who fear death turn pale.[1]

INTRODUCTION

Alterations in the skin can give the astute clinician insight into the inner workings of the immune system that may otherwise remain invisible. The skin can be altered in numerous ways via numerous pathologic mechanisms. This review focuses on 2 of those alterations: atopic dermatitis (AD) and allergic urticaria (AU). Although AD and AU are common in themselves, they may also serve to be the presenting sign of an uncommon underlying disease. More specifically, this review focuses on how these 2 conditions may be accompanied by other sentinel symptoms serving to comprise a distinct syndromic phenotype. The presence of the syndromic phenotype may then serve as a clue to the presence of an underlying immune defect. The objective of this review is to provide a differential diagnosis for both conditions as they relate to those immune defects to provide a diagnostic pathway to aid in establishing a diagnosis. Infectious, oncologic, or other causes leading to AD and AU will not be considered here.

This study was supported by the Division of Intramural Research of the NIAID, NIH (ZO1 1ZIAAI001098-02).

National Institute of Allergy and Infectious Diseases, Genetics and Pathogenesis of Allergy Section, 10 Center Drive, Building 10 Room 11N240A, Bethesda, MD 20814, USA
* Corresponding author. 10 Center Drive, NIH Building, 10CRC 5-3950, Bethesda, MD 20892.
E-mail address: jdmilner@niaid.nih.gov

ATOPIC DERMATITIS

AD is a chronic condition characterized by pruritic skin lesions related to epithelial barrier dysfunction with an immunologic involvement. It affects between 10% and 20% of children in developed countries, making it one of the most common diseases of childhood.[2] Adult presentation of AD should prompt consideration of an alternate diagnosis. AD is a complex disorder consisting of a constellation of historical and physical features but lacking a pathognomonic sign or biomarker. As such, diagnostic criteria have been established to support AD as a clinical diagnosis. The modified UK Working Party's Diagnostic Criteria for Atopic Dermatitis[3] (**Box 1**) is widely used and validated.[4] The lesions can affect the scalp, face, and extensor surfaces in infants, whereas the flexor surfaces become more commonly affected in older children and adults. Immunoglobulin E (IgE) and peripheral eosinophilia frequently accompany AD. The loss of skin epithelial barrier integrity is a key concept in understanding the structural defects leading to AD. Genetic studies of AD have been able to provide insights into some of the genes involved in epithelial integrity.[5] Treatment of AD is meant to reestablish epithelial barrier integrity and limit the effects of allergic inflammation.

ALLERGIC URTICARIA

Urticaria can be either acute or chronic and is characterized by mast cell degranulation leading to a raised central wheal with surrounding erythematous flaring. Mast cell degranulation may be prompted by a variety of triggers. As such, urticarial lesions may be due to physical, allergic, or autoimmune causes. Physical urticarias cause direct mast cell degranulation and comprise 20% to 30% of chronic urticaria.[6] Stimuli can include heat, cold, and vibration even in the absence of specific antigens. In addition, autoantibodies are associated with 30% to 50% of chronic urticaria.[7] Acute urticarial lesions may develop as a result of IgE-mediated responses of mast cells to a specific antigen. Treatment of urticaria is aimed at limiting the affects of products released during mast cell degranulation as well as stabilizing or otherwise preventing mast cells from degranulating in the first place. Although physical and autoimmune urticaria needs to be within the differential of chronic urticaria, this review focuses on conditions for which urticaria is feature of a broader syndromic phenotype.

Box 1
Revised criteria for the diagnosis of atopic dermatitis

- Pruritis

Plus 3 or more of the following:

- History of flexural dermatitis (front of elbows, back of knees, front of ankles, neck, around the eyes) or involvement of cheeks and/or extensor surfaces in children aged less than 18 months
- Visible flexural dermatitis involving the skin creases (or the cheeks and/or extensor surfaces in children aged <18 months)
- History of a dry skin in the past year
- History of asthma or hay fever (or atopic disease in a first degree relative in children <4 years of age)
- Onset less than 2 years of age (for children aged ≥4 years at time of diagnosis)

ALARM SIGNS

Given that both AD and AU are common conditions affecting both children and adults alike, there must be distinguishing features that can alert the clinician to consider alternative diagnoses that would make the initially observable skin changes secondary to a primary underlying process. The presence of other features, which can be subtle in nature, can serve to create a syndromic pattern when paired with the skin changes common to AD and AU. These features can include age of onset, severity of disease, concomitant infections unrelated to skin disruption serving as an infectious nidus, as well as a variety of other traits uncommon to AD or AU themselves. **Table 1** summarizes these features.

SPECIFIC SYNDROMIC DISEASES GIVING RISE TO ATOPIC DERMATITIS
Omenn Syndrome

Omenn syndrome is characterized by severe erythroderma, lymphadenopathy, eosinophilia, and immunodeficiency from traditional opportunistic pathogens such as pneumocystis as well as cytomegalovirus and parainfluenza. The underlying defect is typically due to hypomorphic mutations in V(D)J recombination, but numerous gene mutations leading to a variety of changes have been identified, including changes in IL7Ralpha,[8] IL2Rgamma,[9,10] CHD7,[11] ADA,[12] RMRP,[13] and AK2.[14] These mutations lead to a downstream effect of abnormal T- and B-cell development, which can cause an activated autoreactive T-cell phenotype manifested as T cells infiltrating organs, including the skin, and the formation of autoantibodies. Thymic biopsies show distorted architecture and gene expression with limited FOXP3+ cells leading to a lack of central tolerance.[15]

Atypical Complete DiGeorge Syndrome

DiGeorge syndrome is manifested by congenital cardiac abnormalities, hypoparathyroidism, and patients who have very low T cells from the lack of thymic tissue can have complete DiGeorge syndrome. Patients with atypical complete DiGeorge syndrome can develop symptoms similar to Omenn syndrome. In addition, although they are more likely to have an itchy rash, and there is a strong trend that they acquire the diagnosis of AD more frequently than controls, one review of patients found that this was not statistically significant.[16] The severe AD can often have a later onset than other manifestations of DiGeorge syndrome.

Autosomal-Dominant Hyperimmunoglobulin E with Recurrent Infections Syndrome

Autosomal-dominant hyperimmunoglobulin E with recurrent infections syndrome (AD-HIES; Jobs syndrome) leads to an AD-like rash,[17] skin abscesses, pneumonia with pneumatocele formation, skeletal abnormalities including scoliosis, retained primary teeth, abnormal facies, and a characteristically elevated IgE level. The dermatitis is notable in that it frequently occurs immediately after birth and nearly always within 4 weeks of life. Its distribution is less typical than other forms of AD and occurs behind the scalp, ears, back, and buttocks. The phenotype is due to dominant negative mutations in STAT3.[18,19] STAT3 is a gene encoding for a protein involved in a myriad of intracellular signaling functions. The mutation seen in AD-HIES leads to specific findings of increased serum IgE, decreased T- and B-cell populations, decreased Th17 cells, and decreased Th17 cytokines,[20,21] but the mechanism behind which many of these clinical features are caused remains obscure.

Table 1
Immunodeficiencies with Atopic Features

AD	Clinical Features Seen in Addition to Skin Manifestations	Gene Mutation	Laboratory Changes	Estimated Prevalence if Known
Netherton syndrome	Trichorrhexis invaginatum, recurrent infections, failure to thrive, food allergy, angioedema	SPINK5	High IgE	1–9/1,000,000
Omenn syndrome	Lymphadenopathy, recurrent infections, eosinophilia	SCID Genes	Lymphopenia, hypogammaglobulinemia	<1/1,000,000
Autosomal-dominant hyper-IgE syndrome	Skin abscesses, pneumatoceles, joint hypermobility, abnormal facies, retained primary teeth, coronary artery aneurysms	STAT3	High IgE	1–9/100,000
DOCK8 deficiency	Viral skin infections, food allergy, asthma, malignancy	DOCK8	Lymphopenia, low IgM, high IgE	<1/1,000,000
WAS	Bleeding diatheses, recurrent infections, autoimmunity	WASP	Thrombocytopenia, microplatelets	1–9/1,000,000
IPEX	Polyendocrinopathy, chronic diarrhea	FOXP3	High IgE	<1/1,000,000
DiGeorge syndrome	Congenital heart defects, abnormal facies, hypoparathyroidism	chr22q11	T-cell lymphopenia	1/2000–4000 live births
PGM3 deficiency	myoclonus, neurocognitive impairment, recurrent Epstein-Barr virus and sinopulmonary infections leading to bronchiectasis	PGM3	Lymphopenia, high IgE	

SAM syndrome	Severe atopy, metabolic wasting, hypotrichosis, microcephaly	DSG	High IgE	<1/1,000,000
AU				
PLAID	Cold urticaria, recurrent infections, granulomatous disease, autoimmunity	PLCG2	Decreased B cells, NK cells, increased IgE	<1/1,000,000
Familial vibratory urticaria	Lifelong vibratory urticaria, obesity	ADGRE2		
Nonallergic "urticarias"				
Neutrophilic dermatoses (formerly called urticaria)				
FCAS	Cold urticaria, fevers, arthritis, conjunctivitis	NLRP3	Neutrophilia, thrombocytosis, increased acute phase reactants, increased serum amyloid A	
MWS	Urticaria, fevers, arthritis, conjunctivitis, sensorineural hearing loss	NLRP3	Neutrophilia, thrombocytosis, increased acute phase reactants, increased serum amyloid A	
NOMID	Urticaria, fevers, arthritis, conjunctivitis, sensorineural hearing loss, cognitive impairment	NLRP3	Neutrophilia, thrombocytosis, increased acute phase reactants, increased serum amyloid A	

DOCK8 Deficiency

DOCK8 deficiency may appear similar to AD-HIES with an elevated serum IgE and associated skin findings, but includes a more atopic signal with asthma and food allergy. There is also an increased susceptibility to cutaneous viral infections. As opposed to AD-HIES, DOCK8 deficiency has an autosomal-recessive inheritance pattern. In addition to the atopic and infectious manifestations of DOCK8 deficiency, the underlying risk of malignancy from either lymphoma or squamous cell carcinomas is the major risk to life and the impetus for bone marrow transplantation in the treatment of this disease. DOCK8 is part of the family that is implicated in cytoskeletal arrangements important for cell adhesion, migration, and structure.[22] DOCK8 expression is largely limited to cells of the immune system. It serves as a Rho GTPase activating CDC42. The mutation leads to profound effects on T-cell differentiation and survival[23] and cause a specific defect in lymphocyte migration to the skin, potentially explaining the predilection toward cutaneous infection.[24]

Wiskott-Aldrich Syndrome

Wiskott-Aldrich syndrome (WAS) is an X-linked deficiency of the WASP protein, which leads to poor actin polymerization and resulting dysfunction of hematopoietic cells, including immune cells and platelets. There may be an analogous mechanism between the cytoskeletal defects seen in DOCK8 deficiency and WAS, which are both involved in immune dysfunction. Poor actin polymerization leads to a variety of effects across many of the hematopoietic lineages. Myeloid cells fail to phagocytose properly, and their chemotaxis is impaired. Lymphoid cells including T cell and NK cells have difficulty forming effective immunologic synapses, and B-cell function is impaired due to poor T-cell function. Platelets are small and poorly functional leading to bleeding as a prominent clinical feature. The autoimmunity seen in WAS may be due to abnormal Treg function.[25,26]

PGM3 Deficiency

Patients with PGM3 deficiency can present with AD, atopy of any kind, increased serum IgE, myoclonus, neurocognitive impairment associated with dysmyelination, and recurrent EBV and sinopulmonary infections leading to bronchiectasis.[27] The mutations in PGM3 lead to dysfunctional protein glycosylation due to impaired Pgm3 and underproduction of intracellular UDP-GlcNAc, a basic building block of n- and o-linked glycosylation.[28] The exact mechanism as to why alterations in protein glycosylation would result in this phenotype is unclear, but these patients demonstrate and increase in Th2 and Th17 cytokine production.[29]

Immune Dysregulation Polyendocrinopathy Enteropathy X-Linked

Immune dysregulation polyendocrinopathy enteropathy X-linked (IPEX) is a dysregulation of the immune system that leads to multiple autoimmune manifestations and prominent AD. The underlying dysfunction is the loss of function of FOXP3 and resultant absence of regulatory T cells (Treg). Treg cells play a critical role in the prevention of autoimmune disease and self-reactivity,[30] and indeed discovering the loss of Treg cells in IPEX played a critical role as an "experiment of nature" in defining their role. The AD is an early manifestation of the disease and occurs early in infancy. It may be accompanied by other skin manifestations of autoimmune disease such as alopecia universalis.[31] Although enteropathy and chronic watery diarrhea are a constant feature of IPEX, the typical sentinel feature of the disease leading to its diagnosis is autoimmune phenomenon, such as early type I diabetes. End organ manifestations also include thyroiditis, autoimmune cytopenias, hepatitis, interstitial lung disease, and adrenal failure. IgE-mediated food allergy is an additional feature of the atopic character of IPEX.[32]

Netherton and Severe Dermatitis-Multiple Allergies-Metabolic Wasting Syndrome

Mutations in structural skin proteins can also lead to severe AD. Netherton syndrome is characterized by a severe ichthyosis, atopic disease, and pathognomonic changes in the hair shaft resembling bamboo and known as trichorrhexis invaginatum.[33] Food allergy, asthma, and angioedema can accompany the skin disease. Immunodeficiency is also a feature of the disease with patients having an increased rate of respiratory and gastrointestinal infections. The underlying defect is in a mutation in SPINK5, which leads to loss of function of LEKTI.[34] SPINK5 is associated with skin epithelial barrier function, which is thought to be relevant in developing ichthyosis associated with SPINK5 mutations, but patients also have poor vaccine responses. Subsequent initiation of immunoglobulin replacement therapy has been shown to help both the rate of infections and the skin integrity.[35]

Mutations in DSG1 and DSP, both skin junctional barrier proteins, can lead to severe dermatitis-multiple allergies-metabolic wasting (SAM) syndrome, associated with severe atopy and metabolic wasting, and can also be associated with other congenital malformations such as microcephaly and structural heart defects, among others.

SPECIFIC DISEASES GIVING RISE TO ALLERGIC URTICARIA
Phospholipase Cγ2–Associated Antibody Deficiency

Patients with phospholipase Cγ2-associated antibody deficiency (PLAID) were discovered in the context of familial cold urticaria that was life long.[36] Typical cold-induced urticaria, by contrast, is later onset and transient. Further elucidation of the phenotype led to an understanding that it can include antibody deficiency, frequent infections, autoimmunity, and granulomatous disease.[37] The cold urticaria is universal, whereas the other traits are seen to a lesser degree. This phenotype is caused by mutations in PLCG2 leading to alterations in the function of PLCγ2.[38] These mutations lead to a complex effect on intracellular signaling, which is at least partially dependent on temperature. The PLCG2 mutations in PLAID patients are deletions in an autoregulatory unit of the protein, which, when absent, renders the protein more constitutively active, more so in the cold. This activity actually leads to activation of the mast cell at lower temperatures, which accounts for the cold urticaria observed in these patients. The active enzyme paradoxically leads to impaired signaling at physiologic temperatures.

Vibratory Urticaria due to ADGRE2 Mutations

Physical causes of mast cell degranulation are well known, but at least one form of physical urticaria has been associated with a specific mutation affecting mast cell function. Vibratory urticaria inherited in an autosomal-dominant pattern has been shown to be due to mutations in ADGRE2. ADGRE2 is a membrane-bound autoinhibitory unit on the mast cell. Mutations in this protein cause structural fragility, which when disrupted by mechanical stress leads to easy mast cell activation with vibratory stimuli.[39]

Autoinflammatory Syndromes

Autoinflammatory syndromes are a series of disease entities that are caused by abnormal inflammatory responses not caused by antibody or cellular attacks on self. In some cases, mutations in genes involved in the formation of the inflammasome, an intracellular complex that responds to activated pattern recognition receptors in order to induce inflammation through interleukin-1β (IL-1β) and IL-18,[40] can lead to phenotypes with a variety of manifestations, including what appear to be urticarial lesions. These lesions have historically been described as urticarial; however, they are due to neutrophils, not mast cells, and do not result from immediate hypersensitivity. At least 3 such disorders are accompanied by urticarial manifestations: familial cold autoinflammatory syndrome (FCAS), Muckle-Wells syndrome (MWS), and neonatal onset multisystem inflammatory syndrome (NOMID). Quite different from the AU described above, the syndromes are also accompanied by periodic fever, arthritis, conjunctivitis, and other organ-specific and systemic inflammation.

SUMMARY

AD and AU are commonly seen in clinical practice, but when coupled to unusual features, they may constitute a syndrome distinctive for an immunologic defect. These rare syndromes have been able to disclose many mechanisms within the immune system that otherwise would remain obscure. New modes of treatment have been implemented that can modulate the immune dysfunction. In some cases, these immune defects necessitate replacing the immune compartment with a hematopoietic stem cell transplant. Through both mechanistic discovery and patient care, these syndromes present a unique opportunity for the observant physician.

REFERENCES

1. Barnes J. Aristotle, Nichomachean Ethics. Princeton (NJ): Princeton University Press; 1984.
2. Williams H, Robertson C, Stewart A, et al. Worldwide variations in the prevalence of symptoms of atopic eczema in the International Study of Asthma and Allergies in Childhood. J Allergy Clin Immunol 1999;103:125–38.
3. Williams HC, Burney PG, Hay RJ, et al. The U.K. Working Party's Diagnostic Criteria for Atopic Dermatitis. Br J Dermatol 1994;131:383–96.
4. Brenninkmeijer EE, Schram ME, Leeflang MM, et al. Diagnostic criteria for atopic dermatitis: a systematic review. Br J Dermatol 2008;158(4):754.
5. Morar N, Willis-Owen SA, Moffat MF, et al. The genetics of atopic dermatitis. J Allergy Clin Immunol 2006;118(1):24–34.
6. Dice JP. Physical urticaria. Immunol Allergy Clin North Am 2004;24(2):22504.
7. Bernstein JA, Lang DM, Khan DA, et al. The diagnosis and management of acute and chronic urticaria: 2014 update. J Allergy Clin Immunol 2014;133:127014.
8. Giliani S, Bonfim C, de Saint Basile G, et al. Omenn syndrome in an infant with IL7RA gene mutation. J Pediatr 2006;148(2):272–4.
9. Shibata F, Toma T, Wada T, et al. Skin infiltration of CD56(bright) CD16(2) natural killer cells in a case of X-SCID with Omenn syndrome-like manifestations. Eur J Haematol 2007;79(1):81–5.
10. Gruber TA, Shah AJ, Hernandez M, et al. Clinical and genetic heterogeneity in Omenn syndrome and severe combined immune deficiency. Pediatr Transplant 2009;13(2):244–50.
11. Gennery AR, Slatter MA, Rice J, et al. Mutations in CHD7 in patients with CHARGE syndrome cause T-B + natural killer cell + severe combined immune deficiency and may cause Omenn-like syndrome. Clin Exp Immunol 2008;153(1):75–80.

12. Roifman CM, Zhang J, Atkinson A, et al. Adenosine deaminase deficiency can present with features of Omenn syndrome. J Allergy Clin Immunol 2008;121(4): 1056–8.

13. Roifman CM, Gu Y, Cohen A. Mutations in the RNA component of RNase mitochondrial RNA processing might cause Omenn syndrome. J Allergy Clin Immunol 2006;117(4):897–903.

14. Henderson LA, Frugoni F, Hopkins G, et al. First reported case of Omenn syndrome in a patient with reticular dysgenesis. J Allergy Clin Immunol 2013; 131(4):1227–30.

15. Cassani B, Poliani PL, Moratto D, et al. Defect of regulatory T cells in patients with Omenn syndrome. J Allergy Clin Immunol 2010;125(1):209–16.

16. Staple L, Andrews T, McDonald-McGinn D, et al. Allergies in patients with chromosome 22q11.2 deletion syndrome (DiGeorge syndrome/velocardiofacial syndrome) and patients with chronic granulomatous disease. Pediatr Allergy Immunol 2005;16(3):226–30.

17. Eberting CL, Davis J, Puck JM, et al. Dermatitis and the newborn rash of hyper-IgE syndrome. Arch Dermatol 2004;140(9):1119–25.

18. Holland SM, DeLeo FR, Elloumi HZ, et al. STAT3 mutations in the hyper-IgE syndrome. N Engl J Med 2007;18:1608–19.

19. Minegishi Y, Saito M, Tsuchiya S, et al. Dominant negative mutations in the DNA-binding domain of STAT3 cause hyper IgE syndrome. Nature 2007;448:1058–62.

20. Milner JD, Brenchley JM, Laurence A, et al. Impaired Th17 cell differentiation in subjects with autosomal dominant hyper-IgE syndrome. Nature 2008;452:773–6.

21. DeBeaucoudrey L, Puel A, Filipe-Santos O, et al. Mutations in STAT3 and IL12RB1 impair the development of human IL-17 producing cells. J Exp Med 2008;205: 1543–50.

22. Meller N, Merlot S, Guda C. CZH proteins: a new family of Rho-GEFs. J Cell Sci 2005;118:4937–46.

23. Su HC, Jing H, Zhang Q. DOCK8 deficiency. Ann New York Acad Sci 2011;1246: 26–33.

24. Zhang Q, Dove CG, Hor JL, et al. DOCK8 regulates lymphocyte shape integrity for skin antiviral immunity. J Exp Med 2014;211(13):2549–66.

25. Maillard MH, Cotta-de-Almeida V, Takeshima F, et al. The Wiskott-Aldrich syndrome protein is required for the function of CD4(+)CD25(+)Foxp3(+) regulatory T cells. J Exp Med 2007;204:381–91.

26. Marangoni F, Trifari S, Scaramuzza S, et al. WASP regulates suppressor activity of human and murine CD4(+)CD25(+)FOXP3(+) natural regulatory T cells. J Exp Med 2007;204:369–80.

27. Hay BN, Martin JE, Karp B, et al. Familial immunodeficiency with cutaneous vasculitis, myoclonus, and cognitive impairment. Am J Med Gene A 2004; 125A(2):145–51.

28. Zhang Y, Yu X, Ichikawa M, et al. Autosomal recessive phosphoglucomutase 3 (PGM3) mutations link glycosylation defects to atopy, immune deficiency, autoimmunity, and neurocognitive impairment. J Allergy Clin Immunol 2014;133(5): 1400–9.

29. Yang L, Fliegauf M, Grimbacher B. Hyper-IgE syndromes: reviewing PGM3 deficiency. Curr Opin Pediatr 2014;26(6):697–703.

30. Josefowicz SZ, Lu LF, Rudensky AY. Regulatory T cells: mechanisms of differentiation and function. Annu Rev Immunol 2012;30:531–64.

31. Nieves DS, Phipps RP, Pollock SJ, et al. Dermatologic and immunologic findings in the immune dysregulation, polyendocrinopathy, enteropathy, X-linked syndrome. Arch Dermatol 2004;140(4):466–72.

32. Torgerson TR, Linane A, Moes N, et al. Severe food allergy as a variant of IPEX syndrome caused by a deletion in a noncoding region of the FOXP3 gene. Gastroenterology 2007;132(5):1705–17.

33. Wilkinson RD, Curtis GH, Hawk WA. Netherton's disease; trichorrhexis invaginata (bamboo hair), congenital ichthyosiform erythroderma and the atopic diathesis: a histopathologic study. Arch Dermatol 1964;89:46–54.

34. Chavanas S, Bodemer C, Rochat A, et al. Mutations in SPINK5, encoding a serine protease inhibitor, cause Netherton syndrome. Nat Genet 2000;25:141–2.

35. Renner ED, Hartl D, Rylaarsdam S, et al. Comèl-Netherton syndrome defined as primary immunodeficiency. J Allergy Clin Immunol 2009;124(3):536–43.

36. Gandhi C, Healy C, Wanderer AA, et al. Familial atypical cold urticaria: description of a new hereditary disease. J Allergy Clin Immunol 2009;124:1245–50.

37. Milner JD. PLAID: a Syndrome of Complex Patterns of Disease and Unique Phenotypes. J Clin Immunol 2015;35(6):527–30.

38. Ombrello MJ. Cold urticaria, immunodeficiency, and autoimmunity related to PLCG2 deletions. N Engl J Med 2012;366(4):330–8.

39. Boyden SE, Desai A, Cruse G, et al. Vibratory urticaria associated with a missense variant in ADGRE2. N Engl J Med 2016;374:656–63.

40. Dinarello CA. Immunological and inflammatory functions of the interleukin-1 family. Annu Rev Immunol 2009;27:519–50.

Differential Diagnosis of Atopic Dermatitis

Meagan Barrett, MD[a],*, Minnelly Luu, MD[b]

KEYWORDS

- Atopic dermatitis • Eczema • Mimickers • Differential diagnosis

KEY POINTS

- Atopic dermatitis (AD) is a common inflammatory condition of the skin that has a broad clinical spectrum leading to frequent misdiagnosis.
- The characteristic features of AD, including age of onset, distribution, severe pruritus, xerosis, lichenification, and association with atopy, can help distinguish AD from common mimickers.
- The differential diagnosis of AD in children and adults includes seborrheic dermatitis, psoriasis, allergic contact dermatitis, molluscum dermatitis, tinea corporis, mycosis fungoides, dermatomyositis, pityriasis lichenoides chronica, Langerhans cell histiocytosis, polymorphous light eruption, actinic prurigo, and nutritional deficiency.

INTRODUCTION

Atopic dermatitis (AD) is a chronic inflammatory disorder characterized by severe pruritus and an eczematous dermatitis. The estimated prevalence in the United States is approximately 20%,[1] rendering it the most common chronic skin disease in children. Clinically patients with AD can present with mild to severe disease, and lesions can range from weepy erythematous papules and plaques to lichenified xerotic plaques. The characteristic clinical features and distribution tend to evolve based on the patient's age (**Table 1**).

Occasionally, patients who carry a diagnosis of AD may display atypical clinical features that prompt the clinician to broaden the differential diagnosis. When the diagnosis is unclear, both knowledge of clinical findings seen in association with AD (**Table 2**) and recognition of potential alternative diagnoses are important for patient care because management and prognosis may differ. This article provides an overview of the dermatologic conditions that can potentially mimic AD. Although patients

Disclosure Statement: The authors have nothing to disclose.
[a] Department of Dermatology, Keck School of Medicine of USC, 1200 North State Street, Clinic Tower A7D, Los Angeles, CA 90033, USA; [b] Department of Dermatology, Children's Hospital Los Angeles, Keck School of Medicine of USC, 4650 Sunset Boulevard, Los Angeles, CA 90027, USA
* Corresponding author.
E-mail address: meagan.barrett@med.usc.edu

Immunol Allergy Clin N Am 37 (2017) 11–34
http://dx.doi.org/10.1016/j.iac.2016.08.009
0889-8561/17/© 2016 Elsevier Inc. All rights reserved.

immunology.theclinics.com

Table 1
Characteristic features of atopic dermatitis by age

	Infantile	Childhood	Adolescent or Adult
Age Range	Birth to 6 mo	6 mo to 12 y	>12 y of age
Lesions	Exudative erythematous weepy papules and plaques	Weepy erythematous papules and plaques intermixed with lichenified plaques, particularly in flexural areas	Erythematous papules and plaques with xerotic scale and crust Lichenified plaques in flexural areas
Distribution	Scalp, face, trunk, extensor surfaces	Flexural surfaces, including antecubital and popliteal fossa, wrist, and neck	Hands, flexural surfaces, upper trunk

Data from Saeki H, Nakahara T, Tanaka A, et al. Clinical practice guidelines for the management of atopic dermatitis 2016. J Dermatol 2016. [Epub ahead of print]; and Eichenfield LF, Tom WL, Chamlin SL, et al. Guidelines of care for the management of atopic dermatitis: section 1. Diagnosis and assessment of atopic dermatitis. J Am Acad Dermatol 2014;70(2):338–51.

with immunodeficiency, autoimmune, or genetic syndromes, such as hyper-IgE syndrome, immune dysregulation polyendocrinopathy X-linked syndrome (IPEX), Wiskott-Aldrich, and Netherton syndrome can also present with clinical features of AD, this article mainly focuses on primary dermatologic disorders and their distinguishing morphologic features.

SEBORRHEIC DERMATITIS

Seborrheic dermatitis is a common inflammatory condition of the skin with 2 peaks in incidence during early infancy (weeks 2–10) and adulthood.[2,3] Sebaceous gland stimulation and hypersensitivity to yeast, particularly *Malassezia*, have been implicated in the pathogenesis of seborrheic dermatitis.[3,4]

Table 2
Associated features of atopic dermatitis

Features	Clinical
Pityriasis alba	Hypopigmented patches on face, upper trunk, upper extremities
Keratosis pilaris	Follicular hyperkeratosis of outer arms, lateral cheeks, buttocks, thighs
Dennie-Morgan fold (atopic pleat)	Extra line on lower eyelid
Allergic shiners	Violaceous to gray color of infraorbital area
Allergic salute	Transverse linear crease on nose
Hyperlinear palms	Increased and exaggerated skin markings on palms
Ichthyosis vulgaris	Scaling of extensor extremities, fish-scale appearance of extensor leg
Hertoghe sign	Loss of lateral eyebrows
White dermatographism	Blanching of skin after stroking
Circumoral pallor	Pallor of perioral area
Nummular dermatitis	Sharply circumscribed thick coin-shaped scaly plaques

Infants with seborrheic dermatitis often present with adherent yellow greasy scale over the scalp, at times with background erythema, commonly known as cradle cap (**Fig. 1**A). Additional sites of scaling include the retroauricular folds, ears, and eyebrows. Commonly, patients may present with erythema of intertriginous areas, including neck, axillae, and inguinal folds. Some infants may develop a more diffuse eruption on trunk and extremities, usually consisting of salmon-pink fine papules coalescing into poorly defined plaques with variable greasy scaling.

Rarely, infants with seborrheic dermatitis develop extensive involvement with erythroderma and scaling (**Fig. 1**B). Some patients, especially those with more fulminant presentations, may be difficult to distinguish from AD (**Table 3**). However, they may also exist on a continuum, with resolution of seborrheic dermatitis as clinical features of AD becomes more prominent. In a retrospective review by Alexopoulos and colleagues,[4] the prevalence of AD in patients with infantile seborrheic dermatitis was significantly higher than the rate reported in the general population. The relationship between infantile seborrheic dermatitis and AD can at times make the distinction difficult.

Seborrheic dermatitis can also be seen in school-aged children but is far less common. Adolescents can develop adult-form seborrheic dermatitis at any time after puberty. Adolescent or adult seborrheic dermatitis of the scalp is commonly referred to as dandruff, and can present with fine flaky scale. Greasy scale overlying an erythematous base can also be seen. The glabella, eyebrows, nasolabial folds, retroauricular folds, and upper chest are additional sites of involvement, corresponding to a high density of sebaceous glands. In adolescent or adult patients, treatment-refractory or extensive disease can be seen in the setting of human immunodeficiency virus.[5]

PSORIASIS

Psoriasis is a common inflammatory condition, with an estimated prevalence of 1% to 3% in the general population.[6,7] There are 2 peaks in incidence: late adolescence (teens to 20s) and middle age (50s to 60s); however, psoriasis can present at any age, from infancy to late adulthood. In contrast to AD, which is typically a T helper (Th)-2 predominant condition, psoriasis is characterized by a Th1 and Th17 immune milieu. Increased levels of interferon gamma, interleukin (IL)-2, IL-17, IL-22, and IL-23 lead to a robust dermal inflammatory response and proliferation of keratinocytes.[6]

In both pediatric and adult psoriasis, numerous clinical variants exist, including chronic plaque psoriasis, guttate psoriasis, erythrodermic psoriasis, pustular psoriasis, and inverse psoriasis (**Table 4**). Plaque psoriasis, the most common clinical subtype in both children and adults,[8] presents with well-demarcated, pink plaques with adherent silvery scale commonly located over extensor surfaces (**Fig. 2**A). Besides the knees and elbows, psoriasis has a predilection for the scalp, retroauricular creases, gluteal cleft, lower back, and periumbilical area. Occasionally, psoriasis affects the seborrheic areas of the face and scalp, closely mimicking seborrheic dermatitis, a condition sometimes termed sebopsoriasis (see **Table 3**). Nail findings can be a helpful clue to the diagnosis of psoriasis and include irregular pitting, salmon patches, oil spots, thickening, yellowing, and distal onycholysis (**Fig. 2**B).[9]

Guttate psoriasis occurs more frequently in children than adults, and usually presents with an acute onset widespread eruption of subcentimeter thin, pink, scaly papules, and plaques (**Fig. 2**C).[10] Infectious triggers, particularly streptococcal pharyngitis, have been reported in up to two-thirds of patients with acute onset guttate psoriasis.[11] A history of a preceding respiratory tract infection or sore throat 1 to 2 weeks before an outbreak can help substantiate the diagnosis.[9]

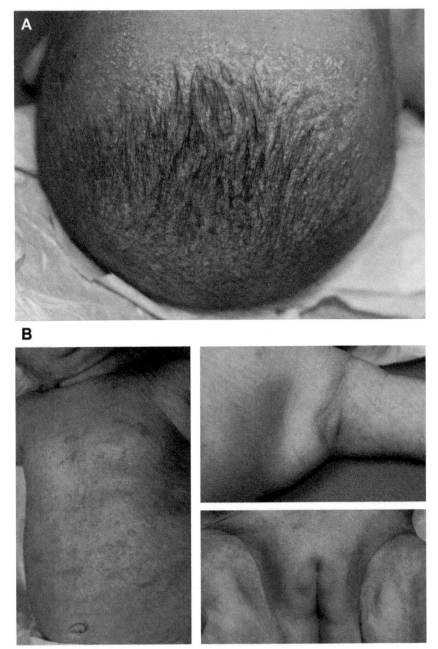

Fig. 1. (A) Classic infantile seborrheic dermatitis. Yellow crust and scale overlying a faintly erythematous base on the scalp. (B) Infantile seborrheic dermatitis. Generalized salmon pink, poorly defined scaly papules with involvement of the folds.

Table 3
Comparing seborrheic dermatitis, psoriasis, and atopic dermatitis

Features	AD	Seborrheic Dermatitis	Psoriasis
Onset	First 5 y of life, usually onset after 1 mo of age	2–10 wk, adolescence-adulthood	All ages
Face	Cheeks, periorbital and perioral areas	Eyebrows, ears, nasolabial fold	Uncommon on face except for seborrheic dermatitis-like eruption
Scalp	Dry scaling	Greasy yellow scaling	Pink plaques with white-silver adherent scale, scalp plaques may cross hairline
Extremities	Extensor surfaces in infants, flexural surfaces in children	Folds of arms and legs	Extensor surface of joints (elbows, knees) and extremities
Folds or groin	Antecubital and popliteal fossae	Retroauricular folds, neck, axillae, inguinal folds	Retroauricular folds, axillae, umbilicus, diaper area, inguinal folds, genitalia, gluteal cleft
Nails	Dystrophy with periungual eczema, pitting		Pitting, thickening, yellowing, distal onycholysis, dystrophy, oil spots
Shape	Poorly circumscribed	Poorly circumscribed	Sharply circumscribed
Color	Red	Salmon-pink	Pink
Scale	Fine, dry	Yellow, moist or greasy	White-silver, micaceous
Symptoms	Severe pruritus	Absent to mild-moderate pruritus	Mild-moderate pruritus

Inverse psoriasis, defined by predilection for intertriginous areas, including axilla, inguinal folds, intergluteal cleft, and umbilicus, can be an isolated subtype or present in conjunction with other morphologies of psoriasis. It is a useful clue to the diagnosis of psoriasis in general. In the folds, psoriasis tends to display a bright pink-red color and well-defined borders but lack scaling due to moisture. In infants, the diaper eruption of psoriasis is distinct in appearance, presenting as a large sharply demarcated bright red plaque affecting the buttock and inguinal folds (**Fig. 2**D). Commonly referred to as napkin dermatitis, this is the most common presentation of psoriasis in the infant.[12] Psoriasis of the diaper should be considered in patients with recalcitrant diaper dermatitis.

Anti-tumor necrosis factor (TNF)-α agents, which are used to treat a variety of immune-mediated conditions, including inflammatory bowel disease, rheumatologic disorders, and psoriasis, have been implicated in triggering psoriasiform eruptions, and should be considered on the differential diagnosis in the correct patient population.[13]

Although the skin is the primary site of involvement, psoriasis is a systemic inflammatory disease process that also commonly affects the joints and may affect the vasculature. The reported prevalence of psoriatic arthritis among patients with psoriasis ranges from 7% to 84%; however, more recent studies estimate that 20% to 30% of patients with psoriasis have psoriatic arthritis.[14,15] Psoriasis has also been associated with an increased risk of metabolic syndrome; cardiovascular events; malignancy, particularly lymphoma; and a small decrease in life expectancy.[16]

Table 4
The subtypes of psoriasis

	Chronic Plaque	Guttate	Inverse	Erythrodermic	Pustular
Lesion	Well-demarcated pink-red plaques with silver-white scale	Thin, annular, less than 1 cm, pink papules and plaques	Brightly erythematous sharply demarcated plaques	Diffuse erythema	Erythematous plaques studded with pinpoint pustules
Distribution	Scalp, extensor surfaces, gluteal cleft, posterior auricular crease	Trunk	Diaper area, axilla, gluteal cleft, inguinal folds	Generalized	Generalized, also palmoplantar variant
Predominant age	Adolescents, middle age	School-aged children and adolescents	All ages, common in infants	All ages	All ages
Additional features	Most common variant, may see overlap with other variants	Commonly triggered by preceding infection, usually streptococcus	Lacks classic scale	Lacks characteristic plaques or scale, look for nail or scalp findings	When generalized, patients are systemically ill usually requiring hospitalization

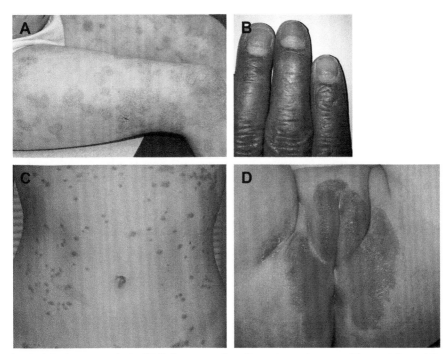

Fig. 2. (*A*) Plaque psoriasis. Well demarcated erythematous plaques with overlying white-silver micaceous scale. (*B*) Psoriatic nails. Irregular pits, distal onycholysis, and oil spots. (*C*) Guttate psoriasis. Multiple discrete small pink papules. (*D*) Inverse psoriasis of the diaper area. A confluent bright red plaque with sharply defined borders and relative lack of scale.

Although classic psoriasis is usually readily differentiated from AD based on morphology and distribution, some patients may exhibit intermediate morphology that can render diagnosis more challenging. This is particularly true for infants and young children. Although psoriasis is usually a clinical diagnosis, a skin biopsy can be performed to confirm the diagnosis and differentiate it from eczema. Histologic examination shows regular acanthosis, parakeratosis, thinning of the suprapapillary plate, capillary dilatation, a mononuclear cellular infiltrate, and collections of neutrophils in the epidermis.[17] Clinically atypical psoriasis frequently lacks a diagnostic biopsy specimen, which is often the case in the setting of erythrodermic psoriasis.

ALLERGIC CONTACT DERMATITIS

Allergic contact dermatitis (ACD) is a type IV delayed hypersensitivity reaction that requires prior sensitization before an allergen will elicit an inflammatory response. Contact dermatitis is characterized by geometric, well-demarcated, erythematous plaques with overlying vesiculation in the acute phase and xerotic crust in the subacute to chronic phase (**Fig. 3**A). However, frequently the inflammation extends beyond the area of exposure, which can make the geometric pattern less discernable. The distribution of lesions may serve as a clue to the potential allergen (**Table 5**).

A few days to weeks following a highly inflammatory eczematous dermatitis, most frequently ACD, a widespread symmetric eczematous eruption can develop distant from the initial site of involvement, known as autoeczematization or an id reaction

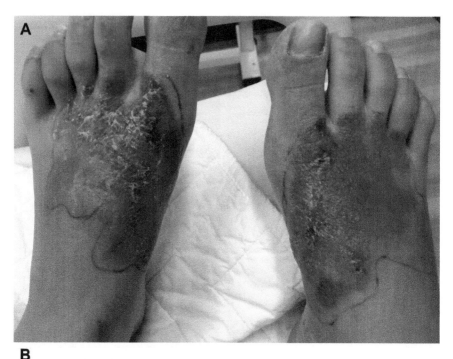

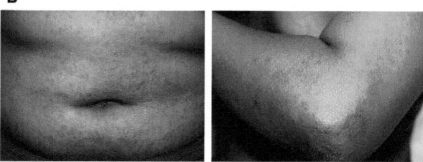

Fig. 3. (*A*) Contact dermatitis. Well-demarcated weepy erythematous plaque localized to the dorsal aspect of the foot is characteristic of a contact dermatitis to chromate found in leather in shoes. (*B*) Id reaction. Symmetric edematous erythematous papules on the trunk and extremities developed in the setting of a contact dermatitis to nickel.

(**Fig. 3**B). The severe pruritus and eczematous nature of the reaction can be difficult to distinguish from AD; however, the acute onset, symmetric distribution, and history of a preceding contact reaction can be used to distinguish the 2 conditions.

ACD may be mistaken for chronic AD, or it may complicate AD. Products used in the treatment of AD may be implicated in ACD.[18] In addition, common sites of involvement in ACD, including lips, eyelids, hands, neck, and flexural areas, frequently overlap with AD.[19] Certain allergens have been found to have higher rates of sensitization among AD patients when compared with nonatopic patients, including formaldehyde releasers,[20] metal allergens,[21] cocamidopropyl betaine (a surfactant),[22] and fragrances.[23] ACD may be considered in patients with treatment refractory AD.[24]

Table 5
Common allergens and their distribution

Allergen	Products	Distribution
Nickel Sulfate	Nickel-containing jewelry	Ear lobes, periumbilical
Methylchloroisothiazolinone or methylisothiazolinone	Preservative in personal care products	Nonspecific
Cobalt chloride	Jewelry (cosensitized with nickel)	Ear lobes, periumbilical
Fragrance mix	Cosmetics, personal care products (PCP)	Face, neck, axilla common
Neomycin or bacitracin	Topical antibiotic agents	Around cuts or wounds
Balsam of Peru	Fragrance in cosmetics, personal care products	Face, neck, axilla common
Formaldehyde	Preservative in PCP	Nonspecific
Formaldehyde releasers[a]	PCP	Nonspecific
Lanolin or wool alcohols	Emollient (Aquaphor, Beiersdorf Inc., CT)	Nonspecific
Potassium dichromate	Tanned leather	Foot dermatitis
Cocamidopropyl betaine	Shampoo and body wash	Posterior auricular, upper neck and back
Decyl glucoside	Shampoo and body wash	Posterior auricular, upper neck and back
Corticosteroids	Medications	Treated areas
Propylene glycol	PCP	Nonspecific

[a] Formaldehyde releasers include quaternium-15, dimethyl-dimethyl (DMDM), hydantoin, imidazolidinyl urea, diazolidinyl urea, and 2-bromo-2-nitropropane-1,3-diol (bronopol).
Data from Militello G, Jacob SE, Crawford GH. Allergic contact dermatitis in children. Curr Opin Pediatr 2006;18(4):385–90.

The gold standard for diagnosis of ACD is patch testing. There are several methods for patch testing, including prepackaged allergen panels, such as the thin-layer rapid use epicutaneous patch test (TRUE test), or customized trays usually performed at a tertiary referral center. Patch test results should be interpreted with clinical context because not all positive results are clinically relevant. This is particularly important in children because allergen panels are developed based on commonly reported allergens in adults; however, children are exposed to a different array of products and thus a close review of their products and environment before patch testing is crucial to increase the diagnostic yield.[25]

SCABIES

Scabies is caused by a cutaneous infection with the mite *Sarcoptes scabiei*, an obligate human parasite. Transmission of scabies is primarily through skin-to-skin contact, with increased outbreaks in crowded living conditions, such as nursing homes, prisons, and hospitals.[26]

Scabies infection usually presents with pinpoint, pruritic, erythematous papules that can range from few to many (**Fig. 4**A) associated with intractable pruritus. Visualization of a burrow, subcentimeter linear erythematous scaly tracks, helps to solidify the diagnosis. In infants and children the development of papulopustules and nodules is common (**Fig. 4**B). Rarely, bullous lesions may be seen, particularly in infants. Secondary

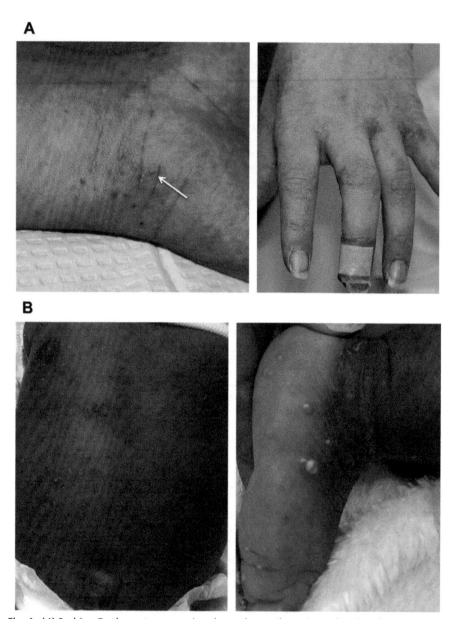

Fig. 4. (*A*) Scabies. Erythematous excoriated papules on the wrist and within the interdigital web spaces. A linear burrow is visualized (*white arrow*). (*B*) Scabies. The presence of papulopustular lesions in young children is characteristic.

skin changes due to severe pruritus are common, including excoriations, eczematization, and crusts, which can mimic AD.[27]

Sites of involvement can help prompt the clinician to consider the diagnosis of scabies. In adolescents and adults, interdigital spaces, wrists, axillae, waist, umbilicus, and nipples are commonly involved. In infants or children, involvement of the palms and soles, dorsal feet, genitalia, and diaper area are common.[28] Crusted scabies, characterized by hyperkeratotic scale and erythema, is secondary to an extremely high mite burden, and develops in patients who are unable to mount an effective immune response. It may be mistaken for psoriasis given its hyperkeratosis.

Scabies mites burrow under the stratum corneum and definitive diagnosis can be made by visualization of the mite, eggs, or excrement (scybala) under the microscope using a mineral oil preparation. Because an individual patient may harbor only 10 to 15 mites, false negatives may occur. Skin biopsy may reveal the scabies mite or its associated elements in addition to an eosinophilic inflammatory infiltrate.

MOLLUSCUM DERMATITIS

Molluscum contagiosum (MC) is a viral infection of the skin caused by the MC virus seen primarily in children. It can also be seen in adults, usually in the setting of sexual transmission. An increased burden has been associated with swimming and a personal history of eczema.[29] Autoinoculation and spread of lesions can occur from scratching.

Although translucent flesh-colored papules with an umbilicated core are pathognomonic for molluscum infection (**Fig. 5**A), inflammatory reactions associated with MC, commonly known as molluscum dermatitis, may obscure the characteristic papules (**Fig. 5**B). Patients present with pruritic eczematous eruptions, usually around the molluscum lesions but, at times, on uninvolved sites as well. These cases may be mistaken for AD or contact dermatitis, especially because many patients may already have pre-existing AD. Close examination and identification of the classic papules can secure the diagnosis.

Inflammation of molluscum lesions is thought to correspond with recognition of the virally infected cells by the immune system and thus has been associated with clearance of the eruption.[30] Although generally unnecessary, if the diagnosis is in question, a biopsy of a molluscum papule will show papillomatosis with central umbilication and viral inclusion bodies known as Henderson-Patterson bodies.

TINEA CORPORIS AND TINEA CAPITIS

Tinea corporis is caused by infection of the epidermis by dermatophytes, a large group of related fungi that can infect human hair, skin, and nails.[31] *Trichophyton rubrum* is the most common cause of tinea corporis worldwide.

Characteristically, a superficial dermatophyte infection is composed of an annular erythematous patch with central clearing and peripheral advancing erythema and scale (**Fig. 6**). Multiple plaques can coalesce to form a polycyclic configuration.

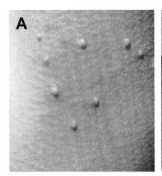
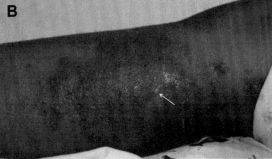

Fig. 5. (A) MC. Flesh-colored translucent papules. (B) Molluscum dermatitis. An ill-defined weepy erythematous plaque, which could be mistaken for AD or contact dermatitis, can be diagnosed by identifying the central molluscum papule (*white arrow*).

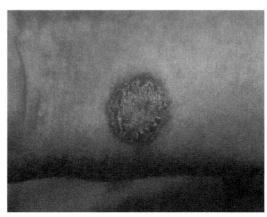

Fig. 6. Tinea corporis. Annular red plaque with peripheral accentuation of scale and central clearing is typical.

However, it is not uncommon for patients to display subtle morphology, resulting in misdiagnosis as AD, nummular eczema (**Fig. 7**), or pityriasis rosea.[32] Partial treatment with topical corticosteroids, known as tinea incognito, commonly leads to alteration in these clinical features and increases the likelihood of misdiagnosis (**Fig. 8**).[33] If suspected, tinea corporis should be ruled out before starting topical corticosteroids.

Tinea capitis, a dermatophyte infection of the scalp, is commonly seen in children, particularly of African American descent, and is very rarely seen in adults. Findings can range from subtle with a fine noninflammatory scaling, which can be mistaken for seborrheic dermatitis or AD, to exuberant with inflammatory boggy alopecic scaly plaques. The presence of diffuse or patchy alopecia, pustules, broken hairs, or posterior auricular lymphadenopathy warrants a work-up for tinea capitis before considering alternative diagnoses.

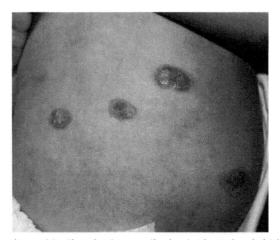

Fig. 7. Nummular dermatitis. Sharply circumscribed coin-shaped red thick exudative scaly plaques. Nummular morphology may be seen in patients with AD, as in this case.

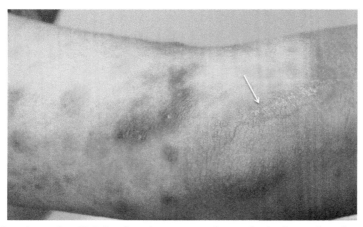

Fig. 8. Tinea incognito. Ill-defined erythematous scaly papules in the setting of steroid use may render diagnosis of tinea challenging. However, the presence of a subtle classic arcuate plaque with peripheral scale (*white arrow*) aids in the diagnosis of tinea corporis.

In-office potassium-hydroxide wet-mount preparations can be performed to confirm the diagnosis. Scraping of the scale can also be sent for fungal culture.[34] Alternatively, a skin biopsy can be performed with PAS staining, which will highlight the presence of fungal elements in the stratum corneum.

MYCOSIS FUNGOIDES

Mycosis fungoides (MF) is the most common form of cutaneous T-cell lymphoma, and typically affects adults with a median age of 55 to 60 years but can rarely be seen in childhood and adolescence.[35–37] Among the diagnosed cases of MF, approximately 4% to 11% are children.[38] Early in the disease course, the diagnosis of MF is frequently delayed due to clinical similarity to more benign dermatoses, such as AD, the latter of which is a reported prior diagnosis in up to one-third of patients with MF.[39]

Typically, patients present with ill-defined erythematous patches, papules, or plaques with faint scale. Subtle morphologic clues may alert the astute clinician to consider the diagnosis of MF early in the disease course. MF has a predilection for photoprotected sites, in particular the buttock, lower trunk, thighs, breasts, and groin, the so-called bathing suit distribution.[36] Lesions display fine scaling and poikiloderma (atrophy, subtle wrinkling, telangiectasias, pigmentary alteration), and are often arranged in a polycyclic or annular configuration (**Fig. 9**).

Hypopigmented MF is a common variant seen in children, especially those with darker skin types, Fitzpatrick skin types III-VI.[36] Hypopigmented MF is characterized by ill-defined hypopigmented macules and patches with fine scaling. Hypopigmented lesions of MF frequently resembles pityriasis alba; however, the lack of pruritus, involvement of the bathing suit distribution, and fine scale can help distinguish hypopigmented MF.

A skin biopsy is required to confirm the diagnosis of MF and will demonstrate a dermal infiltrate composed of lymphocytes with hyperchromatic and irregularly contoured nuclei with epidermotropism.[39] These findings are often subtle and serial biopsies may be required if there is a high index of suspicion.

Immunohistochemical studies showing a CD4+ predominant infiltrate with loss of CD7+ staining can help verify the diagnosis of MF. The infiltrate in hypopigmented

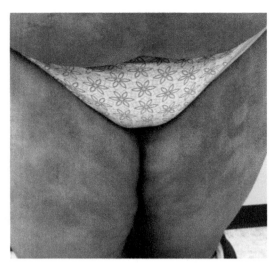

Fig. 9. MF. Ill-defined erythematous patches with overlying poikilodermatous change in a characteristic bathing suit distribution.

MF may be composed predominantly of CD8+ T cells rather than CD4+ T cells.[39] T-cell rearrangement studies are performed on tissue to confirm clonality.

Lymph nodes, peripheral blood, and/or visceral organs may be clinically involved. All patients warrant a complete physical examination with palpation for lymph nodes, complete blood count with differential, comprehensive metabolic panel, and lactate dehydrogenase. Tumor stage of the disease is considered the most important predictor of disease-specific survival.[40] Disease prognosis and response to treatment in childhood is not well described.[41]

DERMATOMYOSITIS

Dermatomyositis (DM) is a complex immune-mediated condition seen in adults at an estimated rate of 5 to 11 cases per 100,000 per year,[42] and children at an estimated rate of 2 to 3 children per million per year.[43] The mean age of onset of juvenile DM is slightly greater than 7 years of age.[44]

Classic DM is characterized by an inflammatory myopathy with associated cutaneous findings, which frequently precede muscle involvement and thus represent an opportunity for early diagnosis.[42] Violaceous to erythematous flat-topped papules with fine scale overlying the elbows and knees (Gottron sign) and distal and proximal interphalangeal joints (Gottron papules) are the most common cutaneous manifestation seen in DM (**Fig. 10**).[45] Early in the disease course, these lesions are often mistaken for AD due to their extensor distribution and morphology composed of scaly erythematous papules. Nail bed changes, including cuticular fraying and periungual telangiectasias, can serve as a clinical clues to the diagnosis of DM. In addition, the erythema in DM tends to be more violaceous. A violaceous hue and edema of the periorbital skin, termed the heliotrope rash, may be present. Additional diagnostic clinical features include poikilodermatous change commonly over the upper chest and shoulders (Shawl sign) and lateral thighs (Holster sign). In darker skin types in particular, poikilodermatous change can be mistaken for erythema associated with AD (**Fig. 11**).

The presence of the pathognomonic cutaneous findings with 2 to 3 clinical signs of myositis (progressive symmetric proximal muscle weakness, muscle biopsy with

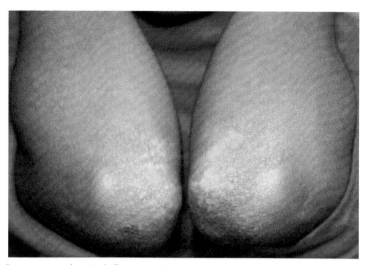

Fig. 10. Gottron papules. Pink flat-topped papules over the elbows in a patient with DM.

evidence of myositis, elevation of muscle-derived serum enzyme levels, and/or evidence of myopathy on MRI) secures the diagnosis.

PITYRIASIS LICHENOIDES CHRONICA

Pityriasis lichenoides chronica (PLC) is an idiopathic, generally benign, T-cell lymphoproliferative disorder that exists on a clinical spectrum with pityriasis lichenoides et varioliformis acuta (PLEVA), the more acute form, and febrile ulceronecrotic Mucha-Habermann disease (FUMHD), which is more severe, generalized, and associated with systemic symptoms.[46] Approximately 20% of cases of PLC are seen in children, with a peak incidence between 5 to 10 years of age.[47,48]

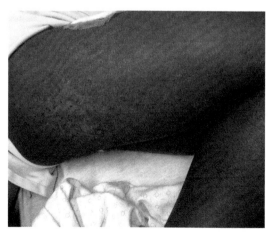

Fig. 11. DM. Violaceous erythema and poikiloderma, characterized by atrophy, telangiectasias, and pigmentary alteration. The presence of these changes over the lateral thigh is also known as the holster sign.

PLC is characterized by recurrent crops of multiple small erythematous to red-brown papules and plaques with central scale that have a predilection for the trunk and proximal extremities (**Fig. 12**A). Individual lesions spontaneously regress over weeks, leaving behind macules of hyperpigmentation and hypopigmentation without scarring (**Fig. 12**B).[46]

On histopathology, PLC demonstrates more subtle but similar features to PLEVA, with parakeratosis, acanthosis, a wedge-shaped perivascular lymphocytic infiltrate, subtle vacuolar interface with variable necrotic keratinocytes, and erythrocyte extravasation.[49]

In most cases, PLC is a benign, self-limited, condition that may last for years but usually spontaneously resolves. However, there are reports, more commonly in adults, of PLC in association with cutaneous T-cell lymphoma, thus requiring regular clinical monitoring in these patients.[46] The presence of poikiloderma in patients with PLC has been associated with increased risk of MF.

LANGERHANS CELL HISTIOCYTOSIS

Langerhans cell histiocytosis (LCH) is a rare clonal proliferative disorder that classically encompasses 4 conditions: Letterer-Siwe, Hand-Schuller-Christian, eosinophilic granuloma, and congenital self-healing reticulohistiocytosis. However, more recently, LCH has been classified as a single disease entity with a wide clinical spectrum, ranging from solitary skin or bone lesions to severe, progressive, multisystem disease. Although the cause is unknown, up to 50% of patients harbor a BRAFV600E mutation pointing to a neoplastic cause.[50]

Cutaneous findings in LCH are variable; however, patients typically develop erythematous to flesh-colored papules and thin plaques with a predilection for the scalp, flexural areas of the neck, inguinal folds, perineum, and lower trunk. The presence of petechiae, ecchymoses, and fissuring in a characteristic seborrheic distribution (**Fig. 13**) can distinguish LCH from conditions with a similar distribution, such as seborrheic dermatitis and AD.

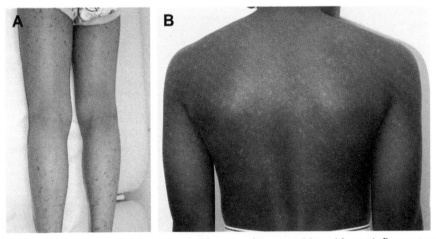

Fig. 12. (*A*) PLC. Crops of red brown papules over the extremities with postinflammatory dyschromia. (*B*) PLC. Residual postinflammatory hypopigmentation is commonly seen and may be the prominent feature.

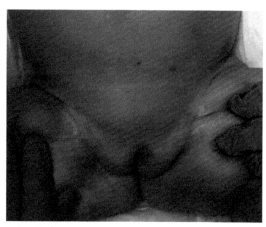

Fig. 13. LCH. Although subtle, petechiae and crusted red brown papules can be appreciated on the waist and in the inguinal folds.

Skin biopsy can be performed to confirm the diagnosis. On histopathology there is a proliferation of Langerhans cells in the dermis (CD1a+, S100+, Langerin+).

POLYMORPHOUS LIGHT ERUPTION

Polymorphous light eruption (PMLE) is the most common photodermatosis, affecting up to 20% of the general population, and is thought to be due to a delayed-type hypersensitivity response to an unknown photoinduced antigen.[51] PMLE is induced by UV-A; less commonly, UV-B; and, rarely, visible light. A young woman in the second to third decade of life is the prototypical patient.

Within hours to days after exposure to light, erythematous papules and papulovesicles distributed over photoexposed areas erupt. The eruption typically begins in the spring, summer, or during a vacation when usually photoprotected sites, such as the chest and arms, are exposed to sunlight. Areas of the body that are consistently exposed to sunlight year-round, such as the face and dorsal hands, are usually spared, a phenomenon known as hardening. Associated pruritus is common.

The history and clinical morphology is usually sufficient to make the diagnosis; however, a skin biopsy can be performed and will show spongiosis, superficial and deep perivascular dermatitis with papillary dermal edema, and scattered neutrophils and eosinophils.

Although topical and oral steroids may acutely alleviate the eruption and pruritus, the mainstay of treatment is sun protection. Photoprovocation testing can be performed to determine the action spectrum (UV-A, UV-B, visible, or combination) that elicits the clinical eruption to enable targeted photoprotection. Leading up to springtime or vacation, a patient may undergo hardening of the skin with phototherapy 2 to 3 times per week for 4 to 5 weeks, which allows for desensitization of the skin and reduces the presence or severity of the reaction.

ACTINIC PRURIGO

Actinic prurigo is a rare photodermatoses that has been linked to a genetic predisposition with several identified HLA antigen alleles. It is seen more commonly in people of Mestizo ancestry, with an estimated prevalence of 0.1% to 3.5%, depending on the population being studied.[52] Onset of actinic prurigo is between 4 to 5 years of age.

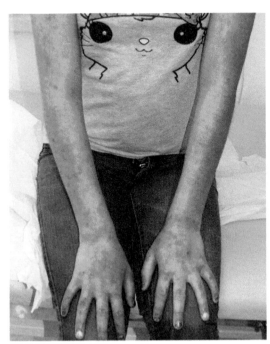

Fig. 14. Actinic prurigo. Erythematous papules and lichenified papules on photoexposed sites.

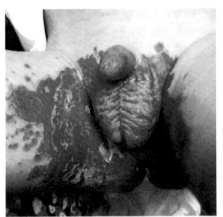
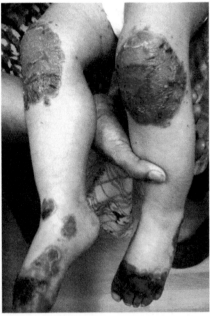

Fig. 15. Zinc deficiency. Sharply circumscribed bright red eroded plaque of the diaper region, as well as psoriasiform crusted plaques of the knees and distal feet.

Table 6
Mimickers of atopic dermatitis

Disorder	Age	Morphology	Distribution	Other Clinical Features
ACD	Any age, incidence increases with age	Geometric erythematous eczematous weepy plaques	Based on exposure (see **Table 4**)	Severe pruritus
Scabies	Any age	Poorly defined erythematous papules, nodules, burrows, pustules, and vesicles in infants	Wrists, interdigital spaces, axillae, umbilicus, nipples, diaper area, scrotum	Severe recalcitrant pruritus
Molluscum dermatitis	Childhood	Flesh-colored translucent umbilicated papules surrounded by erythematous eczematous plaques	Asymmetric, irregularly scattered	
Tinea corporis	Any age	Annular or polycyclic erythematous plaque with peripheral leading edge of erythema and scale	Asymmetric, irregularly scattered on trunk, extremities, face	Steroid treatment may blunt characteristic features
MF	More common in adulthood (50s–60s)	Poorly defined erythematous patches, papules, or plaques with subtle scale; polycyclic or annular	Bathing suit distribution: buttock, lower trunk, thighs, breasts, and groin	Overlying poikiloderma More recalcitrant to topical steroids
Hypopigmented MF	More common in children	Ill-defined hypopigmented patches, often with fine scaling	Bathing suit distribution: buttock, lower trunk, thighs, breasts, and groin	Lack classic features AD (see **Table 1**)
DM	2 peaks: childhood and middle age	Violaceous scaly papules Poikiloderma	Small joints of hands and elbows V-distribution on upper trunk and lateral thighs (shawl and holster sign, respectively)	• Myositis • Cuticular dystrophy • Periorbital violaceous edema • Calcinosis cutis • Malignancy (adult DM) • Visceral involvement (interstitial lung disease, cardiac, esophageal)

(continued on next page)

Table 6
(continued)

Disorder	Age	Morphology	Distribution	Other Clinical Features
Pityriasis lichenoides Chronica	More common in children and young adults	Crops of discrete erythematous to red-brown papules and plaques with central scale, hypopigmented macules	Trunk and proximal extremities	• Usually spontaneously regresses (y) • Rare cases associated with MF (adults)
LCH	More common in infancy and childhood	Wide range of clinical features: erythematous to flesh-colored papules and thin plaques, fissuring, crusting, petechiae	Scalp, posterior auricular fold, neck, axilla, perineum, trunk	• Solitary or multiple osteolytic lesions • Exophthalmos • Diabetes insipidus • Hepatosplenomegaly
PMLE	Adolescence to early adulthood	Erythematous papules and papulovesicles	Photoexposed areas; however, often sparing the face and hands	Worsening in spring or summer
Actinic prurigo	Early childhood	Erythematous papules and lichenified plaques	Photoexposed areas, including face and lips Photoprotected areas can also be involved	• Cheilitis • Conjunctivitis • Mestizo ancestry
Macronutrient deficiency	Any age	Erythematous plaques with superficial desquamation, flaky paint dermatitis	Diffuse	• Peripheral edema • Hepatomegaly • Splenomegaly • Sparse, brittle hair • Dyschromia • Alopecia
Zinc deficiency	Infancy, any age	Sharply circumscribed erythematous with overlying shiny brown crust	Perioral, intertriginous and acral sites	• Low serum alkaline phosphatase • Poor wound healing • Increased cutaneous infections

Erythematous papules and lichenified plaques in a photodistribution are characteristic (**Fig. 14**) of actinic prurigo; however, involvement of photoprotected areas can be seen in up to 35% to 40% of patients.[52] Due to the eczematous and lichenified morphology, misdiagnosis as AD, particularly early in the disease course is common. The presence of cheilitis and/or ocular findings, including conjunctivitis, hyperemia, photophobia, increased lacrimation, and pseudopterygium, can differentiate actinic prurigo from more common dermatoses, such as AD.[53] Patch and photopatch testing are usually negative.

NUTRITIONAL DEFICIENCY

Inadequate intake, absorption, or utilization of calories, protein, or micronutrients can result in clinical manifestations of nutritional deficiency. Nutritional deficiency can affect individuals of all ages but is estimated to affect up to 30% of children worldwide.[54] In industrialized countries, genetic syndromes, eating disorders, illness, gastrointestinal surgery, and alcoholism are frequent contributors to malnutrition.

Cutaneous manifestations of macronutrient deficiency includes large erythematous plaques with fine superficial desquamation, known as flaky paint dermatitis, xerosis, wrinkling of the skin, poor wound healing, dyspigmentation, and alteration in hair pigmentation. In mild to moderate deficiencies, the clinical manifestations are often subtle, and can be mistaken for more common dermatoses, such as AD. More severe cases are defined by the presence of peripheral edema, hepatosplenomegaly, muscle wasting, stunted growth, and immunodeficiency. The presence of psoriasiform epidermal hyperplasia, epidermal pallor and ballooning, and dermal edema can corroborate the diagnosis.[54]

Deficiency in micronutrients (ie, vitamins and trace minerals) can result in a spectrum of systemic and dermatologic findings, including scaly eczematous eruptions that may mimic AD early on. Most notably, zinc deficiency is associated with characteristic sharply circumscribed erythematous scaly plaques with overlying thin shiny brown crust primarily on acral sites and in intertriginous areas (**Fig. 15**). Additional morphologies may include psoriasiform, vesiculobullous, and pustular presentations. Several other deficiencies, in particular biotin, essential fatty acids, vitamin B_6 (pyridoxine), and vitamin B_2 (riboflavin), may also produce a similar clinical picture.[55]

SUMMARY

AD is a common chronic inflammatory skin disorder seen in all ages but most commonly during childhood. Rarely, patients may present with skin eruptions that mimic AD, which are reviewed in **Table 6**. Knowledge of the distinguishing features of both AD and alternative diagnoses is useful for clinicians caring for AD.

REFERENCES

1. Totri CR, Diaz L, Eichenfield LF. 2014 update on atopic dermatitis in children. Curr Opin Pediatr 2014;26(4):466–71.
2. Foley P, Zuo Y, Plunkett A, et al. The frequency of common skin conditions in preschool-aged children in Australia: seborrheic dermatitis and pityriasis capitis (cradle cap). Arch Dermatol 2003;139(3):318–22.
3. Borda LJ, Wikramanayake TC. Seborrheic dermatitis and dandruff: a comprehensive review. J Clin Investig Dermatol 2015;3(2):1–22.
4. Alexopoulos A, Kakourou T, Orfanou I, et al. Retrospective analysis of the relationship between infantile seborrheic dermatitis and atopic dermatitis. Pediatr Dermatol 2014;31(2):125–30.

5. Forrestel AK, Kovarik CL, Mosam A, et al. Diffuse HIV-associated seborrheic dermatitis - a case series. Int J STD AIDS 2016. [Epub ahead of print].

6. Shah KN. Diagnosis and treatment of pediatric psoriasis: current and future. Am J Clin Dermatol 2013;14(3):195–213.

7. Napolitano M, Megna M, Balato A, et al. Systemic treatment of pediatric psoriasis: a review. Dermatol Ther (Heidelb) 2016;6(2):125–42.

8. Morris A, Rogers M, Fischer G, et al. Childhood psoriasis: a clinical review of 1262 cases. Pediatr Dermatol 2001;18(3):188–98.

9. Leman J, Burden D. Psoriasis in children: a guide to its diagnosis and management. Paediatr Drugs 2001;3(9):673–80.

10. Verbov J. Psoriasis in childhood. Arch Dis Child 1992;67(1):75–6.

11. Fry L, Baker BS. Triggering psoriasis: the role of infections and medications. Clin Dermatol 2007;25(6):606–15.

12. Burden-Teh E, Thomas KS, Ratib S, et al. The epidemiology of childhood psoriasis: a scoping review. Br J Dermatol 2016;174(6):1242–57.

13. Nguyen K, Vleugels RA, Velez NF, et al. Psoriasiform reactions to anti-tumor necrosis factor α therapy. J Clin Rheumatol 2013;19(7):377–81.

14. López Estebaránz JL, Zarco-Montejo P, Samaniego ML, et al. Prevalence and clinical features of psoriatic arthritis in psoriasis patients in Spain. Limitations of PASE as a screening tool. Eur J Dermatol 2015;25(1):57–63.

15. Pedersen OB, Svendsen AJ, Ejstrup L, et al. The occurrence of psoriatic arthritis in Denmark. Ann Rheum Dis 2008;67(10):1422–6.

16. Balato A, Scalvenzi M, Cirillo T, et al. Psoriasis in children: a review. Curr Pediatr Rev 2015;11(1):10–26.

17. Johnson MA, Armstrong AW. Clinical and histologic diagnostic guidelines for psoriasis: a critical review. Clin Rev Allergy Immunol 2013;44(2):166–72.

18. Thyssen JP, McFadden JP, Kimber I. The multiple factors affecting the association between atopic dermatitis and contact sensitization. Allergy 2014;69(1): 28–36.

19. Aquino M, Fonacier L. The role of contact dermatitis in patients with atopic dermatitis. J Allergy Clin Immunol Pract 2014;2(4):382–7.

20. Shaughnessy CN, Malajian D, Belsito DV. Cutaneous delayed-type hypersensitivity in patients with atopic dermatitis: reactivity to topical preservatives. J Am Acad Dermatol 2014;70(1):102–7.

21. Malajian D, Belsito DV. Cutaneous delayed-type hypersensitivity in patients with atopic dermatitis. J Am Acad Dermatol 2013;69(2):232–7.

22. Shaughnessy CN, Malajian D, Belsito DV. Cutaneous delayed-type hypersensitivity in patients with atopic dermatitis: reactivity to surfactants. J Am Acad Dermatol 2014;70(4):704–8.

23. Herro EM, Matiz C, Sullivan K, et al. Frequency of contact allergens in pediatric patients with atopic dermatitis. J Clin Aesthet Dermatol 2011;4(11):39–41.

24. Militello G, Jacob SE, Crawford GH. Allergic contact dermatitis in children. Curr Opin Pediatr 2006;18(4):385–90.

25. de Waard-van der Spek FB, Darsow U, Mortz CG, et al. EAACI position paper for practical patch testing in allergic contact dermatitis in children. Pediatr Allergy Immunol 2015;26(7):598–606.

26. Hengge UR, Currie BJ, Jäger G, et al. Scabies: a ubiquitous neglected skin disease. Lancet Infect Dis 2006;6(12):769–79.

27. Heukelbach J, Feldmeier H. Scabies. Lancet 2006;367(9524):1767–74.

28. Boralevi F, Diallo A, Miquel J, et al. Clinical phenotype of scabies by age. Pediatrics 2014;133(4):e910–6.

29. Olsen JR, Piguet V, Gallacher J, et al. Molluscum contagiosum and associations with atopic eczema in children: a retrospective longitudinal study in primary care. Br J Gen Pract 2016;66(642):e53–8.

30. Berger EM, Orlow SJ, Patel RR, et al. Experience with molluscum contagiosum and associated inflammatory reactions in a pediatric dermatology practice: the bump that rashes. Arch Dermatol 2012;148(11):1257–64.

31. Kelly B. Superficial fungal infections. Pediatr Rev 2012;33(4):e22–37.

32. Atzori L, Pau M, Aste N. Dermatophyte infections mimicking other skin diseases: a 154-person case survey of tinea atypica in the district of Cagliari (Italy). Int J Dermatol 2012;51(4):410–5.

33. Alston SJ, Cohen BA, Braun M. Persistent and recurrent tinea corporis in children treated with combination antifungal/corticosteroid agents. Pediatrics 2003; 111(1):201–3.

34. Levitt JO, Levitt BH, Akhavan A, et al. The sensitivity and specificity of potassium hydroxide smear and fungal culture relative to clinical assessment in the evaluation of tinea pedis: a pooled analysis. Dermatol Res Pract 2010;2010:764843.

35. Fink-Puches R, Chott A, Ardigó M, et al. The spectrum of cutaneous lymphomas in patients less than 20 years of age. Pediatr Dermatol 2004;21(5):525–33.

36. Onsun N, Kural Y, Su O, et al. Hypopigmented mycosis fungoides associated with atopy in two children. Pediatr Dermatol 2006;23(5):493–6.

37. Jawed SI, Myskowski PL, Horwitz S, et al. Primary cutaneous T-cell lymphoma (mycosis fungoides and Sézary syndrome): part I. Diagnosis: clinical and histopathologic features and new molecular and biologic markers. J Am Acad Dermatol 2014;70(2):205.e1-16 [quiz: 221–2].

38. Pope E, Weitzman S, Ngan B, et al. Mycosis fungoides in the pediatric population: report from an international childhood registry of cutaneous lymphoma. J Cutan Med Surg 2010;14(1):1–6.

39. Boulos S, Vaid R, Aladily TN, et al. Clinical presentation, immunopathology, and treatment of juvenile-onset mycosis fungoides: a case series of 34 patients. J Am Acad Dermatol 2014;71(6):1117–26.

40. Agar NS, Wedgeworth E, Crichton S, et al. Survival outcomes and prognostic factors in mycosis fungoides/Sézary syndrome: validation of the revised International Society for Cutaneous Lymphomas/European Organisation for Research and Treatment of Cancer staging proposal. J Clin Oncol 2010;28(31):4730–9.

41. Laws PM, Shear NH, Pope E. Childhood mycosis fungoides: experience of 28 patients and response to phototherapy. Pediatr Dermatol 2014;31(4):459–64.

42. Iaccarino L, Ghirardello A, Bettio S, et al. The clinical features, diagnosis and classification of dermatomyositis. J Autoimmun 2014;48-49:122–7.

43. Almeida B, Campanilho-Marques R, Arnold K, et al. Analysis of published criteria for clinically inactive disease in a large juvenile dermatomyositis cohort shows that skin disease is underestimated. Arthritis Rheumatol 2015;67(9):2495–502.

44. Wedderburn LR, Rider LG. Juvenile dermatomyositis: new developments in pathogenesis, assessment and treatment. Best Pract Res Clin Rheumatol 2009;23(5): 665–78.

45. Hung CH. Treatment and clinical outcome of juvenile dermatomyositis. Pediatr Neonatol 2015;56(1):1–2.

46. Bowers S, Warshaw EM. Pityriasis lichenoides and its subtypes. J Am Acad Dermatol 2006;55(4):557–72 [quiz: 573–6].

47. Brazzelli V, Carugno A, Rivetti N, et al. Narrowband UVB phototherapy for pediatric generalized pityriasis lichenoides. Photodermatol Photoimmunol Photomed 2013;29(6):330–3.

48. Geller L, Antonov NK, Lauren CT, et al. Pityriasis lichenoides in childhood: review of clinical presentation and treatment options. Pediatr Dermatol 2015;32(5): 579–92.

49. Khachemoune A, Blyumin ML. Pityriasis lichenoides: pathophysiology, classification, and treatment. Am J Clin Dermatol 2007;8(1):29–36.

50. Badalian-Very G, Vergilio JA, Degar BA, et al. Recurrent BRAF mutations in Langerhans cell histiocytosis. Blood 2010;116(11):1919–23.

51. Hönigsmann H. Polymorphous light eruption. Photodermatol Photoimmunol Photomed 2008;24(3):155–61.

52. Valbuena MC, Muvdi S, Lim HW. Actinic prurigo. Dermatol Clin 2014;32(3): 335–44, viii.

53. Hojyo-Tomoka MT, Vega-Memije ME, Cortes-Franco R, et al. Diagnosis and treatment of actinic prurigo. Dermatol Ther 2003;16(1):40–4.

54. Lee LW, Yan AC. Skin manifestations of nutritional deficiency disease in children: modern day contexts. Int J Dermatol 2012;51(12):1407–18.

55. Lakdawala N, Grant-Kels JM. Acrodermatitis enteropathica and other nutritional diseases of the folds (intertriginous areas). Clin Dermatol 2015;33(4):414–9.

Clinical Measures of Chronic Urticaria

Karsten Weller, MD*, Frank Siebenhaar, MD, Tomasz Hawro, MD,
Sabine Altrichter, MD, Nicole Schoepke, MD, Marcus Maurer, MD

KEYWORDS

- Urticaria • Angioedema • Patient reported outcome • Disease activity
- Disease control • Quality of life

KEY POINTS

- Because of the fluctuating nature of chronic urticaria symptoms, physicians almost never see a representative picture of patients' disease and objective and specific biomarkers are not yet established. Accordingly, patient reported outcome instruments and other clinical measures are required to determine the patient's disease status.
- There are various validated and reliable clinical measures to assess patients with chronic urticaria, that is, recurrent wheals that itch, angioedema, or both.
- Disease activity can be determined by the Urticaria Activity Score, the Angioedema Activity Score, the Cholinergic Urticaria Activity Score, and, for all chronic inducible urticarias, the measurement of critical trigger thresholds.
- Disease control is determined by the Urticaria Control Test, and the impairment of health-related quality of life can be assessed by use of the Chronic Urticaria Quality of Life Questionnaire and the Angioedema Quality of Life Questionnaire.
- These clinical measures may support treatment decisions and improve the detection and documentation of treatment responses. In addition, these measures facilitate, improve, and standardize medical record keeping and, at the same time, provide new insights into patients' disease burden.

Conflicts of Interest: K. Weller is or recently was a speaker, investigator, and/or consultant for Dr R. Pfleger, Essex pharma (now MSD), FAES, Novartis, Shire, UCB, Uriach, Viropharma, and Moxie. F. Siebenhaar is or recently was a speaker, grant recipient, and/or advisor for BioCryst, Novartis, Moxie, Patara, and Uriach. T. Hawro is or recently was a speaker for Moxie. S. Altrichter is or recently was a speaker for Moxie. N. Schoepke is or recently was a speaker for Moxie. M. Maurer is or recently was a speaker, grant recipient, and/or advisor for BioCryst, Courage & Khazaka, FAES, Genentech, Moxie, Novartis, Sanofi, Shire, and/or Uriach.
Financial Support and Sponsorship: None.
Department of Dermatology and Allergy, Allergie-Centrum-Charité, Charité – Universitätsmedizin Berlin, Chariteplatz 1, 10117 Berlin, Germany
* Corresponding author. Department of Dermatology and Allergy, Allergie-Centrum-Charité, Charité – Universitätsmedizin Berlin, Charitéplatz 1, 10117 Berlin, Germany.
E-mail address: karsten.weller@charite.de

INTRODUCTION

Chronic urticaria is a common skin disorder[1] with a high relevance in dermatologic and allergological patient care.[2,3] It is defined by the occurrence of transient itchy wheals (hives), angioedema, or both for more than 6 weeks.[4]

Chronic urticaria is divided into chronic spontaneous urticaria (CSU) and chronic inducible urticarias (CIndUs) (**Table 1**).[4] In CSU, wheals and/or angioedema occur suddenly and unpredictably without a specific trigger. The intake of nonsteroidal anti-inflammatory drugs or specific foods, stress, and physical triggers, such as heat, can prompt exacerbations in some patients; but these triggers are not specific, that is, their presence does not reproducibly lead to wheals or angioedema and wheals and angioedema also occur without these triggers. In contrast, CIndUs are characterized by specific triggers, which are required for urticaria signs and symptoms to occur and which reproducibly induce them. The development of wheals and angioedema in patients with CIndU is typically but not always limited to the areas of exposure, for example, to areas of cold contact in cold urticaria. Both CSU and CIndUs frequently cause a major impairment of patients' health-related quality of life (HR-QoL).[5–8]

As of yet, there are no established, objective, reliable, and specific biomarkers to measure the disease activity and disease control in patients with CSU and CIndU. In addition, there are no biomarkers available to assess changes of these disorders over time, for example, before and after treatment adjustment. Accordingly, clinical measures are currently the only way to assess these features as well as to assess the disease burden.

This review gives an overview of the currently available clinical measures for chronic urticaria. In addition, the authors provide information on how to best use these measures in clinical practice and the evaluation and interpretation of their results.

CLINICAL MEASURES OF CHRONIC SPONTANEOUS URTICARIA AND CHRONIC INDUCIBLE URTICARIAS

It is not trivial to determine the disease status in patients with chronic urticaria. CSU is a strongly fluctuating disorder. Many patients have daily or almost-daily symptoms;

Table 1 Classification of chronic urticaria	
CSU	**CIndU**
Spontaneous appearance of wheals, angioedema, or both ≥6 wk due to known or unknown causes	Symptomatic dermographism (also known as urticaria factitia)
	Cold urticaria (also known as cold contact urticaria)
	Delayed pressure urticaria (also known as pressure urticaria)
	Solar urticaria
	Heat urticaria (also known as heat contact urticaria)
	Vibratory angioedema
	Cholinergic urticaria
	Contact urticaria
	Aquagenic urticaria

Adapted from Zuberbier T, Aberer W, Asero R, et al. The EAACI/GA(2) LEN/EDF/WAO guideline for the definition, classification, diagnosis, and management of urticaria: the 2013 revision and update. Allergy 2014;69(7):871; with permission.

but the timing of their occurrence, their severity, and duration can change considerably from day to day. In addition, symptom episodes occur particularly often during the evening, nighttime, and early morning.[9] Accordingly, many patients do not have visible wheals or angioedema at the time of appointments with their doctors or they show up with signs and symptoms, but these are not representative for what they usually have.[10] In addition, itch is not objectively assessable,[10] although it is a key symptom and major driver of patients' disease burden.[11]

In CIndUs, there is an additional factor that makes it difficult to assess the disease status: patients with CindU usually avoid the triggers of their urticaria as best as they can. This avoidance may lead to little or mild urticaria symptoms, and patients, therefore, may falsely be categorized as suffering from only mild disease, although their disease burden remains high and their CIndU is only poorly under control.

The best way to address these problems is to implement standardized, valid, and reliable clinical measures, that is, patient-reported outcome tools (PROs) and critical trigger threshold (CTT) measurements, to determine patients' disease activity, disease control, and HR-QoL impairment in routine care. In addition, the availability and use of these measures are important to improve and standardize outcome assessment in clinical studies.

PROs are questionnaires that obtain all relevant information directly from the affected patients.[12] They are typically designed to gather information on one specific topic or for one specific purpose. PROs usually result in total scores and/or several subscores that subsequently need to be interpreted by the administering health care professional.

CTTs are assessed by standardized, provocation tests that expose patients with CIndU to the specific trigger of their urticaria in graded intensity.[13] Subsequently, patients are monitored for the occurrence of urticaria signs and symptoms. The lowest trigger intensity that still induces symptoms is the individual CTT and indicates patients' disease activity.

This article focuses on the available and specific PRO measure to determine disease activity, disease control, and HR-QoL impairment in CSU and CIndUs (**Tables 2 and 3**). In addition, it provides a short overview of ways to determine CTTs.

CLINICAL MEASURES OF DISEASE ACTIVITY IN CHRONIC SPONTANEOUS URTICARIA
Urticaria Activity Score

The Urticaria Activity Score (UAS) is the broadly accepted gold standard to assess disease activity in CSU and is recommended by the current guidelines.[4] It has been used

Table 2
Relevant patient-reported outcome measures in chronic spontaneous urticaria and areas of use

	CSU		
	Patients with Wheals (Hives)	Patients with Wheals (Hives) and Angioedema	Patients with Angioedema
Disease activity	UAS	UAS[a] and AAS[b]	AAS
Disease control	UCT	UCT	UCT
HR-QoL	CU-Q$_2$oL	CU-Q$_2$oL and AE-QoL	AE-QoL

Abbreviations: AAS, Angioedema Activity Score; AE-QoL, Angioedema Quality of Life Questionnaire; CU-Q$_2$oL, Chronic Urticaria Quality of Life Questionnaire; UAS, Urticaria Activity Score; UCT, Urticaria Control Test.
[a] The Urticaria Activity Score does not assess angioedema.
[b] The Angioedema Activity Score does not assess wheals (hives).

Table 3
Characteristics and availability of relevant patient-reported outcome measures in chronic urticaria

	UAS	AAS	UCT	CU-Q2oL	AE-QoL
Original or source publication	[4]	[22]	[39]	[43]	[52]
Number of items (questions)	2 (everyday)	1-6 (everyday)	4 (once)	23 (once)	17 (once)
Recall period	1 d	1 d	4 wk	2 wk	4 wk
Applicable in CSU	+[a]	+[b]	+	+[a]	+[b]
Applicable in CIndU	−	+[b]	+	−	+[b]
Results available directly after administration (retrospective assessment)	−	−	+	+	+
Results available only in the future (prospective, diary-type assessment)	+	+	−	−	−
High level of patient compliance required	+	+	−	−	−
Scoring and evaluation fast and simple	+	+	+	−	−
Cutoff values published	−	−	+	−	−
Minimal important difference published	+	+	+	+	+

Cost-free use in routine patient management and investigator-initiated clinical research	+	+	+	+	+
Cost-free use in industry-driven projects and studies	+	–	–	–	–
Different language versions available[f]	+[c]	+[d] (German, American-English, Spanish, French, Portuguese, Azeri, Swedish, Hungarian, Romanian, Greek, Polish, Dutch, Russian, Canadian-French, Danish, Italian, Mexican, Japanese, UK-English, Canadian-English, Hebrew, Macedonian, Turkish, Brazilian-Portuguese)	+[d] (German, American-English, Spanish, French, Turkish, Thai, Greek, Polish, Dutch, Russian, Canadian-English, Danish, Mexican, Portuguese, Brazilian-Portuguese, Finish)	+[e] Italian, German, Greek, Spanish, Polish, Turkish, Persian, Thai	+[d] (German, American-English, Spanish, French, Portuguese, Turkish, Azeri, Swedish, Hungarian, Hebrew, Romanian, Greek, Polish, Dutch, Russian, Canadian-English, Danish, Italian, Mexican, Japanese, Canadian-French, US-Spanish, Brazilian-Portuguese, Macedonian, Arabic (Jordan), Hebrew, Slovakian)

Abbreviations: AAS, Angioedema Activity Score; AE-QoL, Angioedema Quality of Life Questionnaire; CU-Q$_2$oL, Chronic Urticaria Quality of Life Questionnaire; UAS, Urticaria Activity Score; UCT, Urticaria Control Test.

[a] Results may not provide an accurate picture in patients with CSU in whom recurrent angioedema is a major factor.

[b] Applicable in those patients with CSU and CIndU who display recurrent angioedema, with or without wheals.

[c] Availability in several languages. Original source is the urticaria guideline.[4] Because of its easy structure, the Urticaria Activity Score is usually translated but not formally linguistically validated.

[d] Availability may be checked at Moxie.[36]

[e] Availability may be checked at original author team.[43]

[f] Additional language versions may be or are in preparation (for more details with regard to the Angioedema Activity Score, Urticaria Control Test, and Angioedema Quality of Life Questionnaire versions, the corresponding author can be contacted).

in many clinical trials as an outcome parameter, including the recent studies on the efficacy and safety of omalizumab,[14–18] when it once again demonstrated its high value and usefulness as a PRO measure.

The UAS focuses on 2 key symptoms of CSU, that is, wheals and itch. It is a diary-type tool that asks the patients once daily for numbers of wheals and severity of itch during the past 24 hours (**Table 4**). The answers related to each symptom are rated from 0 to 3 points, that is, the minimum and maximum daily score are 0 and 6 points, respectively, with higher values indicating stronger disease activity. Because of the considerable fluctuation of symptoms from day to day, data of at least 4 subsequent days should be collected to obtain a good picture of patients' current disease activity.[19] In clinical studies and daily care it has been found most useful to collect and sum up the UAS from 7 days in a row (UAS7, range 0–42 points), which is now established and recommended by the European Academy of Allergology and Clinical Immunology/Global Allergy and Asthma European Network/European Dermatology Forum/World Allergy Organization's urticaria guideline (see **Table 4**).[4]

For the interpretation of PRO measure results, it is very important to know which score changes over time are really clinically meaningful to patients, that is, what is the minimal important difference (MID) (also known as minimal important change)? Currently, the MID of the guideline-recommended UAS7 is not known; but studies examining the MID are underway. In addition, it is important to know which scores represent mild, moderate, and severe disease activity. As of yet, there are no commonly accepted UAS7 score ranges or cutoff values available. In the recent phase III trials on omalizumab in CSU,[14–18] a criterion for inclusion was a UAS7 of 16 points or greater during the baseline assessment; it has been promoted that a UAS7 less than 16 points indicates mild CSU, whereas a UAS7 of 16 points or greater indicates moderate to severe CSU. However, this cutoff value remains to be formally validated against appropriate anchors.

It may cause confusion that, during the past years, a different version of the UAS has been used in adults,[20] with different categories for wheal numbers (no wheals, 1–6 wheals, 7–12 wheals, >12 wheals) and a different frequency of documentation (twice daily instead of once daily).[20] For this UAS, an MID of around 10 points has been established.[20] At the time being, it is not fully clear how the scores of both UAS tools correspond to each other, which hampers the comparison and meta-analysis of studies that applied different UAS versions.

Table 4
Urticaria Activity Score

Score	Wheals	Pruritus
0	None	None
1	Mild (<20 wheals during last 24 h)	Mild (present but not annoying or troublesome)
2	Moderate (20–50 wheals during last 24 h)	Moderate (troublesome but does not interfere with normal daily activity or sleep)
3	Intense (>50 wheals or large confluent areas of wheals during last 24 h)	Intense (severe pruritus that is sufficiently troublesome to interfere with normal daily activity or sleep)

Adapted from Zuberbier T, Aberer W, Asero R, et al. The EAACI/GA(2) LEN/EDF/WAO guideline for the definition, classification, diagnosis, and management of urticaria: the 2013 revision and update. Allergy 2014;69(7):871; with permission.

In a recent randomized controlled trial on the efficacy and safety of the second-generation antihistamine rupatadine in chronic spontaneous urticaria, an additional children-adapted version of the UAS7 was applied. For this study, the guideline-recommended UAS was slightly modified by an adjusted documentation of wheal numbers to no wheals, 1 to 9 wheals, 10 to 30 wheals, and greater than 30 wheals, because of the lower body surface area of children.[21] However, this UAS remains to be formally validated.

The major strength of the UAS7 is that it provides a fairly exact picture of the current frequency and severity of CSU symptoms because the short recall period of 24 hours for each entry and the summing up of 7 days in a row make sure that the provided information is accurate and fluctuations of the disease are leveled out. However, the UAS7 also has several limitations: (1) it only works prospectively, that is, results are not instantly available, for example, at a patient's first appointment; (2) it requires good patient compliance and documentation discipline (its results may become inaccurate or are lost in case patients forget to document their symptoms or forget to bring the documentation to the next appointment); (3) it only works in CSU but not patients with CIndU; (4) it is only validated for use in adults; (5) score ranges representing low, medium, or high disease activity have yet to be established; and finally (6) it does not include angioedema, although angioedema is a key symptom and major driver of disease burden in many patients. For these angioedema patients, different tools, such as the Angioedema Activity Score (AAS), are required. An overview of the characteristics and the availability of the UAS and other urticaria-relevant PRO measures is shown in **Table 3**.

Angioedema Activity Score

The AAS has been developed as the first symptom-specific PRO measure to assess angioedema activity in patients with all forms of recurrent angioedema (RA).[22] RA can be histamine mediated (in CSU and CIndU) or bradykinin mediated (RA due to C1-inhibitor deficiency and RA caused by intake of angiotensin-converting enzyme inhibitors).[10]

As the UAS, the AAS is a prospective, diary-type tool. It asks the patients to once daily document if angioedema occurred during the past 24 hours or not. If angioedema was present, the AAS asks 5 additional questions to determine the severity and impact of this episode, each with answer options that are scored from 0 to 3 points. Accordingly, the minimum and maximum daily score is 0 and 15 points. To get a sufficient picture of patients' disease activity, it is usually recommended to collect data from 4 weeks (AAS28).[22] The AAS is particularly useful in patients with RA without wheals and in patients where angioedema is a predominant factor.

In its original validation study, the AAS was found to have a one-dimensional structure and excellent internal consistency.[22] Its levels of validity and test-retest reliability were shown to be good.[22] In addition, the AAS was demonstrated to be sensitive to changes of angioedema activity over time, and a MID of 8 points for the 7-day cumulative AAS (AAS7) is established.[22] Finally, the AAS also has been applied successfully in recent randomized controlled trials in CSU[23] but also in RA due to C1-inhibitor deficiency.[24] The available language versions as well as their terms of use are shown in **Table 3**.

Because the UAS and AAS are both diary-type tools with a comparable structure and scoring, their strengths and limitations are also comparable (see **Table 3**): As the UAS, the AAS provides an exact picture of the current frequency and severity of angioedema episodes; but, on the other hand, it also only works prospectively; ad hoc results are not available; AAS28 score ranges that can be regarded to represent low, moderate, or high angioedema activity have yet to be established. However, the original validation study already provides information on AAS7 values of patients with different disease activities, that is, a mean AAS7 standard deviation of 6.5 ±6.9 was found in patients with angioedema globally self-rating their disease activity as mild; a value of 15.4 ±10.1 was found in patients indicating their angioedema activity to be moderate; a score of 21.2 ±11.3 was determined in patients who reported their angioedema activity to be severe.[22]

If the AAS is used in patients with CSU with wheals and angioedema, it should be made sure that patients do not confuse the two. Otherwise, the AAS results may not correctly capture angioedema-related disease activity.

CLINICAL MEASURES OF DISEASE ACTIVITY IN CHRONIC INDUCIBLE URTICARIAS
Cholinergic Urticaria Activity Score

In CIndUs, an assessment of the quality and quantity of symptoms alone does not provide a reliable picture of the patients' disease activity. As mentioned earlier, the avoidance behavior of patients with CIndU strongly influences the frequency and severity of their symptoms. Accordingly, in a PRO measure, the actual exposure to triggers would need to be evaluated as well. As of yet, the only CindU for which such an activity score has been established is cholinergic urticaria. Here, the cholinergic UAS (CholUAS) has been developed and was found to be a valuable outcome parameter in a clinical trial.[25] The CholUAS is a modification of the UAS and collects data, once daily, on the intensity of wheals (not wheal numbers) and pruritus as well as the intensity of exposure to individually relevant symptom elicitors during the past 24 hours.[25] As in case of the UAS7, it makes sense to sum up 7 consecutive days in order to obtain a more reliable picture of the patients' current disease activity.

Critical Trigger Threshold Assessment

For CIndUs other than cholinergic urticaria, there are, as of yet, no comparable PRO tools available. However, the inducibility of symptoms opens up the possibility for an objective assessment of disease activity by determining CTTs. CTTs have also been found to be sensitive to changes, for example, during successful treatment.[26–29] Examples for standardized CTT measurements are the assessment of the critical temperature threshold in patients with cold urticaria by using the Peltier-element-based TempTest,[13,30–32] the standardized application of graded shear forces in symptomatic dermographism by using FricTest,[33,34] or the standardized pulse-controlled ergometry provocation test in cholinergic urticaria.[35] For more details on available CTT test devices and measurement of CTTs in CIndUs, the authors would like to refer to the recent review of Magerl and colleagues.[13]

CLINICAL MEASURES OF DISEASE CONTROL

The treatment of CSU has improved strongly during the past years. The currently most widely accepted treatment algorithm suggests using second-generation antihistamines in the licensed dose as the first-line therapy, an updosing of second-generation antihistamines to up to 4 times the licensed dose as second-line treatment, and the addition of omalizumab, cyclosporin, or montelukast as third-line options.[4] However, most of these treatment options are off-label (updosing of second-generation antihistamines, cyclosporin, montelukast), associated with an unfavorable long-term safety profile (cyclosporin), or go along with considerable costs (omalizumab). Accordingly, it is important that treatment decisions are made carefully and that they are ideally based on and backed by a standardized, valid, and reliable documentation of the patients' current disease status.

Urticaria Control Test

The currently easiest way to assess the patients' disease status is to apply the Urticaria Control Test (UCT). The UCT was specifically developed and validated to determine disease control, in all forms of chronic urticaria (CSU and CIndU), that is, to determine the level of disease control but also to give a clear answer to the question of whether the urticaria is well-controlled or not, and thereby to aid and back treatment decisions. Several different language versions are available,[36–39] and their terms of use are presented in **Table 3**.

The UCT is a retrospective PRO measure with a recall period of 4 weeks that consists of only 4 questions. The answer options to each question are scored from 0 to 4 points and subsequently added up to the UCT score with a minimum and maximum value of 0 and 16 points, respectively. A score of 11 points or less points toward poorly controlled urticaria, whereas a score of 12 or higher indicates well-controlled disease.

The original publication of the UCT proved that the UCT strongly correlates with the UAS but also with the HR-QoL impairment in patients with chronic urticaria.[39] It was found to have good levels of validity, an excellent reliability, and a high screening accuracy to identify patients with insufficiently controlled disease.[39] The MID of the UCT was found to be 3 points in 2 independent studies[38,40]; a change of a least 3 points can be regarded as a change that is meaningful to patients.

The major strengths of the UCT are its retrospective approach, short and simple structure, and its easy scoring system. It is possible to use the UCT at any patient presentation; its results are instantly available after completion; its clear cutoff value of 12 points enables a direct evaluation of the disease status. In addition, the UCT is applicable in all forms of chronic urticaria. These properties make the UCT an ideal PRO measure for daily patient management. However, one of its major strengths, its shortness, is also its limitation. Although UCT results are accurate, the information obtained by the UCT is not very detailed. If one wants to know exactly which symptoms currently occur and which areas of HR-QoL are impaired, the UCT is not a suitable tool to provide this information.

CLINICAL MEASURES OF HEALTH-RELATED QUALITY-OF-LIFE IMPAIRMENT

CSU causes major impairment of patients' HR-QoL[5–7] for several reasons. The symptoms usually occur unpredictably and vary strongly with regard to their frequency and intensity. Accordingly, many patients have major problems planning their daily life. Symptoms, including chronic itch, often occur during the nights, and interference with sleep, difficulties concentrating during the next day, and a reduced ability to handle daily activities, including a reduced performance at work and school, are common. In addition, recurrent angioedema, which occurs in around 50% of patients with CSU with a preference of the face and upper respiratory tract,[23] commonly leads to disfigurement and fear of suffocation.

In order to better understand and assess the full extent of urticaria-related disease burden and/or its changes over time, it is not sufficient to just evaluate the frequency and severity of symptoms.[41] For this purpose, disease-specific, patient-centered tools focusing on patients' HR-QoL are required. These tools should be preferred over generic HR-QoL instruments, unless a comparison of chronic urticaria with other disorders is intended because they are usually more robust and sensitive in obtaining meaningful QoL data[42] as well as their changes over time.

Chronic Urticaria Quality of Life Questionnaire

The Chronic Urticaria Quality of Life Questionnaire (CU-Q$_2$oL) is the first disease-specific tool to assess HR-QoL impairment in patients with CSU.[43] It contains 23 questions and has a recall period of 2 weeks. Each question has 5 answer options that are scored from 0 to 4 points. The CU-Q$_2$oL may be applied as an index instrument to assess the overall CSU-related QoL impairment (total score assessment), but it may also be used to examine the profile of impairment by computing its domain scores. The total score is generated by summing up all 23 question scores and by subsequently transferring the score to a 0 to 100 scale to limit the influence of missing items.[43] Higher values indicate a higher HR-QoL impairment. The domain scores are computed similarly, with the exception that for each domain only the scores of that domain are considered.

Several language versions are available and have been validated.[6,43–49] Although the CU-Q$_2$oL total score of all language versions is similarly computed and may be compared, the CU-Q$_2$oL domain structure varies between different versions, for example, between the original Italian version[43] and the German version,[6] thus, limiting the possibility for comparisons or joint analyses of the domain scores.

In the original publication[43] and subsequent validation studies, the CU-Q$_2$oL has been found to have good levels of validity and reliability. In addition, a recent Korean study found a good sensitivity to change and suggested an MID of 15 points for the CU-Q$_2$oL total score.[47] Moreover, the CU-Q$_2$oL was found to be more sensitive in comparison with other, non–disease-specific HR-QoL measures, such as the Dermatology Quality of Life Index.[50] The CU-Q$_2$oL has been used in many clinical studies, including pharmacologic randomized controlled trials.[15,23,51]

Major limitations of the CU-Q$_2$oL are (1) that it is only applicable in CSU but not in CIndUs (CIndUs disease-specific HR-QoL measures are not available yet and strongly needed); (2) that good information on which CU-Q$_2$oL scores indicate mild, moderate, and severe HR-QoL impairment are missing (however, studies to determine this are currently underway); (3) that because of the relatively complicated scoring system, the CU-Q$_2$oL is not ideally suited for routine patient management (here only a rough estimation of the total score is realistic rather than an exact evaluation of the total and all domain scores); and (4) that the CU-Q$_2$oL questions are not well tailored for patients with CSU predominantly with angioedema (although angioedema is part of the CU-Q$_2$oL symptoms domain). For the last limitation, the Angioedema Quality of Life Questionnaire (AE-QoL) was developed.

Angioedema Quality of Life Questionnaire

The AE-QoL is the first symptom-specific PRO measure to assess HR-QoL in RA.[52] As the AAS, it is applicable for all subforms of RA and has a recall period of 4 weeks.[52] With regard to its characteristics, structure, and scoring, the AE-QoL is closely related to the CU-Q$_2$oL. It consists of 17 questions with 5 answer options each that are all scored from 0 to 4 points.

In the original publication on its development and validation, the AE-QoL has been found to have a 4-dimensional structure with good levels of internal consistency as well as a valid total score.[52] The question scores can be summed up to a total score but also grouped together to 4 different domain scores (functioning, fatigue/mood, fears/shame, food), which are each displayed on a 0 to 100 scale.[52] Accordingly, the AE-QoL may serve as an index or a profile instrument for RA-related QoL impairment.

In addition to the original publication, in a recent study, the authors were able to confirm the good convergent validity of the AE-QoL: they found its total scores to correlate well with the frequency of angioedema attacks, that is, to be higher in patients with higher frequency of attacks. In addition, the authors were able to prove the AE-QoL's sensitivity to change as well as to determine its MID, which is 6 points.[53]

Although only published in 2012, the AE-QoL is available in many different language versions already (see **Table 3**) and has been applied in different randomized controlled clinical trials in CSU and hereditary angioedema with good results.[23,24]

Major limitations of the AE-QoL are comparable with those of the CU-Q$_2$oL: (1) it has relatively complicated scoring system, which may hamper its broad application in routine patient management; (2) in patients with CSU or CIndU with wheals and angioedema, it provides only a picture of the angioedema-related component of HR-QoL impairment; and (3) it will not yield accurate results in patients with CSU who confuse wheals and angioedema.

In addition to the CU-Q$_2$oL and the AE-QoL, there is a tool available to assess HR-QoL in patients with chronic itch, the ItchyQoL.[11,54] This PRO instrument is particularly interesting for physicians and researchers who want to focus specifically on pruritus and its impact.

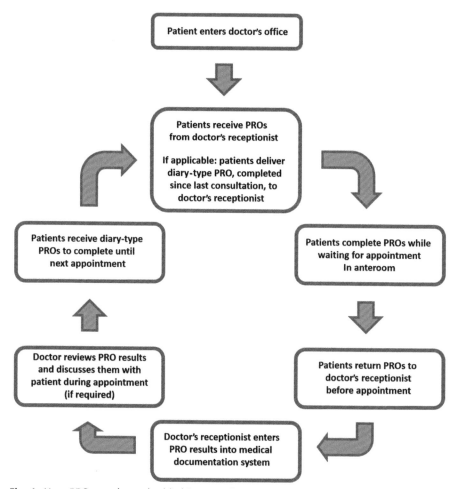

Fig. 1. How PROs can be embedded into routine patient management.

SUMMARY

The use of standardized, valid, and reliable clinical measures is an important component of modern patient-centered care. In addition, the availability of these measures is essential for the quality and performance of clinical trials.

In the last years, several new and well-developed clinical measures became available in CSU and CIndUs, that is, PRO instruments to determine disease activity, disease control, and HR-QoL impairment as well as CTT test devices. These measures strongly improved the understanding, assessment, and evaluation of these disorders. Some even became approachable by studies for the first time.

In routine patient management, the presented clinical measures can help aid and back treatment decisions, provide better insights into the patients' disease burden, and facilitate, improve, and standardize the increasingly important documentation work. In addition, clinical measures may serve to better determine changes in patients' disease status over time. This is particularly relevant in times of both limited resources and high costs for modern treatment options, which require careful decisions on the best individual therapy approaches.

The clinical measures described in this review have already proven their high value in daily patient care and clinical studies. Most of them are self-explaining, easy to administer, and simple to score and evaluate. If well embedded into daily routines (**Fig. 1**), they may help save valuable time for a longer and more intensive communication with patients because an important part of the required documentation work is done by those who are the center of our efforts, the patients themselves.

ACKNOWLEDGMENTS

The authors would like to thank the Urticaria Network e.v. (UNEV), the Global Allergy and Asthma European Network (GA²LEN), as well as the International Center for Angioedema Research (iCARE) for supporting PRO research in urticaria and recurrent angioedema during the last years. The authors also thank all physicians of the Charité urticaria clinic, a GA²LEN Urticaria Center of Reference and Excellence (UCARE, www.ga2len.net/ucare), for their support and helpful discussions.

REFERENCES

1. Maurer M, Weller K, Bindslev-Jensen C, et al. Unmet clinical needs in chronic spontaneous urticaria. A GA(2)LEN task force report. Allergy 2011;66(3):317–30.

2. Weller K, Schoepke N, Krause K, et al. Selected urticaria patients benefit from a referral to tertiary care centres–results of an expert survey. J Eur Acad Dermatol Venereol 2013;27(1):e8–16.

3. Weller K, Viehmann K, Brautigam M, et al. Cost-intensive, time-consuming, problematical? How physicians in private practice experience the care of urticaria patients. J Dtsch Dermatol Ges 2012;10(5):341–7.

4. Zuberbier T, Aberer W, Asero R, et al. The EAACI/GA(2) LEN/EDF/WAO guideline for the definition, classification, diagnosis, and management of urticaria: the 2013 revision and update. Allergy 2014;69(7):868–87.

5. Lewis V, Finlay AY. 10 years experience of the Dermatology Life Quality Index (DLQI). J Investig Dermatol Symp Proc 2004;9(2):169–80.

6. Mlynek A, Magerl M, Hanna M, et al. The German version of the chronic urticaria quality-of-life questionnaire: factor analysis, validation, and initial clinical findings. Allergy 2009;64(6):927–36.

7. O'Donnell BF, Lawlor F, Simpson J, et al. The impact of chronic urticaria on the quality of life. Br J Dermatol 1997;136(2):197–201.
8. Schoepke N, Mlynek A, Weller K, et al. Symptomatic dermographism: an inadequately described disease. J Eur Acad Dermatol Venereol 2015;29(4):708–12.
9. Maurer M, Ortonne JP, Zuberbier T. Chronic urticaria: an Internet survey of health behaviours, symptom patterns and treatment needs in European adult patients. Br J Dermatol 2009;160(3):633–41.
10. Weller K, Zuberbier T, Maurer M. Clinically relevant outcome measures for assessing disease activity, disease control and quality of life impairment in patients with chronic spontaneous urticaria and recurrent angioedema. Curr Opin Allergy Clin Immunol 2015;15(3):220–6.
11. Krause K, Kessler B, Weller K, et al. German version of ItchyQoL: validation and initial clinical findings. Acta Derm Venereol 2013;93(5):562–8.
12. U.S. Department of Health and Human Services FDA Center for Drug Evaluation and Research, U.S. Department of Health and Human Services FDA Center for Biologics Evaluation and Research, U.S. Department of Health and Human Services FDA Center for Devices and Radiological Health. Guidance for industry: patient-reported outcome measures: use in medical product development to support labeling claims: draft guidance. Health Qual Life Outcomes 2006;4:79.
13. Magerl M, Altrichter S, Borzova E, et al. The definition, diagnostic testing, and management of chronic inducible urticarias - The EAACI/GA(2) LEN/EDF/UNEV consensus recommendations 2016 update and revision. Allergy 2016;71(6): 780–802.
14. Kaplan A, Ledford D, Ashby M, et al. Omalizumab in patients with symptomatic chronic idiopathic/spontaneous urticaria despite standard combination therapy. J Allergy Clin Immunol 2013;132(1):101–9.
15. Maurer M, Altrichter S, Bieber T, et al. Efficacy and safety of omalizumab in patients with chronic urticaria who exhibit IgE against thyroperoxidase. J Allergy Clin Immunol 2011;128(1):202–9 e5.
16. Maurer M, Rosen K, Hsieh HJ, et al. Omalizumab for the treatment of chronic idiopathic or spontaneous urticaria. N Engl J Med 2013;368(10):924–35.
17. Saini S, Rosen KE, Hsieh HJ, et al. A randomized, placebo-controlled, dose-ranging study of single-dose omalizumab in patients with H1-antihistamine-refractory chronic idiopathic urticaria. J Allergy Clin Immunol 2011;128(3): 567–73.e1.
18. Saini SS, Bindslev-Jensen C, Maurer M, et al. Efficacy and safety of omalizumab in patients with chronic idiopathic/spontaneous urticaria who remain symptomatic on H1 antihistamines: a randomized, placebo-controlled study. J Invest Dermatol 2015;135(1):67–75.
19. Mlynek A, Zalewska-Janowska A, Martus P, et al. How to assess disease activity in patients with chronic urticaria? Allergy 2008;63(6):777–80.
20. Mathias SD, Crosby RD, Zazzali JL, et al. Evaluating the minimally important difference of the urticaria activity score and other measures of disease activity in patients with chronic idiopathic urticaria. Ann Allergy Asthma Immunol 2012; 108(1):20–4.
21. Potter P, Mitha E, Barkai L, et al. Rupatadine is effective in the treatment of chronic spontaneous urticaria in children aged 2-11 years. Pediatr Allergy Immunol 2016; 27(1):55–61.
22. Weller K, Groffik A, Magerl M, et al. Development, validation, and initial results of the Angioedema Activity Score. Allergy 2013;68(9):1185–92.

23. Staubach P, Metz M, Chapman-Rothe N, et al. Effect of omalizumab on angioedema in H1 -antihistamine-resistant chronic spontaneous urticaria patients: results from X-ACT, a randomized controlled trial. Allergy 2016;71(8):1135–44.

24. Aygoren-Pursun E, Magerl M, Graff J, et al. Prophylaxis of hereditary angioedema attacks: a randomized trial of oral plasma kallikrein inhibition with avoralstat. J Allergy Clin Immunol 2016;138:934–6.e5.

25. Koch K, Weller K, Werner A, et al. Antihistamine updosing reduces disease activity in difficult-to-treat cholinergic urticaria. J Allergy Clin Immunol 2016. [Epub ahead of print]. http://dx.doi.org/10.1016/j.jaci.2016.05.026.

26. Krause K, Spohr A, Zuberbier T, et al. Up-dosing with bilastine results in improved effectiveness in cold contact urticaria. Allergy 2013;68(7):921–8.

27. Metz M, Scholz E, Ferran M, et al. Rupatadine and its effects on symptom control, stimulation time, and temperature thresholds in patients with acquired cold urticaria. Ann Allergy Asthma Immunol 2010;104(1):86–92.

28. Maurer M, Schütz A, Weller K, et al. Omalizumab is effective in symptomatic dermographism - results of a randomized, placebo controlled trial. J Allergy Clin Immunol 2016.

29. Metz M, Schütz A, Weller K, et al. Omalizumab is effective in cold urticaria - results of a randomized, placebo controlled trial. J Allergy Clin Immunol 2016.

30. Magerl M, Abajian M, Krause K, et al. An improved Peltier effect-based instrument for critical temperature threshold measurement in cold- and heat-induced urticaria. J Eur Acad Dermatol Venereol 2015;29(10):2043–5.

31. Siebenhaar F, Staubach P, Metz M, et al. Peltier effect-based temperature challenge: an improved method for diagnosing cold urticaria. J Allergy Clin Immunol 2004;114(5):1224–5.

32. Magerl M, Pisarevskaja D, Staubach P, et al. Critical temperature threshold measurement for cold urticaria: a randomized controlled trial of H(1) -antihistamine dose escalation. Br J Dermatol 2012;166(5):1095–9.

33. Mlynek A, Vieira dos Santos R, Ardelean E, et al. A novel, simple, validated and reproducible instrument for assessing provocation threshold levels in patients with symptomatic dermographism. Clin Exp Dermatol 2013;38(4):360–6 [quiz: 366].

34. Schoepke N, Abajian M, Church MK, et al. Validation of a simplified provocation instrument for diagnosis and threshold testing of symptomatic dermographism. Clin Exp Dermatol 2015;40(4):399–403.

35. Altrichter S, Salow J, Ardelean E, et al. Development of a standardized pulse-controlled ergometry test for diagnosing and investigating cholinergic urticaria. J Dermatol Sci 2014;75(2):88–93.

36. Available at: http://moxie-gmbh.de/medical-products/. Accessed September 29, 2016.

37. Garcia-Diez I, Curto-Barredo L, Weller K, et al. Cross-cultural adaptation of the urticaria control test from German to Castilian Spanish. Actas Dermosifiliogr 2015;106(9):746–52.

38. Kulthanan K, Chularojanamontri L, Tuchinda P, et al. Validity, reliability and interpretability of the Thai version of the urticaria control test (UCT). Health Qual Life Outcomes 2016;14(1):61.

39. Weller K, Groffik A, Church MK, et al. Development and validation of the Urticaria Control Test: a patient-reported outcome instrument for assessing urticaria control. J Allergy Clin Immunol 2014;133(5):1365–72, 1372.e1–6.

40. Ohanyan T, Schoepke N, Bolukbasi B, et al. Responsiveness and minimal important difference of the Urticaria Control Test (UCT). J Allergy Clin Immunol 2016.

41. Baiardini I, Braido F, Bindslev-Jensen C, et al. Recommendations for assessing patient-reported outcomes and health-related quality of life in patients with urticaria: a GA(2) LEN taskforce position paper. Allergy 2011;66(7):840–4.
42. Siebenhaar F, von Tschirnhaus E, Hartmann K, et al. Development and validation of the mastocytosis quality of life questionnaire: MC-QoL. Allergy 2016;71(6): 869–77.
43. Baiardini I, Pasquali M, Braido F, et al. A new tool to evaluate the impact of chronic urticaria on quality of life: chronic urticaria quality of life questionnaire (CU-QoL). Allergy 2005;60(8):1073–8.
44. Brzoza Z, Badura-Brzoza K, Mlynek A, et al. Adaptation and initial results of the Polish version of the GA(2)LEN chronic urticaria quality of life questionnaire (CU-Q(2)oL). J Dermatol Sci 2011;62(1):36–41.
45. Kocaturk E, Weller K, Martus P, et al. Turkish version of the chronic urticaria quality of life questionnaire: cultural adaptation, assessment of reliability and validity. Acta Derm Venereol 2012;92(4):419–25.
46. Koti I, Weller K, Makris M, et al. Disease activity only moderately correlates with quality of life impairment in patients with chronic spontaneous urticaria. Dermatology 2013;226(4):371–9.
47. Kulthanan K, Chularojanamontri L, Tuchinda P, et al. Minimal clinical important difference (MCID) of the Thai Chronic Urticaria Quality of Life Questionnaire (CU-Q2oL). Asian Pac J Allergy Immunol 2016;34:137–45.
48. Tavakol M, Mohammadinejad P, Baiardini I, et al. The Persian version of the chronic urticaria quality of life questionnaire: factor analysis, validation, and initial clinical findings. Iran J Allergy Asthma Immunol 2014;13(4):278–85.
49. Valero A, Herdman M, Bartra J, et al. Adaptation and validation of the Spanish version of the Chronic Urticaria Quality of Life Questionnaire (CU-Q2oL). J Investig Allergol Clin Immunol 2008;18(6):426–32.
50. Weller K, Church MK, Kalogeromitros D, et al. Chronic spontaneous urticaria: how to assess quality of life in patients receiving treatment. Arch Dermatol 2011; 147(10):1221–3.
51. Metz M, Weller K, Neumeister C, et al. Rupatadine in established treatment schemes improves chronic spontaneous urticaria symptoms and patients' quality of life: a prospective, non-interventional trial. Dermatol Ther 2015;5(4):217–30.
52. Weller K, Groffik A, Magerl M, et al. Development and construct validation of the angioedema quality of life questionnaire. Allergy 2012;67(10):1289–98.
53. Weller K, Magerl M, Peveling-Oberhag A, et al. The Angioedema Quality of Life Questionnaire (AE-QoL) - assessment of sensitivity to change and minimal clinically important difference. Allergy 2016;71:1203–9.
54. Desai NS, Poindexter GB, Monthrope YM, et al. A pilot quality-of-life instrument for pruritus. J Am Acad Dermatol 2008;59(2):234–44.

Current and Future Biomarkers in Atopic Dermatitis

Judith L. Thijs, MD, Marjolein S. de Bruin-Weller, MD, PhD,
DirkJan Hijnen, MD, PhD*

KEYWORDS

- Biomarkers • Atopic dermatitis • Biologicals • Personalized medicine • Stratification
- Heterogeneity • Disease severity

KEY POINTS

- Technological advances now allow clinicians to determine large numbers of biomarkers in small volumes of body fluids.
- This enables better characterization and stratification of patients with AD and will result in objective outcome measures, allowing better comparison of current and new treatments.
- We hypothesize that in the near future patients with AD will be stratified based on biomarker expression levels in body fluids, tissue, genetic variants, or composite biomarker scores.
- This will lead to better identification of patients that can benefit from new highly specific, but expensive treatments.
- Biomarkers are essential in moving forward to predictive, personalized, preventive, and participatory medicine.

INTRODUCTION

Atopic dermatitis (AD) is the most common chronic inflammatory skin disease world-wide. It affects children and adults. Living with AD has a great impact on the quality of life of patients. AD is a complex disease, thought to be the result of genetic and environmental factors, resulting in immunologic and barrier dysfunctions.[1]

AD is known to be a heterogeneous disease and many attempts have been made to define subsets of patients based on clinical characteristics. However, the current

Disclosure Statement: The authors have nothing to disclose.
Department of Dermatology & Allergology, University Medical Center Utrecht, Heidelberglaan 100, Utrecht 3584 CX, The Netherlands
* Corresponding author.
E-mail address: D.J.HIJNEN@UMCUTRECHT.NL

Immunol Allergy Clin N Am 37 (2017) 51–61
http://dx.doi.org/10.1016/j.iac.2016.08.008
0889-8561/17/© 2016 Elsevier Inc. All rights reserved.

immunology.theclinics.com

characterization of patients with AD might not adequately reflect the pathophysiologic diversity within patients with AD. Biomarkers may help in better defining heterogeneity and contribute to personalized medicine. This is one of many applications for biomarkers in AD.

Two main groups of biomarkers are discussed in this review: biomarkers for selection/stratification of patient groups and biomarkers for monitoring of patients (**Fig. 1**).

WHAT ARE BIOMARKERS?

The term "biomarker" is used in a broad sense to include almost any measurement reflecting an interaction between a biologic system and an environmental agent, which may be chemical, physical, or biologic. Two definitions of biomarkers are commonly used in literature. The World Health Organization definition of a biomarker is as follows: "any substance, structure or process that can be measured in the body or its products and influence or predict the incidence of outcome or disease. Biomarkers can be classified into markers of exposure, effect and susceptibility."[2] The other definition is largely overlapping and was proposed by the National Institutes of Health biomarkers definitions group, defining a biomarker as "a characteristic that is objectively measured and evaluated as an indicator of normal biological processes, pathogenic processes, or pharmacologic responses to a therapeutic intervention."[3]

BIOMARKER TYPES AND THEIR CLINICAL APPLICATION

Two biomarker categories with several subtypes are distinguished based on these definitions. The first category represents biomarkers that are used for selection or stratification of patients. Biomarkers in this category are used for screening and diagnosis, but also include the subcategory of prognostic and predictive biomarkers. Prognostic biomarkers help to estimate the likely course of disease and the patient's future risks to, for example, clinical end points, such as hospitalization.[4] A predictive biomarker identifies subpopulations of patients that are most likely to respond to a given therapy.

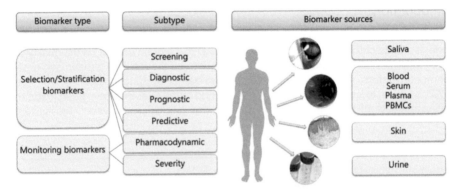

Fig. 1. Biomarker types and sources. This figure summarizes the different types of biomarkers and potential biomarker sources. Biomarkers can broadly be separated into two categories. The first category comprises biomarkers that are used to identify persons at risk to develop a disease, patients with active disease, and populations of patients that are most likely to benefit from a given therapy. The second category includes biomarkers for monitoring treatment effects. PBMCs, peripheral blood mononuclear cells.

The second category comprises biomarkers for monitoring the clinical response to a given therapy or intervention. This category includes biomarkers that measure disease severity and can function as a surrogate end point in clinical trials. This category also includes pharmacodynamic biomarkers. An overview of the different types of biomarkers is given in **Fig. 1**.

WHY ARE BIOMARKERS NEEDED FOR ATOPIC DERMATITIS?

There are many possible uses for biomarkers. Three main reasons for using biomarkers in AD research and clinical trials are discussed in more detail.

Biomarkers for Stratification of Patients to Unravel Disease Heterogeneity

AD is highly heterogeneous with regard to clinical characteristics and natural history of the disease. Many attempts have been made to stratify patients based on clinical characteristics.[5–7] Patients have been divided into clinical phenotypes based on age of onset, severity, and history of bacterial or viral infections. Classically, AD was divided into intrinsic and extrinsic, based on serum IgE levels. Despite high IgE levels in patients with extrinsic AD, suggesting increased expression of Th2-related genes, Suarez-Farinas and coworkers[8] recently found that intrinsic and extrinsic AD patient groups showed similar expression levels of Th2-related genes. This suggests that intrinsic and extrinsic AD are more overlapping in terms of underlying pathomechanisms than was previously thought based on clinical characteristics. This confirms that current characterization of patients with AD does not adequately reflect the pathophysiologic diversity within patients with AD. Biomarkers may help in defining subsets of patients, also called endotypes, related to underlying disease mechanisms, as was previously suggested by the PRACTALL collaboration platform.[9]

Patients with AD are currently being treated with relatively nonspecific treatments, including (topical) steroids and cyclosporine A (CsA). So far, no correlation has been found between clinical phenotypes and treatment response, which may be explained by the relative broad immune suppression with these drugs. With new targeted biologic therapies (ie, dupilumab, anti-interleukin [IL]-4R; and lebrikizumab, anti-IL-13) becoming available, identification of patients with specific immune pathway polarity is of particular importance. This so-called precision medicine will not only be of benefit to the individual patient, but will also be of essence in controlling health care expenditures.

Predicting Treatment Response

Patients with severe, difficult-to-treat AD, not responding to topical treatments are currently being treated with several (mostly off-label) systemic immunosuppressants. In many European countries (but not in the United States) CsA is registered for the treatment of AD. Other off-label immunosuppressants that are frequently used when CsA treatment fails, or when there are contraindications for CsA, include methotrexate, azathioprine (AZA), and mycophenolic acid (MPA).

Besides their possible side effects, a major concern for patients and physicians is the high percentages of treatment failures with these systemic immunosuppressants.[10] In daily practice, these treatments fail in 40% to 50% of patients.[11,12] Feedback from patients with AD focus groups showed that the uncertainty if a patient will respond to a given systemic immunosuppressant is one of their major concerns (personal communication). Biomarkers predicting treatment response for these treatments have not been described so far.

Pharmacogenetics and therapeutic drug monitoring may be used to optimize treatment response to systemic immunosuppressive treatment. Pharmacogenetic biomarkers can play a role in identifying responders and nonresponders to treatment, but can also be used to avoid adverse effects, and to optimize drug dosing.[13,14]

Biomarkers for prediction of therapy response may also be useful with the introduction of new targeted therapies for AD. Stratification based on a serum biomarker has already been proven to be useful in the treatment of asthma, where it was found that patients with asthma with high periostin levels showed a better response to anti-IL-13 (lebrikizumab) treatment, compared with patients with low periostin levels.[15] Periostin is an extracellular matrix protein that is induced by the Th2 cytokines IL-4 and IL-13 in airway epithelial cells and lung fibroblasts. This suggests that the Th2 immune pathway may be more predominant in periostin-high patients, explaining the better response to anti-IL-13 treatment in this subset of patients. Asthma, like AD, is also a highly heterogeneous disease, with many overlapping features to AD. We therefore expect that also in AD a biomarker-based stratification will be essential with the current introduction of new targeted therapies. A biomarker-based selection may even prevent new drugs from failing in early phase clinical trials because they may only be beneficial for a selected patient population as was shown for lebrikizumab in asthma. This treatment effect may be underestimated in an unselected patient population.

Biomarkers as Objective Measures for Disease Severity

Currently, no gold standard for measurement of disease severity in AD exists, and more than 20 different composite indices have been described.[16] A recent systematic review showed that most AD clinical trials used a severity measure (ie, SCORing Atopic Dermatitis; Eczema Area and Severity Index; or six area, six sign AD severity score), but that only 27% of these scales had been previously published.[17] Another review assessed the validity and reliability of the 20 most commonly used severity measures, and found that only three performed adequately.[16] To address these deficiencies in reporting, experts in the field have established the Harmonizing Outcome Measurements in Eczema initiative, an attempt to ensure that investigators use a core set of outcome measures to improve comparability between studies.[18] The Harmonizing Outcome Measurements in Eczema initiative now recommends to use the Eczema Area and Severity Index in AD clinical trials.[19] However, whether this score is preferable over the commonly used SCORing Atopic Dermatitis, even within the Harmonizing Outcome Measurements in Eczema group, is still a matter of debate.[20] The SCORing Atopic Dermatitis not only reports clinical signs, but also assesses subjective symptoms of pruritus and sleep loss with Visual Analogue Scales. We suggest that in addition to improve clinical outcome reporting, biomarkers for monitoring of disease severity would be of great added value. Biomarkers offer reliable and objective outcome measures, and may reflect objective and subjective signs and symptoms. Moreover, the use of biomarkers as a surrogate end point in clinical trials will improve comparisons across trials and facilitate meta-analyses.

CURRENT BIOMARKERS IN ATOPIC DERMATITIS

This section provides a brief overview of currently known biomarkers in AD. Biomarkers are summarized according to their subtype in **Table 1**.

Table 1 Types of biomarkers	
Biomarker Type	**Known Biomarkers in AD**
Screening	Filaggrin gene[52] SPINK5[53] Cord blood IgE[26] Infantile LT-α and FcϵRI-β genotypes[26] TSLP[27]
Diagnostic	No specific biomarkers currently available
Prognostic	Filaggrin gene[23] IgE[54,55] Indoleamine 2,3-dioxygenase-1[28]
Predictive	Not yet identified
Pharmacodynamic	CYP3A4/CYP3A5 tacrolimus[30] CYP3A4/CYP3A5 cyclosporine A[32] UGT1A9 mycophenolic acid[33] Thiopurine methyltransferase, 6-thioguanine nucleotides, 6-6-methylmercaptopurine ribonucleotides, azathioprine[35]
Monitoring	
Serum	TARC[39] CTACK[40] sE-selectin[41] Macrophage-derived chemokine[42] Lactate dehydrogenase[43] Interleukin-18[44]
Skin	Transcriptomic changes after treatment[47]
Itch	Interleukin-31,[56] wearables[51]

Diagnostic Biomarkers

AD is a clinical diagnosis, and there are no biomarkers needed to confirm the diagnosis. Classically, AD was divided into an intrinsic and an extrinsic subtype. Patients with the intrinsic subtype have normal total IgE levels, and are also referred to as nonallergic or nonatopic. Patients with the extrinsic subtype of AD show high levels of IgE and are often sensitized to multiple allergens.[21] Because 20% of the patients have the intrinsic form of AD, without elevated total IgE levels, total serum IgE cannot be used as a diagnostic biomarker for all patients with AD. Moreover, total IgE levels can also be increased in patient with other allergic diseases, such as allergic asthma or allergic rhinitis.

Screening and Prognostic Biomarkers

AD is a highly heritable disease and the best known risk factor for the development of AD is having parents with AD. Because results from a recent trial in a birth cohort suggested that emollient therapy might be effective in the prevention of eczema,[22] it might be helpful to use screening biomarkers to identify and treat the population at risk.

Many genome-wide linkage studies have identified several candidate genes associated with AD. The strongest association was found with filaggrin (FLG) gene mutations.[23] FLG gene mutations are found in about 30% of patients with AD, but not all FLG mutation carriers develop AD.[24] FLG gene mutations are more frequent in patients with severe disease and early onset AD. FLG mutations might therefore be used as a prognostic biomarker,[25] in addition to a screening marker for early onset or severe AD.

We hypothesize that a composite score of genetic factors (ie, FLG) and serum or tissue biomarkers will increase the predictive value of prognostic biomarkers.

Other biomarkers that have been proposed as screening biomarkers include elevated cord blood IgE levels, infantile lymphotoxin-α, and FcϵRI-β genotypes during pregnancy, which were shown to be associated with development of childhood AD.[26] Kim and colleagues[27] recently showed that epidermal TSLP protein expression may also serve as a screening biomarker in children at risk of developing AD. Indoleamine 2,3-dioxygenase-1 is a prognostic candidate biomarker for a specific phenotype (eczema herpeticum) that was proposed by Staudacher and colleagues.[28]

Predictive Biomarkers

Although many attempts have been made to define subsets of patients based on clinical characteristics and biomarkers, such as total serum IgE levels or peripheral blood eosinophils, no predictive biomarkers have been identified so far.

Pharmacodynamic Biomarkers

Pharmacogenetics has been defined as the study of variability in drug response caused by heredity.[29] Pharmacogenetic research explores the effect of pharmacokinetics, pharmacodynamics, efficacy, and safety of drug treatments in relation to genome variations.[13] The most common genetic variations that have been studied are single-nucleotide polymorphisms (SNPs), genetic copy number variations, and genomic insertions and deletions.[14] All of these genetic variations can influence the response of a patient to a specific drug and can be used as biomarkers.

Pharmacodynamic markers are scarcely used in AD treatment. However, we recently showed that pharmacogenetic testing can be used to personalize and optimize treatment with systemic extended-release tacrolimus in patients with AD.[30] Tacrolimus is extensively metabolized by CYP3A4 and CYP3A5. The presence of a C > T SNP in intron 6 of CYP3A4 is associated with intermediate or poor tacrolimus metabolism, resulting in high tacrolimus blood levels. In addition, it was shown that carrying CYP3A5*3 (slow metabolism) and CYP3A5*1 (fast metabolism) alleles also affects tacrolimus metabolism. Expression analysis of SNPs in the genes for CYP3A4 and CYP3A5 now enables classification of patients with AD into poor, intermediate, or extensive metabolizers of tacrolimus.[30] This CYP3A4/CYP3A5 genotype cluster classification is used to tailor dosing of tacrolimus to the individual patient, and to avoid adverse effects.

CsA is frequently used in the treatment of severe AD.[31] Bioavailability and systemic clearance of CsA is also mainly controlled by the isoenzymes CYP3A4 and CYP3A5.[32] Therefore, pharmacogenetic testing of SNPs for CYP3A4 and CYP3A5 may also be of use in the treatment of patients with CsA and needs further investigation.

MPA is used off-label in treatment of patients with AD that failed CsA treatment. Unfortunately, MPA is only effective in around half of the patients.[10,11] Pharmacogenetic biomarkers may be the key to optimizing MPA treatment. In kidney patients, low blood levels of MPA were found to correlate to lower efficacy and acute rejection of the graft.[33,34] Low MPA blood levels also correlate to the presence of SNPs in the gene promotor region of UGT1A9.[33,34] MPA is mainly metabolized by UGT1A9; therefore, increased UGT1A9 activity caused by SNPs could result in lower MPA blood levels. In patients with AD, UGT1A9 SNPs may be used as a pharmacogenetic biomarker to identify patients with nonresponsiveness to MPA. By prescribing higher MPA doses to these patients, the clinical efficacy of MPA in AD treatment may improve.

AZA is another second-line drug in the treatment of AD that also shows a good clinical performance in only half of the patients.[11] The performance of AZA is mainly limited by discontinuation of treatment because of side effects.[11] Studies in inflammatory bowel disease have shown that genetic polymorphisms in thiopurine methyltransferase influence the metabolism of AZA.[35] Genotyping of thiopurine methyltransferase before the start of AZA treatment allows identification of those at increased risk for adverse events.[35] During treatment, monitoring of the AZA metabolites 6-thioguanine nucleotides and 6-methylmercaptopurine ribonucleotides can be used for the risk assessment of myelotoxicity and liver toxicity.[35]

Although pharmacogenetic biomarkers are currently scarcely used in AD treatment, we think that they are of great potential in optimizing and personalizing treatment in AD.

Monitoring Biomarkers

Total serum IgE is the most commonly measured biomarker in AD trials.[36] Although patients with severe disease tend to have higher total serum IgE levels, there is a group of patients with intrinsic AD that do not have increased IgE levels. This suggests that total serum IgE levels are not suitable as a biomarker for monitoring disease severity. In a recent meta-analysis it was shown that total IgE levels only weakly correlate to disease severity during follow-up of patients with AD.[36]

Other serum biomarkers that have been frequently reported for monitoring disease activity in AD include eosinophilic cationic protein,[37] IL-2R,[38] and thymus and activation-regulated chemokine (TARC/CCL17).[39] In a meta-analysis on serum biomarkers for disease severity we found that serum TARC is the most reliable biomarker currently available.[36] Serum TARC levels have been determined in relatively large numbers of patients from different studies, showing pooled correlation coefficients of 0.60 (95% confidence interval, 0.48–0.70) and 0.64 (95% confidence interval, 0.57–0.70) in longitudinal and cross-sectional studies, respectively.[36] Additional biomarkers that showed promising results in this meta-analysis, but require additional research, include serum CTACK,[40] serum sE-selectin,[41] serum macrophage-derived chemokine,[42] serum lactate dehydrogenase,[43] and serum IL-18.[44]

Although TARC strongly correlates with disease activity in individual patients during follow-up, TARC levels vary between patients within cross-sectional cohorts of patients that have similar disease severity scores.[45] The variation in TARC levels between these patients may be the result of the large number of biologic pathways involved in the pathogenesis of AD. The use of a panel of several biomarkers from different biologic pathways, representing different phenotypes/endotypes, may overcome this problem. Indeed, we recently demonstrated that a multivariate signature consisting of TARC, PARC, IL-22, and sIL-2R for serum biomarkers showed a correlation coefficient of 0.86 to disease severity measured by the six area, six sign AD severity score.[46] Even though this panel was designed in a small pilot study, it demonstrates that using a panel of biomarkers may be necessary in a multifactorial, complex disease, such as AD.

Although circulating inflammatory markers are much easier to investigate, most crucial information on the pathogenesis of AD probably has come from investigations of skin biopsies. The group of Emma-Guttman has shown for several treatments, including UVB,[47] CsA,[48] and more recently also for dupilumab[49] that there are large changes on the skin transcriptome. These studies are essential in reporting on differential disease-modifying effects of new treatments, and further contribute to the understanding of disease pathogenesis.

Itch is an important characteristic of the disease and has a great impact on the quality of life of patients. Although several questionnaires for measuring itch have been developed, there are no objective tools available to measure itch. IL-31 has been associated with pruritus, and might be a potential biomarker for itch. Several studies investigated correlations between serum IL-31 levels and disease severity.[50] However, the correlation of IL-31 with pruritus has not yet been investigated. In the era of wearable fitness devices, one would expect that the introduction of a wearable scratching/itching device should not take much longer.[51]

FUTURE PERSPECTIVES

Technologic advances now allow clinicians to determine large numbers of biomarkers in small volumes of body fluids. This will result in better characterization and stratification of patients with AD and will also result in objective outcome measures that will allow better comparison of current and new treatments.

We hypothesize that in the near future patients with AD will be stratified based on biomarker expression levels in body fluids (blood/saliva/tears), tissue (biopsies/skin strips), genetic variants, or combined biomarker expression patterns (composite biomarker scores). With many new targeted therapies currently investigated in phase I to III clinical trials this will lead to better identification of patients that can benefit from these highly specific, but expensive new treatments. Biomarkers will be essential in moving forward to predictive, personalized, preventive, and participatory medicine.

REFERENCES

1. Eyerich K, Novak N. Immunology of atopic eczema: overcoming the Th1/Th2 paradigm. Allergy 2013;68(8):974–82.
2. WHO International Programme on Chemical Safety Biomarkers in Risk Assessment: Validity and Validation. 2001. Available at: http://www.inchem.org/documents/ehc/ehc/ehc222.htm. Accessed July 5, 2016.
3. Biomarkers Definitions Working Group. Biomarkers and surrogate endpoints: preferred definitions and conceptual framework. Clin Pharmacol Ther 2001; 69(3):89–95.
4. Kramer F, Dinh W. Molecular and digital biomarker supported decision making in clinical studies in cardiovascular indications. Arch Pharm (Weinheim) 2016; 349(6):399–409.
5. Garmhausen D, Hagemann T, Bieber T, et al. Characterization of different courses of atopic dermatitis in adolescent and adult patients. Allergy 2013;68(4):498–506.
6. Bieber T. Atopic dermatitis 2.0: from the clinical phenotype to the molecular taxonomy and stratified medicine. Allergy 2012;67(12):1475–82.
7. Guttman-Yassky E, Dhingra N, Leung DY. New era of biologic therapeutics in atopic dermatitis. Expert Opin Biol Ther 2013;13(4):549–61.
8. Suarez-Farinas M, Dhingra N, Gittler J, et al. Intrinsic atopic dermatitis shows similar TH2 and higher TH17 immune activation compared with extrinsic atopic dermatitis. J Allergy Clin Immunol 2013;132(2):361–70.
9. Muraro A, Lemanske RF Jr, Hellings PW, et al. Precision medicine in patients with allergic diseases: airway diseases and atopic dermatitis-PRACTALL document of the European Academy of Allergy and Clinical Immunology and the American Academy of Allergy, Asthma & Immunology. J Allergy Clin Immunol 2016; 137(5):1347–58.
10. Garritsen FM, Roekevisch E, van der Schaft J, et al. Ten years experience with oral immunosuppressive treatment in adult patients with atopic dermatitis in two academic centres. J Eur Acad Dermatol Venereol 2015;29(10):1905–12.

11. van der Schaft J, Politiek K, van den Reek JM, et al. Drug survival for azathioprine and enteric-coated mycophenolate sodium in a long-term daily practice cohort of adult patients with atopic dermatitis. Br J Dermatol 2016;175(1):199–202.
12. Politiek K, van der Schaft J, Coenraads PJ, et al. Drug survival for methotrexate in a daily practice cohort of adult patients with severe atopic dermatitis. Br J Dermatol 2016;174(1):201–3.
13. Crews KR, Hicks JK, Pui CH, et al. Pharmacogenomics and individualized medicine: translating science into practice. Clin Pharmacol Ther 2012;92(4):467–75.
14. Ventola CL. The role of pharmacogenomic biomarkers in predicting and improving drug response: part 2: challenges impeding clinical implementation. P T 2013;38(10):624–7.
15. Corren J, Lemanske RF, Hanania NA, et al. Lebrikizumab treatment in adults with asthma. N Engl J Med 2011;365(12):1088–98.
16. Schmitt J, Langan S, Williams HC. What are the best outcome measurements for atopic eczema? A systematic review. J Allergy Clin Immunol 2007;120(6): 1389–98.
17. Charman C, Chambers C, Williams H. Measuring atopic dermatitis severity in randomized controlled clinical trials: what exactly are we measuring? J Invest Dermatol 2003;120(6):932–41.
18. Schmitt J, Williams H, HOME Development Group. Harmonising outcome measures for eczema (HOME). Report from the First International Consensus Meeting (HOME 1), 24 July 2010, Munich, Germany. Br J Dermatol 2010;163(6):1166–8.
19. Schmitt J, Spuls PI, Thomas KS, et al. The Harmonising Outcome Measures for Eczema (HOME) statement to assess clinical signs of atopic eczema in trials. J Allergy Clin Immunol 2014;134(4):800–7.
20. Flohr C. Third time coming HOME: not just EASI. Br J Dermatol 2014;171(6): 1287–8.
21. Akdis CA, Akdis M. Immunological differences between intrinsic and extrinsic types of atopic dermatitis. Clin Exp Allergy 2003;33(12):1618–21.
22. Simpson EL, Chalmers JR, Hanifin JM, et al. Emollient enhancement of the skin barrier from birth offers effective atopic dermatitis prevention. J Allergy Clin Immunol 2014;134(4):818–23.
23. Kezic S, O'Regan GM, Yau N, et al. Levels of filaggrin degradation products are influenced by both filaggrin genotype and atopic dermatitis severity. Allergy 2011;66(7):934–40.
24. Weidinger S, O'Sullivan M, Illig T, et al. Filaggrin mutations, atopic eczema, hay fever, and asthma in children. J Allergy Clin Immunol 2008;121(5):1203–9.e1.
25. Barker JN, Palmer CN, Zhao Y, et al. Null mutations in the filaggrin gene (FLG) determine major susceptibility to early-onset atopic dermatitis that persists into adulthood. J Invest Dermatol 2007;127(3):564–7.
26. Wen HJ, Wang YJ, Lin YC, et al. Prediction of atopic dermatitis in 2-yr-old children by cord blood IgE, genetic polymorphisms in cytokine genes, and maternal mentality during pregnancy. Pediatr Allergy Immunol 2011;22(7):695–703.
27. Kim J, Kim BE, Lee J, et al. Epidermal thymic stromal lymphopoietin predicts the development of atopic dermatitis during infancy. J Allergy Clin Immunol 2016; 137(4):1282–5.e1-4.
28. Staudacher A, Hinz T, Novak N, et al. Exaggerated IDO1 expression and activity in Langerhans cells from patients with atopic dermatitis upon viral stimulation: a potential predictive biomarker for high risk of Eczema herpeticum. Allergy 2015; 70(11):1432–9.

29. Nebert DW. Pharmacogenetics and pharmacogenomics: why is this relevant to the clinical geneticist? Clin Genet 1999;56(4):247–58.

30. van der Schaft J, van Schaik RH, van Zuilen AD, et al. First experience with extended release tacrolimus in the treatment of adult patients with severe, difficult to treat atopic dermatitis: clinical efficacy, safety and dose finding. J Dermatol Sci 2016;81(1):66–8.

31. Ring J, Alomar A, Bieber T, et al. Guidelines for treatment of atopic eczema (atopic dermatitis) Part II. J Eur Acad Dermatol Venereol 2012;26(9):1176–93.

32. de Jonge H, Naesens M, Kuypers DR. New insights into the pharmacokinetics and pharmacodynamics of the calcineurin inhibitors and mycophenolic acid: possible consequences for therapeutic drug monitoring in solid organ transplantation. Ther Drug Monit 2009;31(4):416–35.

33. Kuypers DR, Naesens M, Vermeire S, et al. The impact of uridine diphosphate-glucuronosyltransferase 1A9 (UGT1A9) gene promoter region single-nucleotide polymorphisms T-275A and C-2152T on early mycophenolic acid dose-interval exposure in de novo renal allograft recipients. Clin Pharmacol Ther 2005;78(4):351–61.

34. van Schaik RH, van Agteren M, de Fijter JW, et al. UGT1A9 -275T>A/-2152C>T polymorphisms correlate with low MPA exposure and acute rejection in MMF/tacrolimus-treated kidney transplant patients. Clin Pharmacol Ther 2009;86(3):319–27.

35. Bloomfeld RS, Bickston SJ, Levine ME, et al. Thiopurine methyltransferase activity is correlated with azathioprine metabolite levels in inflammatory bowel disease patients in clinical gastroenterology practice. J Appl Res 2004;6(4):5.

36. Thijs J, Krastev T, Weidinger S, et al. Biomarkers for atopic dermatitis: a systematic review and meta-analysis. Curr Opin Allergy Clin Immunol 2015;15(5):453–60.

37. Czech W, Krutmann J, Schopf E, et al. Serum eosinophil cationic protein (ECP) is a sensitive measure for disease activity in atopic dermatitis. Br J Dermatol 1992;126(4):351–5.

38. Kagi MK, Joller-Jemelka H, Wuthrich B. Correlation of eosinophils, eosinophil cationic protein and soluble interleukin-2 receptor with the clinical activity of atopic dermatitis. Dermatology 1992;185(2):88–92.

39. Kakinuma T, Sugaya M, Nakamura K, et al. Thymus and activation-regulated chemokine (TARC/CCL17) in mycosis fungoides: serum TARC levels reflect the disease activity of mycosis fungoides. J Am Acad Dermatol 2003;48(1):23–30.

40. Kakinuma T, Saeki H, Tsunemi Y, et al. Increased serum cutaneous T cell-attracting chemokine (CCL27) levels in patients with atopic dermatitis and psoriasis vulgaris. J Allergy Clin Immunol 2003;111(3):592–7.

41. Morita H, Kitano Y, Kawasaki N. Elevation of serum-soluble E-selectin in atopic dermatitis. J Dermatol Sci 1995;10(2):145–50.

42. Leung TF, Ma KC, Hon KL, et al. Serum concentration of macrophage-derived chemokine may be a useful inflammatory marker for assessing severity of atopic dermatitis in infants and young children. Pediatr Allergy Immunol 2003;14(4):296–301.

43. Morishima Y, Kawashima H, Takekuma K, et al. Changes in serum lactate dehydrogenase activity in children with atopic dermatitis. Pediatr Int 2010;52(2):171–4.

44. Yoshizawa Y, Nomaguchi H, Izaki S, et al. Serum cytokine levels in atopic dermatitis. Clin Exp Dermatol 2002;27(3):225–9.

45. Landheer J, de Bruin-Weller M, Boonacker C, et al. Utility of serum thymus and activation-regulated chemokine as a biomarker for monitoring of atopic dermatitis severity. J Am Acad Dermatol 2014;71(6):1160–6.
46. Thijs JL, Nierkens S, Herath A, et al. A panel of biomarkers for disease severity in atopic dermatitis. Clin Exp Allergy 2015;45(3):698–701.
47. Tintle S, Shemer A, Suarez-Farinas M, et al. Reversal of atopic dermatitis with narrow-band UVB phototherapy and biomarkers for therapeutic response. J Allergy Clin Immunol 2011;128(3):583–93.e1-4.
48. Khattri S, Shemer A, Rozenblit M, et al. Cyclosporine in patients with atopic dermatitis modulates activated inflammatory pathways and reverses epidermal pathology. J Allergy Clin Immunol 2014;133(6):1626–34.
49. Hamilton JD, Suarez-Farinas M, Dhingra N, et al. Dupilumab improves the molecular signature in skin of patients with moderate-to-severe atopic dermatitis. J Allergy Clin Immunol 2014;134(6):1293–300.
50. Raap U, Wichmann K, Bruder M, et al. Correlation of IL-31 serum levels with severity of atopic dermatitis. J Allergy Clin Immunol 2008;122(2):421–3.
51. Ebata T, Iwasaki S, Kamide R, et al. Use of a wrist activity monitor for the measurement of nocturnal scratching in patients with atopic dermatitis. Br J Dermatol 2001;144(2):305–9.
52. Seguchi T, Cui CY, Kusuda S, et al. Decreased expression of filaggrin in atopic skin. Arch Dermatol Res 1996;288(8):442–6.
53. Walley AJ, Chavanas S, Moffatt MF, et al. Gene polymorphism in Netherton and common atopic disease. Nat Genet 2001;29(2):175–8.
54. Perkin MR, Strachan DP, Williams HC, et al. Natural history of atopic dermatitis and its relationship to serum total immunoglobulin E in a population-based birth cohort study. Pediatr Allergy Immunol 2004;15(3):221–9.
55. Peters AS, Kellberger J, Vogelberg C, et al. Prediction of the incidence, recurrence, and persistence of atopic dermatitis in adolescence: a prospective cohort study. J Allergy Clin Immunol 2010;126(3):590–5.e1-3.
56. Sonkoly E, Muller A, Lauerma AI, et al. IL-31: a new link between T cells and pruritus in atopic skin inflammation. J Allergy Clin Immunol 2006;117(2):411–7.

The Role of Fungi in Atopic Dermatitis

Martin Glatz, MD[a,b,*], Philipp Bosshard, PhD[c], Peter Schmid-Grendelmeier, MD[a,b]

KEYWORDS

• Atopic dermatitis • Malassezia spp • Sensitization

KEY POINTS

• Malassezia spp is a genus of lipophilic yeasts and the most common fungus on healthy skin.
• Malassezia spp. may contribute to skin inflammation and flares during the course of atopic dermatitis.
• Some Malassezia species release immunogenic proteins (allergens), that elicit an IgE response and react with skin immune cells.
• IgE-mediated sensitization to Malassezia spp. is common in atopic dermatitis patients but rare in healthy individuals.

INTRODUCTION

Atopic dermatitis (AD) is a chronic relapsing inflammatory skin disorder, characterized by intensely itchy eczema. The prevalence of AD has tripled within the last 3 decades, currently affecting up to 30% of children and 10% of adults in industrial countries.[1] The pathogenesis of AD is not fully understood. Besides some other environmental factors, the skin microbiome—the community of microorganisms colonizing the skin—has been attributed a pathogenic role in AD. The altered skin colonization with microorganisms in AD patients versus healthy individuals has been extensively investigated for bacteria, in particular *Staphylococcus aureus*. These aspects are highlighted in the article, (See Sun and Ong's article, "Infectious Complications in Atopic Dermatitis", in this issue). Recently, microbiome research extended the possible pathogenic role of fungi in AD. This research has focused on the commensal lipophilic yeast *Malassezia* spp because (i) AD patients are more frequently sensitized to *Malassezia* spp than healthy individuals, and (ii) AD patients may benefit from an antifungal therapy that is effective against *Malassezia* spp. This research led to the

[a] Allergy Unit, Department of Dermatology, University Hospital of Zurich, Gloriastrasse 31, Zurich 8091, Switzerland; [b] Christine-Kühne Center for Allergy Research and Education CK-CARE, Herman-Burchard-Strasse 1, 7265 Davos Wolfgang, Switzerland; [c] Mycology Laboratory, Department of Dermatology, University Hospital of Zurich, Gloriastrasse 31, Zurich 8091, Switzerland
* Corresponding author. Allergy Unit, Department of Dermatology, University Hospital of Zurich, Gloriastrasse 31, Zurich 8091, Switzerland.
E-mail address: martin.glatz@usz.ch

Immunol Allergy Clin N Am 37 (2017) 63–74
http://dx.doi.org/10.1016/j.iac.2016.08.012
0889-8561/17/© 2016 Elsevier Inc. All rights reserved.

publication of a plethora of studies on the possible role of *Malassezia* spp in the development and course of AD. Several studies applied culture or molecular methods such as polymerase chain reaction (PCR) to assess possible differences in the epidemiology of *Malassezia* spp skin colonization between healthy and diseased skin such as AD. However, these studies obtained variable results presumably owing to methodical inconsistencies such as skin sampling from inconsistent body sites and the use of different cultivation methods or PCR primers. Next-generation sequencing is a molecular method that has been recently introduced into skin microbiome research, because it gives information on skin microbial communities that is complementary to cultivation or PCR. As for the bacterial skin microbiome, next-generation sequencing revealed that the skin fungal microbiome is highly specific for a particular body site.[2] Therefore, comparing the prevalence of *Malassezia* spp between different body sites sampled in different studies will give unreliable results. Also, the epidemiologic studies used different culture media to detect *Malassezia* spp. The authors (Glatz M, unpublished data, 2014) and others have shown that different culture media favor the growth of particular *Malassezia* spp.[3–6] Therefore, the use of only one or a few types of culture media does not necessarily depict the whole spectrum of *Malassezia* spp present in a sample. Surprisingly, studies comparing healthy individuals and AD patients did not reveal a difference in the frequency of skin colonization with *Malassezia* spp between both groups.[6] It therefore appears as a medical conundrum how *Malassezia* spp on the one hand seems to contribute to the pathogenesis of AD patients and on the other hand is a commensal on healthy skin. Recent research at least partially elucidated the possible pathogenetic role of *Malassezia* spp in AD.

EPIDEMIOLOGY

The skin is an ecosystem and harbors diverse and body site–specific microbial communities, which have been termed the skin microbiome. The phylogenetic profiling of the skin microbiome revealed that fungi are part of the normal skin flora at all body sites and comprise 1% to 22% of the phylogenetic composition of the skin microbiome.[7] *Malassezia* spp almost exclusively comprises of the fungal flora of the healthy skin on most body sites. It is therefore the main eukaryotic member of the microbial flora of the skin.[6,7] *Malassezia* spp is a genus of lipophilic yeasts (**Fig. 1**). Most of the *Malassezia* spp lack the genes for fatty acid synthase genes and therefore rely

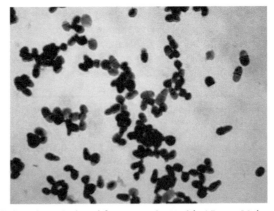

Fig. 1. *M sympodialis* culture isolated from a patient with AD, on *Malassezia* CHROM agar, grown for 72 hours at 32°C. (*From* Glatz M, Bosshard PP, Hoetzenecker W, et al. The role of Malassezia spp. in atopic dermatitis. J Clin Med 2015;4:1219; with permission.)

on exogenous fatty acid sources to satisfy their nutritive requirement.[8] *Malassezia pachydermatis*, a species isolated from dogs and other animals,[9] is the only known *Malassezia* spp that grows in the absence of exogenous lipids.[8] Their need for exogenous lipids explains the predilection of *Malassezia* spp for seborrheic skin sites, such as the head and neck. The taxonomy of *Malassezia* spp has been defined in its current form in 1996, based on morphology, ultrastructure, physiology, and molecular biology.[10] The genus *Malassezia* spp belongs to the phylum Basidiomycota and currently encompasses 14 species that have been isolated from human and animal skin (**Table 1**). Two of these species, *Malassezia globosa* and *Malassezia restricta*, are consistently found on healthy skin of individuals from the United States and Europe and are identified on almost all body sites.[2,6] However, epidemiologic studies indicated a geographic variation in the distribution of particular *Malassezia* spp, presumably owing to climate factors. For example, *Malassezia sympodialis* has been reported in studies from Canada, Russia, and Sweden as the most frequent species, whereas in Japan *Malassezia furfur* was the most common species.[6]

RISK FACTORS FOR SENSITIZATION TO *MALASSEZIA* SPP
Sensitization to Malassezia spp May Correlate with the Severity of Atopic Dermatitis

As *Malassezia* spp is part of the healthy skin flora, it appears reasonable that it regularly interacts with skin immune cells such as dendritic cells or lymphocytes. Accordingly, *Malassezia* spp–specific immunoglobulin G (IgG) and IgM antibodies can be regularly detected in healthy individuals.[8] In contrast, the rate of IgE-mediated sensitization to *Malassezia* spp is very low or even absent among individuals with healthy skin. In contrast, a high proportion of AD patients appears sensitized to this yeast,[14] as demonstrated by positive skin prick tests in up to 80% of adult AD patients.[15–18] Because skin test extracts for *Malassezia* spp are not yet commercially available and standardized, it is nearly impossible to compare the results of different skin prick test studies. Therefore, the detection of *Malassezia* spp–specific serum IgE is

Table 1
Currently identified *Malassezia* species

Malassezia Species	Isolated from Human Skin	Isolated from Animal Skin	Description as Species (Year)
M caprae	—	X	2007
M cuniculi	—	X	2011
M dermatis	X	—	2002
M equina	—	X	2007
M furfur	X	X	1889
M globosa	X	X	1996
M japonica	X	—	2003
M nana	—	X	2004
M obtusa	X	—	1996
M pachydermatis	—	X	1925
M restricta	X	—	1996
M slooffiae	X	X	1996
M sympodialis	X	X	1990
M yamatoensis	X	—	2004

Adapted from Refs.[11–13]

desirable to assess sensitization. Fortunately, a standardized kit (ImmunoCAP m70, Phadia AG, Steinhausen, Switzerland) for the detection of *Malassezia* spp–specific serum IgE is available, which is based on the ATCC strain 42132. Recently, a new test kit (ImmunoCAP m227) has been introduced that contains the antigens of several *Malassezia* spp and therefore is very sensitive.[19] Using these commercial kits, *Malassezia* spp–specific IgE are found in up to one-third of children[15,20–22] and two-thirds of adults with AD.[15,19,22–24] Accordingly, a recent study on 176 adult AD patients found higher rates of IgE-mediated *Malassezia* sensitization among patients with severe compared with moderate AD.[25] These high rates of *Malassezia* spp–specific IgE detection in adult AD patients are consistent with the rates of positive *Malassezia* spp skin prick tests in this population (see above). Interestingly, sensitization rates against *Malassezia* spp are particularly higher in patients with head and neck type of AD.[19] These higher sensitization rates may be attributed to the lipophilic properties and hence the predilection of this yeast for seborrheic skin areas, such as the head and neck region. Therefore, some authors assume that *Malassezia* spp plays a pathogenic role particularly in this clinical subtype of AD.[26]

Pathophysiology

The pathophysiologic mechanisms underlying this high frequency of *Malassezia* spp sensitization in AD patients compared with healthy individuals remain to be elucidated. It appears that several endogenous factors such as the dysfunctional skin barrier or aberrations in the skin immune system of AD patients as well as environmental factors influence the skin colonization with *Malassezia* spp and the IgE-mediated sensitization to this yeast.[27] This sensitization to *Malassezia* spp may correlate to the severity of AD particularly in adults as recently shown in 2 studies on 132 children and 128 adults with AD.[22,28] The lower frequency of *Malassezia* spp sensitization in children compared with adults and therefore the missing correlation between AD severity and *Malassezia* spp–specific IgE in children might owe to the poor growth conditions for *Malassezia* spp in children compared with adults. Children produce low amounts of sebum in their skin, and sebum production increases during puberty and is high until the age of 50.[29] Hence, the growth conditions for *Malassezia* spp on pediatric skin are worse than on adult skin, and this could be the reason that sensitization to *Malassezia* spp preferably occurs in adulthood.[22] Several allergens of *Malassezia* spp elucidate a specific IgE response. To date, at least 14 allergens of 3 *Malassezia* spp, namely *M furfur*, *M sympodialis*, and *M globosa*, are characterized on a molecular basis[30] (**Table 2**), and 13 of these allergens are listed in the official allergen nomenclature list (http://www.allergen. org). These allergens may be released to a higher amount in the environment of atopic skin. For example, the allergen Mala s 12 is released in a higher amount at pH 6.0 that represents conditions of atopic skin, than in the more acidic environment of pH 5.5 of healthy skin.[31] It remains unclear if the IgE response plays a pathogenic role in AD or rather serves as a marker for the severity of AD, but the some possible mechanisms how *Malassezia* spp allergens induce inflammation in atopic skin have been elucidated in recent years and are described in the later discussion.

Malassezia spp Interacts with the Skin Immune System

Prior studies indicated that *Malassezia* spp interacts with various types of human skin and immune cells. This induces a proinflammatory immune response by these immune cells, which seems to contribute to the inflammation during AD flares. It is still unclear how the interaction between *Malassezia* spp cells and host cells occurs, but some different mechanisms have been postulated. First, *Malassezia* spp penetrated the impaired skin barrier, which is typical for AD patients. In the epidermis and dermis,

Table 2
Allergens from *Malassezia* spp and their relevance in atopic dermatitis

Allergen	Source	Mass (kDa)	Function	IgE-Mediated Sensitization (%)	Comment	References
Mala f 2	*M furfur*	21	Peroxisomal membrane protein	72		32
Mala f 3	*M furfur*	20	Peroxisomal membrane protein	70		32
Mala f 4	*M furfur*	35	Mitochondrial malate dehydrogenase	83		33
Mala s 1	*M Sympodialis*	36		Unknown		34
Mala s 5	*M sympodialis*	19		Unknown		35
Mala s 6	*M sympodialis*	18	Cyclophilin	92		35,36
Mala s 7	*M sympodialis*	22		40–60		35,37
Mala s 8	*M sympodialis*	16		40–72		35,37
Mala s 9	*M sympodialis*	11		24–36		35,37
Mala s 10	*M sympodialis*	86	Heat shock protein70	69		38
Mala s 11	*M sympodialis*	23	Manganese superoxide dismutase	43–75	Induces dendritic cell maturation, release of IL-6, IL-8, IL-12p70, TNF-α by dendritic cells, auto-reactive T cells against human homologue	39–42
Mala s 12	*M sympodialis*	67	Glucose-methanol-choline oxidoreductase	62		43
Mala s 13	*M sympodialis*	13	Thioredoxin	50	Induces autoreactive T cells against human homologue	44,45
MGL_1304	*M globosa*	17		62	Induces degranulation of mast cells, IL-4 release by basophils	46,47

Malassezia spp is recognized by keratinocytes and immune cells such as Langerhans cells, dermal dendritic cells, natural killer cells, and fibroblasts.[48] A second possible mechanism of *Malassezia* spp–human cell interaction might be mediated by proteins of *Malassezia* spp that are packed and released in nanovesicles.[49] It was demonstrated that these nanovesicles stimulate dendritic cells and mast cells to release of tumor necrosis factor-α (TNF-α), interleukin-6 (IL-6), IL-8, IL-10, and IL-12p70.[40,50] These cytokines may contribute to skin inflammation in AD. Some other investigators suggest that Toll-like receptors (TLRs) such as TLR2 recognize *Malassezia* spp.[51] TLRs are members of the large family of pattern recognition receptors, which play a key role in the innate immune system because they recognize molecules that are commonly shared by pathogens. Some recent findings substantiated the relevance of TLRs for the immune response of human cells against *Malassezia* spp. For example, *Malassezia* spp induces the expression of TLR2 and TLR4 on human keratinocytes[52] and human dendritic cells,[48] inducing the production human beta defensin 2 and CXLC8[53] (**Fig. 2**). Another possible mechanism could be the activation of the NLRP3 inflammasome in skin dendritic cells by *Malassezia* spp. This inflammasome activation leads to the release of

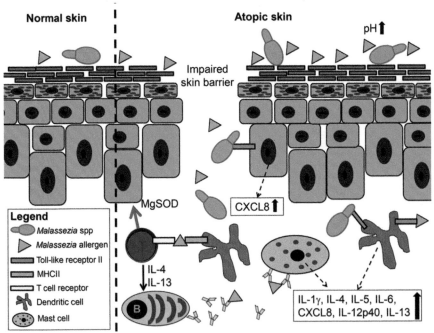

Fig. 2. Proposed mechanisms by which *Malassezia* spp contributes to skin inflammation in AD patients. The increased pH in atopic skin contributes to increased allergen release by *Malassezia* spp. These allergens, supposedly together with whole *Malassezia* spp cells, penetrate the epidermis through the disturbed skin barrier in AD patients. *Malassezia* spp cells and their allergens may be recognized by TLR2 expressed on keratinocytes and dendritic cells that elicit the release of proinflammatory cytokines. *Malassezia* spp components elicit the production of *Malassezia* spp–specific IgE antibodies through the dendritic cell and T-cell–mediated activation of B cells. These IgE antibodies may also contribute, possibly through mast cells, to the inflammation in atopic skin. Finally, autoreactive T cells can cross-react between fungal and human manganese-dependent superoxide dismutase (MgSOD) and hence sustain skin inflammation. (*From* Glatz M, Bosshard PP, Hoetzenecker W, et al. The role of Malassezia spp. in atopic dermatitis. J Clin Med 2015;4:1221; with permission.)

proinflammatory cytokines such as production of IL-1β, and IL-4, IL-5, and IL-13, which are key players in the pathogenesis of AD[54–56] (see **Fig. 2**).

The authors have mentioned the IgE-mediated sensitization to various *Malassezia* spp allergens above. These allergens may also directly stimulate IgE-independent immune mechanisms. For example, Mala s 13 is a fungal thioredoxin that is very similar to its human counterpart (**Fig. 3**). When human CD4$^+$ T cells recognize the fungal thioredoxin, they may cross-react to the human enzyme, which is expressed by human keratinocytes. This cross-reaction will induce a T-cell–mediated skin inflammation, which is commonly seen in AD.[45] A similar induction of autoreactive T cells and T-cell–mediated inflammation was observed for another *Malassezia* spp allergen, Mala s 11, which is a manganese-dependent superoxide dismutase. The significance of these allergens for skin inflammation in AD was substantiated by the strong correlation between AD severity and Mala s 11 sensitization.[41]

Management and Therapeutic Approaches with Antifungals in Atopic Dermatitis

The basis of every effective AD therapy is the use of skin emollients. They rehydrate the skin and repair the impaired skin barrier. In case of clinically manifest skin inflammation during AD flares, an anti-inflammatory treatment is necessary. This treatment most commonly requires topical corticosteroids or calcineurin inhibitors. Another promising therapeutic approach is the identification and elimination of trigger factors such as *Malassezia* spp,[27] for example, by an antifungal therapy. The usefulness of an antifungal therapy for AD has been discussed for many years. Azole antifungals are the most common class of antifungal drugs prescribed for AD patients. In vitro, azole

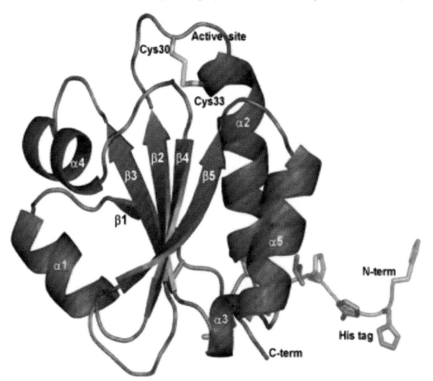

Fig. 3. Crystal structure of the *M sympodialis* thioredoxin Mala s 13. (*Courtesy of* Prof Reto Crameri, PhD, Davos, Switzerland.)

antifungals are effective against *Malassezia* spp,[29,57] but susceptibility testing of *M pachydermatis*, a species most commonly isolated from dogs, showed that strains isolated from dogs with AD were less susceptible to azole antifungals than strains isolated from healthy dogs.[58] In humans, the resistance of *Malassezia* spp to antifungals has not been investigated to date.

Several trials investigated the effects of topical or systemic azole antifungals on AD patients and compared it to placebo. However, these trials gave somehow ambiguous results. As a clinical experience, the topical application of ketoconazole on the face of patients with AD of the head and neck type improved eczema. However, in a placebo-controlled study, the combination of topical miconazole-hydrocortisone cream with ketoconazole shampoo was not superior to hydrocortisone alone in patients with head and neck–type AD.[59] The benefit of a systemic antifungal treatment for the AD patient has been investigated in a randomized, placebo-controlled trial on 36 AD patients treated with ketoconazole versus 39 AD patients treated with placebo. AD severity improved significantly in the ketoconazole group but not in the placebo group.[60] For another trial, a total of 53 AD patients were treated with either 2 different dosages of itraconazole or placebo. The improvement of AD severity was significantly higher in itraconazole-treated patients than in the placebo group.[61] The positive effect of azole antifungals on AD could also owe to the anti-inflammatory properties of ketoconazole or itraconazole, because these drugs inhibit the production of IL-4 and IL-5 by T cells.[62]

The positive effects of antifungals were not confirmed by another study on 15 AD patients treated with ketoconazole versus 14 AD patients treated with placebo. Both treatment groups received topical corticosteroids. Although AD severity improved in both treatment groups, this improvement was not correlated to ketoconazole but rather to the topical corticosteroids.[63] The ambiguous results of these clinical trials might be attributed to a selection bias and low patient numbers. It can be speculated that antifungal therapies are more effective in a particular subgroup of AD, for example in patients with a head and neck type of eczema. More recently published studies were of less quality, for example, they comprised retrospective observations and lacked a standardized scoring system to assess the severity of AD.[64] More randomized, placebo-controlled studies on large patient populations are needed to reliably assess the benefit of an antifungal therapy in AD.

In summary, there is little doubt that *Malassezia* spp plays a role in AD because it may interact with the local skin immune responses and barrier function, and sensitization against this skin-colonizing yeast can correlate with disease activity. Also, antifungal therapy shows beneficial effects in some patients. However, the pathogenetic mechanism and mutual interaction between *Malassezia* spp and AD still remain partly unclear and need further investigation.

REFERENCES

1. Bieber T. Atopic dermatitis. N Engl J Med 2008;358:1483–94.
2. Findley K, Oh J, Yang J, et al. Topographic diversity of fungal and bacterial communities in human skin. Nature 2013;498:367–70.
3. Kaneko T, Makimura K, Abe M, et al. Revised culture-based system for identification of Malassezia spp. J Clin Microbiol 2007;45:3737–42.
4. Kaneko T, Makimura K, Sugita T, et al. Tween 40-based precipitate production observed on modified chromogenic agar and development of biological identification kit for Malassezia spp. Med Mycol 2006;44:227–31.
5. Ashbee HR. Recent developments in the immunology and biology of Malassezia spp. FEMS Immunol Med Microbiol 2006;47:14–23.

6. Gaitanis G, Magiatis P, Hantschke M, et al. The Malassezia genus in skin and systemic diseases. Clin Microbiol Rev 2012;25:106–41.
7. Oh J, Byrd AL, Deming C, et al. Biogeography and individuality shape function in the human skin metagenome. Nature 2014;514:59–64.
8. Saunders CW, Scheynius A, Heitman J. Malassezia fungi are specialized to live on skin and associated with dandruff, eczema, and other skin diseases. PLoS Pathog 2012;8:e1002701.
9. Chen TA, Hill PB. The biology of Malassezia organisms and their ability to induce immune responses and skin disease. Vet Dermatol 2005;16:4–26.
10. Gueho E, Midgley G, Guillot J. The genus Malassezia with description of four new spp. Antonie Van Leeuwenhoek 1996;69:337–55.
11. Harada K, Saito M, Sugita T, et al. Malassezia spp. and their associated skin diseases. J Dermatol 2015;42:250–7.
12. Cabanes FJ. Malassezia yeasts: how many spp. infect humans and animals? Plos Pathog 2014;10:e1003892.
13. Gueho E, Boekhout Y, Begerow D. Biodiversity, phylogeny and ultrastructure. Berlin: Springer; 2010.
14. Johansson C, Sandstrom MH, Bartosik J, et al. Atopy patch test reactions to Malassezia allergens differentiate subgroups of atopic dermatitis patients. Br J Dermatol 2003;148:479–88.
15. Scalabrin DM, Bavbek S, Perzanowski MS, et al. Use of specific IgE in assessing the relevance of fungal and dust mite allergens to atopic dermatitis: a comparison with asthmatic and nonasthmatic control subjects. J Allergy Clin Immunol 1999;104:1273–9.
16. Scheynius A, Johansson C, Buentke E, et al. Atopic eczema/dermatitis syndrome and Malassezia. Int Arch Allergy Immunol 2002;127:161–9.
17. Zargari A, Eshaghi H, Back O, et al. Serum IgE reactivity to Malassezia furfur extract and recombinant M. furfur allergens in patients with atopic dermatitis. Acta Derm Venereol 2001;81:418–22.
18. Johansson C, Eshaghi H, Linder MT, et al. Positive atopy patch test reaction to Malassezia furfur in atopic dermatitis correlates with a T helper 2-like peripheral blood mononuclear cells response. J Invest Dermatol 2002;118:1044–51.
19. Brodska P, Panzner P, Pizinger K, et al. IgE-mediated sensitization to malassezia in atopic dermatitis: more common in male patients and in head and neck type. Dermatitis 2014;25:120–6.
20. Lange L, Alter N, Keller T, et al. Sensitization to Malassezia in infants and children with atopic dermatitis: prevalence and clinical characteristics. Allergy 2008;63:486–7.
21. Kekki OM, Scheynius A, Poikonen S, et al. Sensitization to Malassezia in children with atopic dermatitis combined with food allergy. Pediatr Allergy Immunol 2013;24:244–9.
22. Glatz M, Buchner M, von Bartenwerffer W, et al. Malassezia spp.-specific immunoglobulin E level is a marker for severity of atopic dermatitis in adults. Acta Derm Venereol 2015;95(2):191–6.
23. Sandstrom Falk MH, Faergemann J. Atopic dermatitis in adults: does it disappear with age? Acta Derm Venereol 2006;86:135–9.
24. Ramirez de Knott HM, McCormick TS, Kalka K, et al. Cutaneous hypersensitivity to Malassezia sympodialis and dust mite in adult atopic dermatitis with a textile pattern. Contact Dermatitis 2006;54:92–9.
25. Mittermann I, Wikberg G, Johansson C, et al. IgE sensitization profiles differ between adult patients with severe and moderate atopic dermatitis. PLoS One 2016;11:e0156077.

26. Faergemann J. Atopic dermatitis and fungi. Clin Microbiol Rev 2002;15:545–63.

27. Akdis CA, Akdis M, Bieber T, et al. Diagnosis and treatment of atopic dermatitis in children and adults: European Academy of Allergology and Clinical Immunology/American Academy of Allergy, Asthma and Immunology/PRACTALL Consensus Report. Allergy 2006;61:969–87.

28. Zhang E, Tanaka T, Tajima M, et al. Anti-Malassezia-specific IgE antibodies production in Japanese patients with head and neck atopic dermatitis: relationship between the level of specific IgE antibody and the colonization frequency of cutaneous Malassezia spp. and clinical severity. J Allergy (Cairo) 2011;2011:645670.

29. Darabi K, Hostetler SG, Bechtel MA, et al. The role of Malassezia in atopic dermatitis affecting the head and neck of adults. J Am Acad Dermatol 2009;60:125–36.

30. Matricardi PM, Kleine-Tebbe J, Hoffmann HJ, et al. EAACI molecular allergology user's guide. Pediatr Allergy Immunol 2016;27(Suppl 23):1–250.

31. Selander C, Zargari A, Mollby R, et al. Higher pH level, corresponding to that on the skin of patients with atopic eczema, stimulates the release of Malassezia sympodialis allergens. Allergy 2006;61:1002–8.

32. Yasueda H, Hashida-Okado T, Saito A, et al. Identification and cloning of two novel allergens from the lipophilic yeast, Malassezia furfur. Biochem Biophys Res Commun 1998;248:240–4.

33. Onishi Y, Kuroda M, Yasueda H, et al. Two-dimensional electrophoresis of Malassezia allergens for atopic dermatitis and isolation of Mal f 4 homologs with mitochondrial malate dehydrogenase. Eur J Biochem 1999;261:148–54.

34. Schmidt M, Zargari A, Holt P, et al. The complete cDNA sequence and expression of the first major allergenic protein of Malassezia furfur, Mal f 1. Eur J Biochem 1997;246:181–5.

35. Lindborg M, Magnusson CG, Zargari A, et al. Selective cloning of allergens from the skin colonizing yeast Malassezia furfur by phage surface display technology. J Invest Dermatol 1999;113:156–61.

36. Fluckiger S, Fijten H, Whitley P, et al. Cyclophilins, a new family of cross-reactive allergens. Eur J Immunol 2002;32:10–7.

37. Rasool O, Zargari A, Almqvist J, et al. Cloning, characterization and expression of complete coding sequences of three IgE binding Malassezia furfur allergens, Mal f 7, Mal f 8 and Mal f 9. Eur J Biochem 2000;267:4355–61.

38. Andersson A, Scheynius A, Rasool O. Detection of Mala f and Mala s allergen sequences within the genus Malassezia. Med Mycol 2003;41:479–85.

39. Andersson A, Rasool O, Schmidt M, et al. Cloning, expression and characterization of two new IgE-binding proteins from the yeast Malassezia sympodialis with sequence similarities to heat shock proteins and manganese superoxide dismutase. Eur J Biochem 2004;271:1885–94.

40. Vilhelmsson M, Johansson C, Jacobsson-Ekman G, et al. The Malassezia sympodialis allergen Mala s 11 induces human dendritic cell maturation, in contrast to its human homologue manganese superoxide dismutase. Int Arch Allergy Immunol 2007;143:155–62.

41. Schmid-Grendelmeier P, Fluckiger S, Disch R, et al. IgE-mediated and T cell-mediated autoimmunity against manganese superoxide dismutase in atopic dermatitis. J Allergy Clin Immunol 2005;115:1068–75.

42. Guarneri F, Costa C, Foti C, et al. Frequency of autoallergy to manganese superoxide dismutase in atopic dermatitis patients: experience of three Italian dermatology centers. Br J Dermatol 2015;173:559–62.

43. Zargari A, Selander C, Rasool O, et al. Mala s 12 is a major allergen in patients with atopic eczema and has sequence similarities to the GMC oxidoreductase family. Allergy 2007;62:695–703.
44. Limacher A, Glaser AG, Meier C, et al. Cross-reactivity and 1.4-A crystal structure of Malassezia sympodialis thioredoxin (Mala s 13), a member of a new pan-allergen family. J Immunol 2007;178:389–96.
45. Balaji H, Heratizadeh A, Wichmann K, et al. Malassezia sympodialis thioredoxin-specific T cells are highly cross-reactive to human thioredoxin in atopic dermatitis. J Allergy Clin Immunol 2011;128:92–9.e4.
46. Hiragun M, Hiragun T, Ishii K, et al. Elevated serum IgE against MGL_1304 in patients with atopic dermatitis and cholinergic urticaria. Allergol Int 2014;63:83–93.
47. Hiragun T, Ishii K, Hiragun M, et al. Fungal protein MGL_1304 in sweat is an allergen for atopic dermatitis patients. J Allergy Clin Immunol 2013;132(3): 608–15.e4.
48. Buentke E, Scheynius A. Dendritic cells and fungi. Apmis 2003;111:789–96.
49. Gehrmann U, Qazi KR, Johansson C, et al. Nanovesicles from Malassezia sympodialis and host exosomes induce cytokine responses–novel mechanisms for host-microbe interactions in atopic eczema. PLoS One 2011;6:e21480.
50. Selander C, Engblom C, Nilsson G, et al. TLR2/MyD88-dependent and -independent activation of mast cell IgE responses by the skin commensal yeast Malassezia sympodialis. J Immunol 2009;182:4208–16.
51. Baker BS. The role of microorganisms in atopic dermatitis. Clin Exp Immunol 2006;144:1–9.
52. Brasch J, Morig A, Neumann B, et al. Expression of antimicrobial peptides and toll-like receptors is increased in tinea and pityriasis versicolor. Mycoses 2014; 57:147–52.
53. Baroni A, Orlando M, Donnarumma G, et al. Toll-like receptor 2 (TLR2) mediates intracellular signalling in human keratinocytes in response to Malassezia furfur. Arch Dermatol Res 2006;297:280–8.
54. Novak N, Leung DY. Advances in atopic dermatitis. Curr Opin Immunol 2011;23: 778–83.
55. De Benedetto A, Kubo A, Beck LA. Skin barrier disruption: a requirement for allergen sensitization? J Invest Dermatol 2012;132:949–63.
56. Kistowska M, Fenini G, Jankovic D, et al. Malassezia yeasts activate the NLRP3 inflammasome in antigen-presenting cells via Syk-kinase signaling. Exp Dermatol 2014;23(12):884–9.
57. Sugita T, Tajima M, Ito T, et al. Antifungal activities of tacrolimus and azole agents against the eleven currently accepted Malassezia spp. J Clin Microbiol 2005;43: 2824–9.
58. Watanabe S, Koike A, Kano R, et al. In vitro susceptibility of Malassezia pachydermatis isolates from canine skin with atopic dermatitis to ketoconazole and itraconazole in East Asia. J Vet Med Sci 2014;76:579–81.
59. Broberg A, Faergemann J. Topical antimycotic treatment of atopic dermatitis in the head/neck area. A double-blind randomised study. Acta Derm Venereol 1995;75:46–9.
60. Lintu P, Savolainen J, Kortekangas-Savolainen O, et al. Systemic ketoconazole is an effective treatment of atopic dermatitis with IgE-mediated hypersensitivity to yeasts. Allergy 2001;56:512–7.
61. Svejgaard E, Larsen PO, Deleuran M, et al. Treatment of head and neck dermatitis comparing itraconazole 200 mg and 400 mg daily for 1 week with placebo. J Eur Acad Dermatol Venereol 2004;18:445–9.

62. Kanda N, Enomoto U, Watanabe S. Anti-mycotics suppress interleukin-4 and interleukin-5 production in anti-CD3 plus anti-CD28-stimulated T cells from patients with atopic dermatitis. J Invest Dermatol 2001;117:1635–46.
63. Back O, Bartosik J. Systemic ketoconazole for yeast allergic patients with atopic dermatitis. J Eur Acad Dermatol Venereol 2001;15:34–8.
64. Kaffenberger BH, Mathis J, Zirwas MJ. A retrospective descriptive study of oral azole antifungal agents in patients with patch test-negative head and neck predominant atopic dermatitis. J Am Acad Dermatol 2014;71:480–3.

Infectious Complications in Atopic Dermatitis

Di Sun, MD, MPH[a], Peck Y. Ong, MD[a,b],*

KEYWORDS

- Atopic dermatitis • *Staphylococcal aureus* • Eczema herpeticum • Keratinocytes
- Innate

KEY POINTS

- Atopic dermatitis (AD) and allergic urticaria are common conditions of the skin that can also be the presenting symptoms of uncommon diseases.
- Defects leading to immunodeficiency may be associated with AD or allergic urticaria.
- Unusually severe or otherwise atypical presentations of AD or allergic urticaria may lead to clinical suspicion of an underlying immunodeficiency.

INTRODUCTION

Atopic dermatitis (AD) is a chronic, relapsing inflammatory skin disease with a prevalence of 10% to 20% in children and 1% to 3% in adults in industrialized countries.[1] This common condition arises from the interplay of genetic and environmental factors that culminates in skin barrier defects and an inappropriate immunologic response.[2] Characterized by intensely pruritic lesions that can lead to sleep disruption, AD is associated with inferior school performance, poor self-esteem, and familial stress.[3,4] Despite these sizable comorbidities, the major complication of AD remains infection.

PATHOPHYSIOLOGY OF INFECTIOUS COMPLICATIONS

The infectious complications of AD are rooted in its pathogenesis. The interaction between the immune system, environment, and skin barrier defects initiates an inflammatory cycle that alters the skin's innate immunity and microbiome (**Fig. 1**), leading to infectious complications.

Disclosure: Dr P.Y. Ong has received funding from National Institute of Allergy and Infectious Disease (UAI117673, 20096801) (Atopic Dermatitis Research Network) and Regeneron (Dupilumab).
[a] Department of Pediatrics, Keck School of Medicine, University of Southern California, 1975 Zonal Ave, Los Angeles, CA 90033, USA; [b] Division of Clinical Immunology and Allergy, Children's Hospital Los Angeles, 4650 Sunset Boulevard, MS 75, Los Angeles, CA 90027, USA
* Corresponding author.
E-mail address: pyong@chla.usc.edu

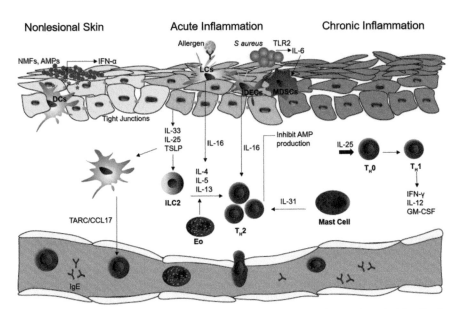

Fig. 1. Pathophysiology of skin infections in AD. ILC2, group 2 innate lymphoid cells. Eo, eosinophil; NMF, natural moisturizing factor.

Skin Barrier Defects

The outermost layer of the epidermis, the stratum corneum (SC), a cornified squamous epithelium that prevents water loss and guards against entry of foreign substances, is defective in AD.[5] A "bricks and mortar" structure, the SC is composed of dead SC cells held by a mortar of cornified cell envelope comprised of a protein/lipid polymer just beneath the cytoplasmic surface of the cells.[6] Defects in the layer are associated with AD: skin in AD patients has significantly thinner SC than healthy controls and transepidermal water loss studies demonstrate increased water loss in affected sites—a hallmark of AD—with increasing transepidermal water loss correlating with increasing AD severity.[7,8]

This skin barrier defect has been linked to mutations in filaggrin gene (*FLG*).[9] Meta-analyses of studies evaluating the association between *FLG* mutations and AD found an odds ratio (OR) of 4.78.[10] This association is likely due to the important role of filaggrin in interacting with the keratin cytoskeleton to excrete lipid lamellae to form the cornified envelope comprising the mortar structure of the SC.[2] Impaired excretion of the envelope results in compromise of the skin barrier. Filaggrin also helps maintain cell-to-cell integrity; those with *FLG* defects have decreased tight junctions and corneodesmosin density—proteins needed to main connections between cells.[11] The filaggrin breakdown products, pyrrolidone carboxylic acid and urocanic acid, are also natural moisturizing factors that maintain skin moisture and acidify skin-surface pH, which prevent activation of serine proteases and kallikrein.[12] Defects in *FLG* thus result in dry skin and activation of these downstream enzymes that inhibit lamellar excretion via activation of protease-activated receptor type 2, degrade tight junctions and corneodesmosomes, and down-regulate ceramide synthesis.[9] The rise in pH also promotes proliferation and adhesion of *Staphylococcus aureus*.[13–16] Moreover, activation of kallikrein produces the pro–helper T-cell (T_H), T_H2, response without allergen priming, thereby interacting with the immune system to promote an inflammatory response.[17]

Despite the association of *FLG* mutations with AD, many individuals with AD do not carry *FLG* mutations and 40% of individuals with *FLG* null mutations do not have AD.[18] This suggests that other gene mutations or mechanisms may result in epidermal barrier dysfunction. Another possible region of interest is the epidermal differentiation complex on chromosome 1q21 that encodes structural proteins in the epidermis.[19] Other barrier genes of interest in AD include claudins of tight junction[11] and *SPINK5*, which is the cause of Netherton syndrome.[20]

Immune Dysregulation

Keratinocytes, which interface between the environment and the dermal immune system, are the primary source of protein and lipid molecules that make up the physical barrier of the skin. In addition, they are capable of mounting a variety of basic immune responses that function in first-line defense and barrier repair. Keratinocytes produce antimicrobial peptides (AMPs), which consists of mainly β-defensins and cathelicidins. These AMP are important in direct killing of microbial pathogens as well as alerting the hematopoietic arm of the immune system to potential threat of infections. Keratinocytes also produce interleukin (IL)-33, IL-25, and thymic stromal lymphopoietin (TSLP),[21–23] which activate group 2 innate lymphoid cells 2, which in turn produce T_H2 cytokines (IL-5 and IL-13) that may be important in tissue repair.[24] Other capabilities of keratinocytes include the production of IL-1, granulocyte-macrophage colony-stimulating factor (GM-CSF), tumor necrosis factor (TNF)-α, and a variety of chemokines. Taken together, keratinocytes are an important member of the cutaneous immune system. They are a prime candidate in the immune dysregulation and barrier defects of AD. These defects are further exaggerated by the intrusion of allergens and infectious agents, which are then processed and presented by dendritic cells (DCs), leading to further T_H2 polarization and inflammation in AD.

The propagation of the inflammation in AD is carried out by key players in adaptive immunity, which is transferrable: hematopoietic stem cell transplant from an atopic donor resulted in development of AD in the recipient.[25] This demonstrates the importance of the interplay between the innate and adaptive immune system in the pathogenesis of AD. In AD lesions, plasmacytoid DCs, which produce interferon (IFN)-α crucial in fighting viral infections, are absent, whereas myeloid DCs—Langerhans cells (LCs) and inflammatory dendritic epidermal cells (IDECs)—predominate.[26,27] In atopic skin, LCs are in the upper layers of the epidermis and penetrate tight junctions to capture outside antigens.[28] Both LC and IDEC overexpress FcεR1, the high-affinity receptor for IgE.[29] Allergen challenge during atopy patch test results in infiltration of LCs and up-regulation of FcεR1.[30] Binding of IgE on LCs results in the production of IL-16, which attracts $CD4^+$ T cells and also aids in T_H2 polarization.[31] The T_H2 response is characterized by production of IL-4, IL-5, IL-10, and IL-13, which contribute to the inflammation and severity of AD.[32] IL-4, IL-13, and more recently TSLP have been shown to affect keratinocytes by reducing the production of AMP.[33] T_H2 cytokine-suppression of the AMP, human β-defensin 2 (hBD-2), has been observed in multiple studies.[34,35] Suppression of inflammation may represent a host mechanism in limiting harmful inflammation and protecting the host from collateral damage.[36] This concept in AD is supported by a more recent study, which showed a significant increased number of myeloid-derived suppressor cells (MDSCs) in AD skin compared with healthy skin.[37] Activation of Toll-like receptor 2 (TLR-2) by *S aureus* leads to production of IL-6, which induces MDSCs, culminating in the suppression of inflammation created by excessive cutaneous immunity.[37] TSLP also enhances the T_H2 response from DCs via regulation of the production of T_H2-cell–attracting thymus and activation-regulated chemokine, TARC/CCL17.[38] Mast cells may also release IL-31 to promote the T_H2 inflammatory response.[39] IL-25 activates T_H2 memory cells with TSLP-activated DCs.[40]

A small number of T_H17 cells have been found in AD skin. T_H17 cells produce IL-17A, which may suppress TSLP and T_H2 cytokines, whereas IL-4 suppresses IL-17A, suggesting a coregulatory model.[41] Mice deficient of IL-17A, however, demonstrate a weakened T_H2 response in the acute phase of AD. In AD patients, Ustekinumab, a monoclonal antibody that blocks IL-12/IL-23 signaling and regulates IL-17, was not found effective, suggesting that IL-17 may be a bystander of the inflammatory state, rather than a key instigator of AD inflammation.[42] In addition, the number of T_H17 cells is relatively low in AD lesions compared with other inflammatory skin diseases, including Sjögren syndrome, systemic lupus erythematosus, and psoriasis vlugaris.[43] These cells are crucial in mucosal immunity and a low number of them in AD, compared with that in psoriasis, is consistent with increased skin infections in AD.

Although the initial recruitment of T cells to atopic lesions may result in a T_H2 response, the later phase of inflammation yields an increase in IFN-γ, IL-12, and GM-CSF, which characterize the T_H1 and T_H0 response.[44] Persistent chronic inflammation results in recruitment of T cells into the skin via chemokines that sustain a combined T_H2, T_H1, T_H0, and T_H22 inflammatory response.[45,46] IL-22, produced by T_H22 and $CD8^+$ T cells, is an important cytokine in the pathogenesis of adult AD.[45] This cytokine causes epidermal hyperplasia. Its expression has been found to be similar or higher in AD lesions compared with that in psoriatic lesions.

Regulatory T cells ($CD25^+$ $FOXP3^+$) are found increased in the circulation of AD patients but are not found in the skin lesions.[47,48] Further studies are needed to determine the role of these cells in AD.

Skin Microbiome

The normal skin microbiome is modulated by skin pH, moisture, and keratinocytes. Although skin flora varies based on skin site, diet, age, and gender, the most commonly detected normal skin flora include *Propionibacterium acnes, S epidermidis*, and *Cornyebacterium*.[49–53] Skin flora are also found within multiple layers of the skin, suggesting that commensal bacteria may play a greater role in immune modulation than previously thought.[54] Maintenance of the skin microbiome has been linked to *S epidermidis*, which interacts with the innate immune system through activation of TLR-2. By promoting binding of its cell wall component, lipoteichoic acid, to TLR-2, *S epidermidis* suppresses TLR-3–dependent inflammation in the skin.[55] TLR-2 activation on keratinocytes also stimulates production of AMP, such as hBD-2 and hBD-3, which increase tight junction expression to improve skin barrier function, and recruit mast cells.[56–58] Activation of the immune response does not affect survival of normal skin flora. In addition, these commensal bacteria, *S epidermidis* and *P acnes* in particular, produce proteins that inhibit the growth of *S aureus*.[59–61] Thus, the maintenance of the skin microbiome requires the growth of normal skin flora, which modulates immune activity without initiating a state of chronic inflammation, and prevents growth of pathogenic bacteria.[62]

Alterations in the skin barrier function and pH as well as suppression of innate immunity by the inflammatory milieu in the skin renders the skin prone to colonization by *S aureus*. In AD, in addition to skin barrier dysfunction and exposure to additional microbes, excessive production of fibronectin and fibrinogen promotes the binding and colonization of *S aureus*.[63,64] Consequently, patients with AD lesions are colonized by *S aureus* 90% of the time versus only 10% in healthy controls.[65] Overall skin microbial diversity is also decreased in AD.[66] AD patients who used topical corticosteroids, however, had a higher microbial diversity compared with AD patients who did not have treatment,[66] supporting the importance of inflammation in altering the microbial composition of AD. In AD patients with increased *S aureus* colonization, *S epidermidis* colonization was also found increased.[66] Because *S epidermidis* is a commensal skin flora and may prevent *S aureus* colonization, it is unclear if this increase is simply a response to increased *S aureus* colonization or if the strain of *S epidermidis* in AD is different from healthy individuals.[62]

BACTERIAL INFECTION
Staphylococcus aureus

The colonization of AD skin with *S aureus* contributes to its being the most common skin infection in AD. Review of the literature demonstrated that *S aureus* can lead to severe and invasive bacterial infections, such as bacteremia, endocarditis, septic arthritis, and osteomyelitis.[67]

The virulence of *S aureus* in AD is partly due to the production of superantigens—staphylococcal enterotoxins (SEs) A, B, C, and D and toxic shock syndrome toxin 1.[68] In 1 study, superantigen-producing *S aureus* was found in 57% of AD patients versus 33% of controls and was associated with higher AD severity (SCORing Atopic Dermatitis: 58 ± 17 in AD vs 41 ± 7 in controls).[69] These superantigens bind to major histocompatibility class II on antigen-presenting cells and activate naïve T cells to produce local and systemic inflammation mediated through TNF-α and IL-1β.[70,71] Staphylococcal enterotoxin B increases IL-31 expression, which suppresses filaggrin and defensin production.[72] Superantigens can also induce the host to produce superantigen-specific IgE, resulting in basophil activation and histamine release.[73]

Although other virulence factors are less well-studied, *S aureus* is also known to produce α-toxins, which form heterodimers that result in a pore in the cell membrane of keratinocytes to induce cell lysis.[74,75] This toxic effect is potentiated by the milieu of T_H2 cytokines, in particular IL-4 and IL-13.[76] Keratinocytes deficient in filaggrin also lack sphingomyelinase, required for cleavage of sphingomyelin, which binds α-toxin and causes them to be more susceptible to lysis.[77] Even low levels of α-toxin can produce increased inflammation without resulting in keratinocyte lysis.[78] δ-Toxin is another potential virulence factor produced by *S aureus* that results in mast cell degranulation, which leads to increased inflammation.[79] Other potential virulence factors of *S aureus* that could play a role in the pathogenesis of AD include V8 and exfoliative toxins A and B, which have been shown to increase desquamation and skin inflammation; protein A promotes TNF-α production and activates TLR; lipoteichoic acids result in downstream inflammation through activation of TLR2 and platelet activating receptor; diacylated lipoproteins may trigger keratinocytes to produce TSLP via TLR2 and TLR6; and phenol-soluble modulins may also promote inflammation.[80–84] One study in Brazil found that the genes that code for staphylococcal toxin Panton-Valentine leukocidin were highly prevalent in moderate to severe AD patients compared with mild AD patients.[85]

The increase in community-associated methicillin-resistant *S aureus* (MRSA) skin and soft tissue infections (SSTIs) have also played a role in AD. AD is a risk factor for MRSA carriage.[86] MRSA produce more superantigens than methicillin-sensitive *S aureus* (MSSA).[87] In AD patients, the prevalence of MRSA colonization ranges from 11% to 34% compared with 1% to 3% in the general population, and MRSA is associated with an increase in SSTIs in AD.[88–91] AD patients colonized with MRSA also tend to be resistant to topical anti-inflammatory agents, such as corticosteroids, leading to a cycle of skin inflammation and infection.[92] In addition to *S aureus*, *Streptococcus pyogenes* is also a common skin infection in AD.[93] Infections caused by *S pyogenes* may also be associated with severe AD and may lead to complications, such as acute glomerulonephritis, hypertension, and posterior reversible encephalopathy syndrome.[94,95]

The Role of Fungi in Atopic Dermatitis

The role of fungal colonization in the pathogenesis of AD is reviewed in detail (See Martin Glatz and colleagues' article, "The Role of Fungi in Atopic Dermatitis," in this issue). In brief, the most common fungi known to colonize AD lesions are the Malassezia species. These fungi may induce AD inflammation via cell-mediated immunity and IgE production.[96]

VIRAL INFECTION
Eczema Herpeticum

Eczema herpeticum (EH), which is caused by an infection with herpes simplex virus (HSV), is a potentially serious complication of AD that leads to disseminated vesicles with skin breakdown, viremia, fever, and lymphadenopathy and can result in the more serious complications of keratoconjunctivitis and meningitis (**Fig. 2**). HSV exposure is common in the general population and is present in 60% of adults and 20% of children. Nevertheless, EH only affects 3% of AD patients, suggesting that immunologic and genetic factors render a subset of AD patients susceptible to EH.[97] Patients with AD who develop EH (ADEH) have more severe AD, earlier onset of AD, and increased risk of atopic disease (food allergies and asthma) compared with AD patients without EH.[98] ADEH patients are more prone to EH are associated with recurrent *S aureus*

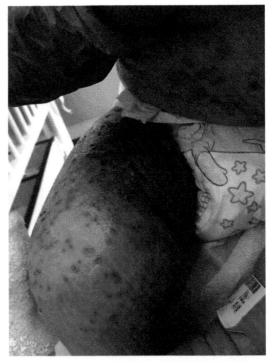

Fig. 2. EH in 15-month-old boy who presented with HSV meningitis.

infections.[98] This may be partly due to the effect of staphylococcal α-toxin in promoting viral replication in skin cells.[99] Because EH can develop in symptomatic or asymptomatic AD patients, identifying the risk factors for EH and understanding the pathogenesis can help prevent against recurrent infections.

The subset of patients with AD who develop EH compared with AD patients without EH also tends to have greater T_H2 polarization characterized by higher total serum IgE, greater eosinophilia, and higher expression of chemokine TARC/CCL17.[98,100] The cytokines involved in the T_H2 response are also known to decrease host antiviral immune responses.[101] In addition, ADEH individuals also tend to have the lowest levels of cathelicidins in the skin.[102]

Various genetic differences have been shown to be associated with the ADEH phenotype.

Polymorphisms in TSLP, which promote the T_H2 response, and signal transducer and activator of transcription 6 (STAT6), a transcription factor implicated in T_H2 response, are associated with ADEH.[103,104]

IFNs are important cytokines in the immunity against HSV. Leung and colleagues[105] evaluated transcription differences in peripheral blood mononuclear cells from ADEH individuals compared with individuals with AD but no history of EH and healthy controls. Genetic variations in type II IFN-α and its receptor are associated with ADEH. Different genetic variants in IFN regulatory factor 2, which blocks IFN-α mediated pathway, were also associated with whites and African Americans with ADEH.[105] IFN-α plays a major role in the immune response against viral infections via the activation of antigen-presenting cells and absence of IFN-α increases susceptibility to HSV infection.

Type III IFN, IL-29, and the gene transcripts of type I IFN-α were found significantly down-regulated in AD patients with history of EH.[106] An increase in indoleamine 2,3-dioxygenase activity in LCs may also be a marker of AD patients who are at risk for EH.[107]

Skin barrier defects have also been associated with ADEH. *FLG* mutations have a stronger association with ADEH patients (OR 10.1) compared with AD patients without EH (OR 3.4).[108] A reduction in a tight junction protein, claudin-1 (CLDN1), correlated with an increase in T_H2 polarization as measured by total serum IgE and eosinophilia.[11] CLDN1 is posited to contribute to the tight junction defect in AD epidermis, which in turn reduces the cell-cell integrity and predisposes AD skin to viral infections.

Eczema Coxsackium

Similar to EH, AD patients who present with coxsackievirus infection, known as eczema coxsackium (EC), can also present with extensive vesicles and skin breakdown.[109,110] EC is not life-threatening, however, and management follows the standard treatments of AD. Although coxsackievirus A16 and enterovirus 71 tend to be associated with hand, foot, and mouth disease, coxsackievirus A6 is associated with more disseminated lesions and tissue destruction.[110] EC is clinically significant in that it may be a differential diagnosis of EH.

Eczema Vaccinatum

Eczema vaccinatum (EV) is a complication of smallpox vaccination that results from infection of AD patients by live vaccinia virus in smallpox vaccine. It is characterized by a vesiculopustular rash. EV can have serious complications with a case fatality rate ranging from 5% to 40%.[111–113] In the era of universal smallpox vaccination, the reported incidence of EV was 10.6 per million in 1968.[114] Since the discontinuation of smallpox vaccination in all but military personnel, there have only been rare cases of EV.[115] This is due to careful screening to exclude patients with AD or history of AD from receiving live smallpox vaccine.

Individuals with AD may be more prone to EV due to the mechanisms (described previously) for EH and due to qualities intrinsic to poxvirus. Vaccinia virus replicates best in injured/inflamed skin, which has hyperplastic keratinocytes with high levels of nucleotides that promote viral infection. Vaccinia virus can also stimulate keratinocytes to enter mitosis through its production of epithelial growth factor.[116] This tendency to favor replication in keratinocytes entering the growth cycle is further substantiated by the finding that in psoriasis patients, who also have skin inflammation but no impairment of keratinocyte maturation, there is no increased risk for vaccinia infection.[117] A mouse model of smallpox prevention using different routes of vaccinia virus vaccinations via intramuscular, subcutaneous, and intradermal injections versus scarification (injured epidermis) showed that only the latter route is protective.[118] This provides support for the primary role of keratinocytes in vaccinia immunity.

Eczema Molluscatum

Patients with AD are also more prone to molluscum contagiosum virus (MCV) infection in both affected and unaffected skin compared with healthy individuals. The infection is characterized by umbilicated, flesh-colored papules. In individuals with AD, the infection can be more severe and widespread with up to hundreds of papules and is known as eczema molluscatum.[119] MCV tends to infect inflamed skin but can spread to nonlesional skin via autoinoculation.[120] Most lesions resolve spontaneously and there are no systemic symptoms, although many lesions resolve quicker with treatment.[120] MCV produces soluble IL-18 binding protein that inhibits IL-18, which stimulates production of IFN-γ.[121] This may to inhibit the immune response and prevent natural killer cell and T-cell activation, both of which are notably absent at the base of MCV papules.[122] The down-regulation of normal antiviral responses in AD may lead to more widespread MCV infection in these individuals.

MANAGEMENT

Prevention of the infectious complications of AD should focus on controlling AD flares and establishment of a routine of maintenance skin care (**Table 1**). To control AD flares, patients should first avoid irritants and allergens that may trigger AD. Common irritants include soaps and detergents with fragrances that are harsh and drying. Instead, AD patients should use fragrance-free gentle cleansers for bathing or showering. Wearing loose, nonabrasive clothing is also useful to prevent trapping of perspiration and to minimize skin irritation. In young children with AD, foods can exacerbate AD with the majority of these food allergens found in cow's milk, egg, soy, and wheat. Identifying these allergens and avoiding them can prevent AD flares. Effects of environmental allergens, such as house dust mites, can also be mitigated with the use of dust mite–proof pillow and mattress covers. Proper control of indoor temperatures to prevent perspiration, skin irritation, and subsequent pruritus is also recommended.

In addition to avoiding allergens, AD patients should maintain their skin hydration. All patients are recommended to shower/bathe in warm water for 15 minutes with a wet towel used to cover areas of the body not covered by water to help seal in moisture. After the bath, patients should pat dry and use a fragrance-free moisturizer using a plastic spoon to avoid contamination of the jar. Although petroleum jelly (Vaseline) seals in water, it does not contain moisturizer and should be used only after hydrating the skin.[123] Moisturizers should be applied multiple times a day and as needed when the skin is dry. Maintenance of adequate skin moisture using a daily regimen can reduce the need for topical corticosteroids. In some cases, a proactive approach of

Table 1
Atopic dermatitis complications and management

Type of Infection	Infectious Complications in Atopic Dermatitis	Management
Bacterial		
S aureus	• SSTIs • Invasive complications include bacteremia, septic arthritis, osteomyelitis, and endocarditis.	• Use topical antibiotics, such as mupirocin for small, localized areas of infections. • Use systemic antibiotics (such as cephalexin) if lesions are widespread. • IV antibiotics are required for invasive infections. • Consider MRSA coverage if there are risk factors (eg, history of MRSA colonization, family members with MRSA infection, etc.).
Viral		
EH	• Disseminated vesicles with skin breakdown, viremia • Serious complications include keratoconjunctivitis and meningitis. • Increased susceptibility to _S aureus_ infections	• Viral culture swab or PCR to identify HSV. • Use oral acyclovir for small, localized lesions. • For extensive, widespread lesions, young children, or if there are systemic symptoms (fever, lethargy), consider hospitalization for IV acyclovir. • Ophthalmology consultation for eye involvement (photophobia, conjunctival erythema, pain, etc.). • For patients with mental status change or seizure, perform a lumbar puncture over nonlesional areas. • Consider antibiotic coverage, because most severe EH patients have secondary bacterial infections.
EC	• Extensive vesicles and skin breakdown • May be difficult to differentiate from EH	• Consider PCR swab for enterovirus. • Treatment is supportive. Monitor for secondary infections. • Continue routine eczema care, including skin hydration, moisturizer and topical corticosteroids.
Eczema vaccinatum	Up to 40% case fatality rate	• History may aid in recognition and diagnosis (eg, patient is a relative of military personnel). • Vaccinia immune globulin from CDC • Isolation from anybody with eczema or history of eczema. • Supportive care and pain control • Investigational drugs: cidofovir, ST-246, and CMX001 (CDC).
Eczema molluscatum	Umbilicated, flesh-colored papules	• Most cases resolve spontaneously. • In severe cases, consider treatment with cryotherapy, curettage, or topical agents (imiquimod).

application of a low-potency to midpotency topical corticosteroid on previously affected skin may be helpful to prevent flares.

During AD flares, the use of at least midpotency topical corticosteroids is necessary. Patient education on the need to continue this medication may be essential in resolution of the AD flare. An alternative to topical corticosteroids, topical calcineurin inhibitors (TCIs), such as tacrolimus (Protopic) and pimecrolimus (Elidel), have been found to effective and safe. A 2015 Cochrane review found that tacrolimus 0.1% was better than low-potency topical corticosteroids, pimecrolimus 1%, and tacrolimus 0.03% by physician assessment of AD lesions.[124] There was no evidence of increased risk of malignancies or skin atrophy with the use of TCIs.[124] The main side effects of TCIs noted were a localized, burning sensation with application.[125]

With AD flares that are resistant to standard treatment, wet wrap therapy is another option (See Noreen Heer Nicol and Mark Boguniewicz's article "Wet Wrap Therapy in Moderate to Severe Atopic Dermatitis," in this issue). This therapy involves applying a layer of topical corticosteroids to affected sites following a bath and placing a layer of wet clothing (cotton long underwear) followed by a layer of dry clothing (cotton sweat suit). The use of wet wraps increases hydration and improves topical corticosteroid efficacy. They are usually left in place overnight or until they dry out in 1 to 2 hours.

AD patients who are on systemic immunosuppressants should be monitored closely, because some are at risk for cytopenias and immunosuppression, which may lead to invasive infections.

When there is widespread bacterial infection of AD lesions, characterized by painful lesions with mucopurulent discharge, an empirical systemic antibiotic, such as cephalexin, is indicated. In addition, a wound culture should be considered to assess antibiotic susceptibility,[126] in case there is a lack of clinical response. In patients with recent history of MRSA colonization or infection, consider using empirical antibiotics that cover MRSA, including trimethoprim-sulfamethoxazole or clindamycin until wound culture and susceptibility are available. The choice of empirical antibiotics for MRSA may depend, however, on the patient population and geographic locations.

AD patients with secondary skin infections and persistent fever or local pain despite systemic antibiotic treatment should raise suspicion for invasive infections, such as bacteremia, endocarditis, or osteomyelitis.

Although it has been well documented that systemic antibiotics can improve the severity and symptoms of AD without the use of anti-inflammatory medications,[127,128] it is not recommended to use antibiotics in noninfected AD due to the potential development of bacterial resistance. Patients with MRSA colonization and recurrent, severe AD exacerbations may require oral antibiotics due to the propensity of these bacterial strains in causing invasive infections and complications. Alternatively, topical antiseptics and antibiotics may be used for decolonization, but their efficacy in AD is a subject of research. A treatment regimen may consist of nasal mupirocin twice daily and chlorhexidine gluconate or diluted bleach baths/shower for 5 to 10 days.[129,130] Decolonization using 4% chlorhexidine gluconate and nasal mupirocin method in a general population of pediatric subjects with both MSSA and MRSA SSTIs does decrease the incidence of reinfections (0.03 infections per month 6 months after decolonization) compared with prior to decolonization (0.84 infections per month 6 months prior to decolonization). Decolonization of household contacts using a similar strategy was also found to decrease the risk of SSTI in both the index cases and their household contacts at the 3-month, 6-month, and 12-month follow-up period compared with decolonization of the index cases alone.[129] This study did not find differences in S aureus eradication at any of these time points. This indicates that there may be other factors that reduce skin infections. Further studies are needed to investigate the mechanisms. Nevertheless, treatment using diluted bleach baths and nasal mupirocin in infected AD patients led to improvement of AD,[131] perhaps through a reduction of S aureus–induced skin inflammation.

Managing viral infections first requires supportive care and identification of the viral agent. In case EH and EC are difficult to differentiate clinically, a viral swab for polymerase chain reaction (PCR) can be used to identify HSV or enterovirus. If EH is suspected with fear of progression to more serious complications, such as keratoconjunctivitis or meningitis, IV acyclovir should be initiated immediately. In less severe EH, oral acyclovir can be used instead. Lumbar puncture should be performed if there is any concern of neurologic findings and the cerebrospinal fluid should be sent for HSV PCR. For severe cases of HSV meningoencephalitis in young children, IV acyclovir dose as high as 60 mg/kg/d for 3 to 6 weeks may be required. In addition, long-term suppressive therapy with oral acyclovir for up to a year may also be required. Monitoring for renal functions and cytopenia is advised during high-dose acyclovir treatment. Ophthalmic involvement should prompt emergent ophthalmology evaluation to prevent corneal involvement.[132] Supportive care includes intravenous (IV) fluids to manage fluid losses, symptomatic management of pain, and pruritus. In most cases, institute anti–S aureus treatments due to the increased risk of secondary bacterial infections.

If EC is suspected, because there are no known agents to treat EC, management is based on supportive care and prevention of secondary infections. The use of topical corticosteroids was shown effective in these lesions.[109]

Most physicians today have not seen EV since universal use of smallpox vaccine was phased out in the early 1970s. Due to the current implementation of smallpox vaccination in military personnel, physicians should be vigilant of EV and be able to recognize it. **Fig. 3** showed a case of pediatric EV that was seen at the authors' institution more than 50 years ago. Although there have only been few recent documented cases of EV, treatment of EV has involved vaccinia immunoglobulin with cidofovir and investigational drugs ST-246 and CMX001.[133] Smallpox vaccine is generally contraindicated in AD patients. Recent Centers for Disease Control and Prevention (CDC) guidelines recommend, however, that AD patients who are at risk for smallpox infection but who are without known exposure to smallpox virus may receive a new attenuated, modified vaccinia Ankara virus vaccine, Imvamune. On the other hand, AD

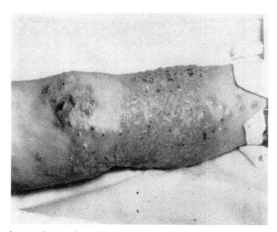

Fig. 3. Umbilicated pustules and vesicles of eczema vaccinatum. (*From* Reynolds AH, Joos HA. Eczema vaccinatum. Pediatrics 1958;22(2):260; with permission.)

patients who are confirmed to have been exposed to smallpox virus should receive the live vaccinia virus vaccine, ACAM2000, because the benefits outweigh the risks.[134]

MCV infection can be managed with observation in mild cases, because most resolve spontaneously. Management of more severe cases involves strategies to reduce scratching, or consideration of cryotherapy, curettage, or topical agents, such as imiquimod.[132]

FUTURE CONSIDERATIONS

AD is a complex disease arising from an interaction of skin barrier defects, environment, and a dysfunctional immune response. This inflammatory cycle also alters the skin microbiome and innate immune system so that pathogenic organisms, such as S aureus, are more likely to colonize and infect the skin. Although preventive treatments rely on daily skin care and anti-inflammatory therapy, a subset of AD patients still suffers from infectious complication despite these treatments. Large-scale studies, such as Atopic Dermatitis and Vaccinia Research Network, aim at identifying the phenotypes and genotypes that predispose to infections.[97–99,102–106] Identification of specific defects may lead to more targeted therapies in the host immune response. Dupilumab, which targets the α receptor of IL-4 and inhibits both IL-4 and IL-13, has been shown effective in decreasing the severity of AD in adult patients.[135] Further studies may evaluate if this monoclonal antibody could decrease AD inflammation, leading to fewer skin infections. Other anti-inflammatory therapy for AD in the research pipeline includes anti-IL-13, anti-IL-22, and anti-IL-31 as well as topical agents, such as phosephodiesterase 4 and janus kinase inhibitors.[136,137] The potential use of microbial skin transplant therapy and topical probiotics in controlling S aureus growth may provide a new paradigm in the management of skin infections in AD, particularly in more virulent strains, such as MRSA.[62,138]

REFERENCES

1. Larsen FS, Hanifin JM. Epidemiology of atopic dermatitis. Immunol Allergy Clin North Am 2002;22(1):1–24.
2. Bieber T. Atopic Dermatitis. N Engl J Med 2008;358:1483–94.
3. Su JC, Kemp AS, Varigos GA, et al. Atopic eczema: its impact on the family and financial cost. Arch Dis Child 1997;76(2):159–62.
4. Chamlin SL, Frieden IJ, Williams ML, et al. Effects of atopic dermatitis on young American children and their families. Pediatrics 2004;114(3):607–11.
5. Grice K, Sattar H, Baker H, et al. The relationship of transepidermal water loss to skin temperature in psoriasis and eczema. J Invest Dermatol 1975;64(5):313–5.
6. Nemes Z, Steinert PM. Bricks and mortar of the epidermal barrier. Exp Mol Med 1999;31(1):5–19.
7. Gupta J, Grube E, Ericksen MB, et al. Intrinsically defective skin barrier function in children with atopic dermatitis correlates with disease severity. J Allergy Clin Immunol 2008;121(3):725–30.e2.
8. Cork MJ, Robinson DA, Vasilopoulos Y, et al. New perspectives on epidermal barrier dysfunction in atopic dermatitis: gene-environment interactions. J Allergy Clin Immunol 2006;118(1):3–21 [quiz: 22–3].
9. Irvine AD, McLean WHI, Leung DYM. Filaggrin mutations associated with skin and allergic diseases. N Engl J Med 2011;365(14):1315–27.
10. van den Oord RAHM, Sheikh A. Filaggrin gene defects and risk of developing allergic sensitisation and allergic disorders: systematic review and meta-analysis. BMJ 2009;339:b2433.

11. De Benedetto A, Rafaels NM, McGirt LY, et al. Tight junction defects in patients with atopic dermatitis. J Allergy Clin Immunol 2011;127(3):773–86.e1-7.
12. Kezic S, O'Regan GM, Yau N, et al. Levels of filaggrin degradation products are influenced by both filaggrin genotype and atopic dermatitis severity. Allergy 2011;66(7):934–40.
13. Thyssen JP, Kezic S. Causes of epidermal filaggrin reduction and their role in the pathogenesis of atopic dermatitis. J Allergy Clin Immunol 2014;134(4):792–9.
14. Hachem J-P, Man M-Q, Crumrine D, et al. Sustained serine proteases activity by prolonged increase in pH leads to degradation of lipid processing enzymes and profound alterations of barrier function and stratum corneum integrity. J Invest Dermatol 2005;125(3):510–20.
15. Schmid-Wendtner M-H, Korting HC. The pH of the Skin Surface and Its Impact on the Barrier Function. Skin Pharmacol Physiol 2006;19(6):296–302.
16. Miajlovic H, Fallon PG, Irvine AD, et al. Effect of filaggrin breakdown products on growth of and protein expression by Staphylococcus aureus. J Allergy Clin Immunol 2010;126(6):1184–90.e3.
17. Briot A, Deraison C, Lacroix M, et al. Kallikrein 5 induces atopic dermatitis-like lesions through PAR2-mediated thymic stromal lymphopoietin expression in Netherton syndrome. J Exp Med 2009;206(5):1135–47.
18. O'Regan GM, Sandilands A, McLean WHI, et al. Filaggrin in atopic dermatitis. J Allergy Clin Immunol 2008;122(4):689–93.
19. Morar N, Willis-Owen SAG, Moffatt MF, et al. The genetics of atopic dermatitis. J Allergy Clin Immunol 2006;118(1):24–34 [quiz: 35–6].
20. Elias PM, Hatano Y, Williams ML. Basis for the barrier abnormality in atopic dermatitis: outside-inside-outside pathogenic mechanisms. J Allergy Clin Immunol 2008;121(6):1337–43.
21. Cevikbas F, Steinhoff M. IL-33: a novel danger signal system in atopic dermatitis. J Invest Dermatol 2012;132(5):1326–9.
22. Hvid M, Vestergaard C, Kemp K, et al. IL-25 in atopic dermatitis: a possible link between inflammation and skin barrier dysfunction? J Invest Dermatol 2011; 131(1):150–7.
23. Kim BS, Siracusa MC, Saenz SA, et al. TSLP elicits IL-33-independent innate lymphoid cell responses to promote skin inflammation. Sci Transl Med 2013; 5(170):170ra16.
24. Pulendran B, Artis D. New paradigms in type 2 immunity. Science 2012; 337(6093):431–5.
25. Bellou A, Kanny G, Fremont S, et al. Transfer of atopy following bone marrow transplantation. Ann Allergy Asthma Immunol 1997;78(5):513–6.
26. Wollenberg A, Wagner M, Günther S, et al. Plasmacytoid dendritic cells: a new cutaneous dendritic cell subset with distinct role in inflammatory skin diseases. J Invest Dermatol 2002;119(5):1096–102.
27. Wollenberg A, Kraft S, Hanau D, et al. Immunomorphological and ultrastructural characterization of Langerhans cells and a novel, inflammatory dendritic epidermal cell (IDEC) population in lesional skin of atopic eczema. J Invest Dermatol 1996;106(3):446–53.
28. Kubo A, Nagao K, Yokouchi M, et al. External antigen uptake by Langerhans cells with reorganization of epidermal tight junction barriers. J Exp Med 2009; 206(13):2937–46.
29. Bruynzeel-Koomen C, van Wichen DF, Toonstra J, et al. The presence of IgE molecules on epidermal Langerhans cells in patients with atopic dermatitis. Arch Dermatol Res 1986;278(3):199–205.

30. Kerschenlohr K, Decard S, Przybilla B, et al. Atopy patch test reactions show a rapid influx of inflammatory dendritic epidermal cells in patients with extrinsic atopic dermatitis and patients with intrinsic atopic dermatitis. J Allergy Clin Immunol 2003;111(4):869–74.

31. Reich K, Heine A, Hugo S, et al. Engagement of the Fc epsilon RI stimulates the production of IL-16 in Langerhans cell-like dendritic cells. J Immunol 2001; 167(11):6321–9.

32. Suarez-Fariñas M, Dhingra N, Gittler J, et al. Intrinsic atopic dermatitis shows similar Th2 and higher Th17 immune activation compared with extrinsic atopic dermatitis. J Allergy Clin Immunol 2013;132(2):361–70.

33. Lee H, Ryu W, Kim J, et al. TSLP downregulates S100A7 and β-defensin2 via the JAK2/STAT3 dependent mechanism. J Invest Dermatol 2016. [Epub ahead of print].

34. Ong PY, Ohtake T, Brandt C, et al. Endogenous antimicrobial peptides and skin infections in atopic dermatitis. N Engl J Med 2002;347(15):1151–60.

35. Onderdijk AJ, Baerveldt EM, Kurek D, et al. IL-4 Downregulates IL-1β and IL-6 and Induces GATA3 in Psoriatic Epidermal Cells: Route of Action of a Th2 Cytokine. J Immunol 2015;195(4):1744–52.

36. Sumpter TL, Falo LD. "Toll"-erance in the skin. Immunity 2014;41(5):677–9.

37. Skabytska Y, Wölbing F, Günther C, et al. Cutaneous innate immune sensing of Toll-like receptor 2-6 ligands suppresses T cell immunity by inducing myeloid-derived suppressor cells. Immunity 2014;41(5):762–75.

38. Soumelis V, Reche PA, Kanzler H, et al. Human epithelial cells trigger dendritic cell mediated allergic inflammation by producing TSLP. Nat Immunol 2002;3(7): 673–80.

39. Otsuka A, Kabashima K. Mast cells and basophils in cutaneous immune responses. Allergy 2015;70(2):131–40.

40. Wang Y-H, Angkasekwinai P, Lu N, et al. IL-25 augments type 2 immune responses by enhancing the expansion and functions of TSLP-DC-activated Th2 memory cells. J Exp Med 2007;204(8):1837–47.

41. Eyerich K, Pennino D, Scarponi C, et al. IL-17 in atopic eczema: linking allergen-specific adaptive and microbial-triggered innate immune response. J Allergy Clin Immunol 2009;123(1):59–66.e4.

42. Samorano LP, Hanifin JM, Simpson EL, et al. Inadequate response to ustekinumab in atopic dermatitis - a report of two patients. J Eur Acad Dermatol Venereol 2016;30(3):522–3.

43. Itoi S, Tanemura A, Tani M, et al. Immunohistochemical Analysis of Interleukin-17 Producing T Helper Cells and Regulatory T Cells Infiltration in Annular Erythema Associated with Sjögren's Syndrome. Ann Dermatol 2014;26(2):203–8.

44. Taha RA, Leung DY, Ghaffar O, et al. In vivo expression of cytokine receptor mRNA in atopic dermatitis. J Allergy Clin Immunol 1998;102(2):245–50.

45. Czarnowicki T, Esaki H, Gonzalez J, et al. Early pediatric atopic dermatitis shows only a cutaneous lymphocyte antigen (CLA)(+) TH2/TH1 cell imbalance, whereas adults acquire CLA(+) TH22/TC22 cell subsets. J Allergy Clin Immunol 2015;136(4):941–51.e3.

46. Homey B, Steinhoff M, Ruzicka T, et al. Cytokines and chemokines orchestrate atopic skin inflammation. J Allergy Clin Immunol 2006;118(1):178–89.

47. Ou L-S, Goleva E, Hall C, et al. T regulatory cells in atopic dermatitis and subversion of their activity by superantigens. J Allergy Clin Immunol 2004;113(4): 756–63.

48. Verhagen J, Akdis M, Traidl-Hoffmann C, et al. Absence of T-regulatory cell expression and function in atopic dermatitis skin. J Allergy Clin Immunol 2006;117(1):176–83.

49. Fitz-Gibbon S, Tomida S, Chiu B-H, et al. Propionibacterium acnes strain populations in the human skin microbiome associated with acne. J Invest Dermatol 2013;133(9):2152–60.

50. Tomida S, Nguyen L, Chiu B-H, et al. Pan-genome and comparative genome analyses of propionibacterium acnes reveal its genomic diversity in the healthy and diseased human skin microbiome. MBio 2013;4(3):e00003–13.

51. Wang Y, Kuo S, Shu M, et al. Staphylococcus epidermidis in the human skin microbiome mediates fermentation to inhibit the growth of Propionibacterium acnes: implications of probiotics in acne vulgaris. Appl Microbiol Biotechnol 2014;98(1):411–24.

52. Kloos WE, Musselwhite MS. Distribution and persistence of Staphylococcus and Micrococcus species and other aerobic bacteria on human skin. Appl Microbiol 1975;30(3):381–5.

53. Belkaid Y, Segre JA. Dialogue between skin microbiota and immunity. Science 2014;346(6212):954–9.

54. Nakatsuji T, Chiang H-I, Jiang SB, et al. The microbiome extends to subepidermal compartments of normal skin. Nat Commun 2013;4:1431.

55. Lai Y, Di Nardo A, Nakatsuji T, et al. Commensal bacteria regulate Toll-like receptor 3-dependent inflammation after skin injury. Nat Med 2009;15(12):1377–82.

56. Lai Y, Cogen AL, Radek KA, et al. Activation of TLR2 by a small molecule produced by Staphylococcus epidermidis increases antimicrobial defense against bacterial skin infections. J Invest Dermatol 2010;130(9):2211–21.

57. Wang Z, MacLeod DT, Di Nardo A. Commensal bacteria lipoteichoic acid increases skin mast cell antimicrobial activity against vaccinia viruses. J Immunol 2012;189(4):1551–8.

58. Yuki T, Yoshida H, Akazawa Y, et al. Activation of TLR2 enhances tight junction barrier in epidermal keratinocytes. J Immunol 2011;187(6):3230–7.

59. Sugimoto S, Iwamoto T, Takada K, et al. Staphylococcus epidermidis Esp degrades specific proteins associated with Staphylococcus aureus biofilm formation and host-pathogen interaction. J Bacteriol 2013;195(8):1645–55.

60. Cogen AL, Yamasaki K, Sanchez KM, et al. Selective antimicrobial action is provided by phenol-soluble modulins derived from Staphylococcus epidermidis, a normal resident of the skin. J Invest Dermatol 2010;130(1):192–200.

61. Shu M, Wang Y, Yu J, et al. Fermentation of Propionibacterium acnes, a commensal bacterium in the human skin microbiome, as skin probiotics against methicillin-resistant Staphylococcus aureus. PLoS One 2013;8(2):e55380.

62. Williams MR, Gallo RL. The role of the skin microbiome in atopic dermatitis. Curr Allergy Asthma Rep 2015;15(11):65.

63. Sinha B, François PP, Nüsse O, et al. Fibronectin-binding protein acts as Staphylococcus aureus invasin via fibronectin bridging to integrin alpha5beta1. Cell Microbiol 1999;1(2):101–17.

64. Cho SH, Strickland I, Boguniewicz M, et al. Fibronectin and fibrinogen contribute to the enhanced binding of Staphylococcus aureus to atopic skin. J Allergy Clin Immunol 2001;108(2):269–74.

65. Leyden JJ, Marples RR, Kligman AM. Staphylococcus aureus in the lesions of atopic dermatitis. Br J Dermatol 1974;90(5):525–30.

66. Kong HH, Oh J, Deming C, et al. Temporal shifts in the skin microbiome associated with disease flares and treatment in children with atopic dermatitis. Genome Res 2012;22(5):850–9.
67. Patel D, Jahnke MN. Serious Complications from Staphylococcal aureus in Atopic Dermatitis. Pediatr Dermatol 2015;32(6):792–6.
68. Ong PY, Leung DYM. The infectious aspects of atopic dermatitis. Immunol Allergy Clin North Am 2010;30(3):309–21.
69. Zollner TM, Wichelhaus TA, Hartung A, et al. Colonization with superantigen-producing Staphylococcus aureus is associated with increased severity of atopic dermatitis. Clin Exp Allergy 2000;30(7):994–1000.
70. Proft T, Fraser JD. Bacterial superantigens. Clin Exp Immunol 2003;133(3):299–306.
71. Hirose A, Ikejima T, Gill DM. Established macrophagelike cell lines synthesize interleukin-1 in response to toxic shock syndrome toxin. Infect Immun 1985;50(3):765–70.
72. van Drongelen V, Haisma EM, Out-Luiting JJ, et al. Reduced filaggrin expression is accompanied by increased Staphylococcus aureus colonization of epidermal skin models. Clin Exp Allergy 2014;44(12):1515–24.
73. Leung DY, Harbeck R, Bina P, et al. Presence of IgE antibodies to staphylococcal exotoxins on the skin of patients with atopic dermatitis. Evidence for a new group of allergens. J Clin Invest 1993;92(3):1374–80.
74. Bantel H, Sinha B, Domschke W, et al. alpha-Toxin is a mediator of Staphylococcus aureus-induced cell death and activates caspases via the intrinsic death pathway independently of death receptor signaling. J Cell Biol 2001;155(4):637–48.
75. Walev I, Martin E, Jonas D, et al. Staphylococcal alpha-toxin kills human keratinocytes by permeabilizing the plasma membrane for monovalent ions. Infect Immun 1993;61(12):4972–9.
76. Brauweiler AM, Goleva E, Leung DYM. Th2 cytokines increase Staphylococcus aureus alpha toxin-induced keratinocyte death through the signal transducer and activator of transcription 6 (STAT6). J Invest Dermatol 2014;134(8):2114–21.
77. Brauweiler AM, Bin L, Kim BE, et al. Filaggrin-dependent secretion of sphingomyelinase protects against staphylococcal α-toxin-induced keratinocyte death. J Allergy Clin Immunol 2013;131(2):421–7.e1-2.
78. Ezepchuk YV, Leung DY, Middleton MH, et al. Staphylococcal toxins and protein A differentially induce cytotoxicity and release of tumor necrosis factor-alpha from human keratinocytes. J Invest Dermatol 1996;107(4):603–9.
79. Nakamura Y, Oscherwitz J, Cease KB, et al. Staphylococcus δ-toxin induces allergic skin disease by activating mast cells. Nature 2013;503(7476):397–401.
80. Hanakawa Y, Selwood T, Woo D, et al. Calcium-dependent conformation of desmoglein 1 is required for its cleavage by exfoliative toxin. J Invest Dermatol 2003;121(2):383–9.
81. Hirasawa Y, Takai T, Nakamura T, et al. Staphylococcus aureus extracellular protease causes epidermal barrier dysfunction. J Invest Dermatol 2010;130(2):614–7.
82. Ladhani S. Understanding the mechanism of action of the exfoliative toxins of Staphylococcus aureus. FEMS Immunol Med Microbiol 2003;39(2):181–9.
83. Syed AK, Reed TJ, Clark KL, et al. Staphlyococcus aureus phenol-soluble modulins stimulate the release of proinflammatory cytokines from keratinocytes and are required for induction of skin inflammation. Infect Immun 2015;83(9):3428–37.

84. Travers JB. Toxic interaction between Th2 cytokines and Staphylococcus aureus in atopic dermatitis. J Invest Dermatol 2014;134(8):2069–71.

85. Cavalcante FS, Abad ED, Lyra YC, et al. High prevalence of methicillin resistance and PVL genes among Staphylococcus aureus isolates from the nares and skin lesions of pediatric patients with atopic dermatitis. Braz J Med Biol Res 2015;48(7):588–94.

86. Daeschlein G, von Podewils S, Bloom T, et al. Risk factors for MRSA colonization in dermatologic patients in Germany. J Dtsch Dermatol Ges 2015;13(10):1015–22.

87. Schlievert PM, Strandberg KL, Lin Y-C, et al. Secreted virulence factor comparison between methicillin-resistant and methicillin-sensitive Staphylococcus aureus, and its relevance to atopic dermatitis. J Allergy Clin Immunol 2010; 125(1):39–49.

88. Klein PA, Greene WH, Fuhrer J, et al. Prevalence of methicillin-resistant Staphylococcus aureus in outpatients with psoriasis, atopic dermatitis, or HIV infection. Arch Dermatol 1997;133(11):1463–5.

89. Suh L, Coffin S, Leckerman KH, et al. Methicillin-resistant Staphylococcus aureus colonization in children with atopic dermatitis. Pediatr Dermatol 2008; 25(5):528–34.

90. Lo W-T, Wang S-R, Tseng M-H, et al. Comparative molecular analysis of meticillin-resistant Staphylococcus aureus isolates from children with atopic dermatitis and healthy subjects in Taiwan. Br J Dermatol 2010;162(5):1110–6.

91. Travers JB, Kozman A, Yao Y, et al. Treatment outcomes of secondarily impetiginized pediatric atopic dermatitis lesions and the role of oral antibiotics. Pediatr Dermatol 2012;29(3):289–96.

92. Hon K-LE, Leung AKC, Kong AYF, et al. Atopic dermatitis complicated by methicillin-resistant Staphylococcus aureus infection. J Natl Med Assoc 2008; 100(7):797–800.

93. Brook I, Frazier EH, Yeager JK. Microbiology of infected atopic dermatitis. Int J Dermatol 1996;35(11):791–3.

94. Hayakawa K, Hirahara K, Fukuda T, et al. Risk factors for severe impetiginized atopic dermatitis in Japan and assessment of its microbiological features. Clin Exp Dermatol 2009;34(5):e63–5.

95. Park JM, Oh SH, Kim J, et al. Atopic dermatitis with group A beta-hemolytic Streptococcus skin infection complicated by posterior reversible encephalopathy syndrome. Arch Dermatol 2009;145(7):846–7.

96. Schmid-Grendelmeier P, Scheynius A, Crameri R. The role of sensitization to Malassezia sympodialis in atopic eczema. Chem Immunol Allergy 2006;91:98–109.

97. Leung DYM. Why is eczema herpeticum unexpectedly rare? Antiviral Res 2013; 98(2):153–7.

98. Beck LA, Boguniewicz M, Hata T, et al. Phenotype of atopic dermatitis subjects with a history of eczema herpeticum. J Allergy Clin Immunol 2009;124(2):260–9, 269.e1–7.

99. Bin L, Kim BE, Brauweiler A, et al. Staphylococcus aureus α-toxin modulates skin host response to viral infection. J Allergy Clin Immunol 2012;130(3): 683–91.e2.

100. Wollenberg A, Zoch C, Wetzel S, et al. Predisposing factors and clinical features of eczema herpeticum: a retrospective analysis of 100 cases. J Am Acad Dermatol 2003;49(2):198–205.

101. Howell MD, Gallo RL, Boguniewicz M, et al. Cytokine milieu of atopic dermatitis skin subverts the innate immune response to vaccinia virus. Immunity 2006; 24(3):341–8.

102. Hata TR, Kotol P, Boguniewicz M, et al. History of eczema herpeticum is associated with the inability to induce human β-defensin (HBD)-2, HBD-3 and cathelicidin in the skin of patients with atopic dermatitis. Br J Dermatol 2010;163(3): 659–61.
103. Gao P-S, Rafaels NM, Mu D, et al. Genetic variants in thymic stromal lymphopoietin are associated with atopic dermatitis and eczema herpeticum. J Allergy Clin Immunol 2010;125(6):1403–7.e4.
104. Howell MD, Gao P, Kim BE, et al. The signal transducer and activator of transcription 6 gene (STAT6) increases the propensity of patients with atopic dermatitis toward disseminated viral skin infections. J Allergy Clin Immunol 2011; 128(5):1006–14.
105. Leung DYM, Gao P-S, Grigoryev DN, et al. Human atopic dermatitis complicated by eczema herpeticum is associated with abnormalities in IFN-γ response. J Allergy Clin Immunol 2011;127(4):965–73.e1-5.
106. Bin L, Edwards MG, Heiser R, et al. Identification of novel gene signatures in patients with atopic dermatitis complicated by eczema herpeticum. J Allergy Clin Immunol 2014;134(4):848–55.
107. Staudacher A, Hinz T, Novak N, et al. Exaggerated IDO1 expression and activity in Langerhans cells from patients with atopic dermatitis upon viral stimulation: a potential predictive biomarker for high risk of Eczema herpeticum. Allergy 2015; 70(11):1432–9.
108. Gao P-S, Rafaels NM, Hand T, et al. Filaggrin mutations that confer risk of atopic dermatitis confer greater risk for eczema herpeticum. J Allergy Clin Immunol 2009;124(3):507–13, 513.e1–7.
109. Johnson VK, Hayman JL, McCarthy CA, et al. Successful treatment of eczema coxsackium with wet wrap therapy and low-dose topical corticosteroid. J Allergy Clin Immunol Pract 2014;2(6):803–4.
110. Mathes EF, Oza V, Frieden IJ, et al. "Eczema coxsackium" and unusual cutaneous findings in an enterovirus outbreak. Pediatrics 2013;132(1):e149–57.
111. Waddington E, Bray PT, Evans AD, et al. Cutaneous complications of mass vaccination against smallpox in South Wales 1962. Trans St Johns Hosp Dermatol Soc 1964;50:22–42.
112. Copeman PW, Wallace HJ. Eczema vaccinatum. Br Med J 1964;2(5414):906–8.
113. Kempe CH, Beneson As. Smallpox and vaccinia. Pediatr Clin North Am 1955;19–32.
114. Lane JM, Ruben FL, Neff JM, et al. Complications of smallpox vaccination, 1968. N Engl J Med 1969;281(22):1201–8.
115. Vora S, Damon I, Fulginiti V, et al. Severe eczema vaccinatum in a household contact of a smallpox vaccinee. Clin Infect Dis 2008;46(10):1555–61.
116. Buller RM, Chakrabarti S, Moss B, et al. Cell proliferative response to vaccinia virus is mediated by VGF. Virology 1988;164(1):182–92.
117. Guttman-Yassky E, Suárez-Fariñas M, Chiricozzi A, et al. Broad defects in epidermal cornification in atopic dermatitis identified through genomic analysis. J Allergy Clin Immunol 2009;124(6):1235–44.e58.
118. Liu L, Zhong Q, Tian T, et al. Epidermal injury and infection during poxvirus immunization is crucial for the generation of highly protective T cell-mediated immunity. Nat Med 2010;16(2):224–7.
119. Wollenberg A, Klein E. Current aspects of innate and adaptive immunity in atopic dermatitis. Clin Rev Allergy Immunol 2007;33(1–2):35–44.
120. Solomon LM, Telner P. Eruptive molluscum contagiosum in atopic dermatitis. Can Med Assoc J 1966;95(19):978–9.

121. Xiang Y, Moss B. Molluscum contagiosum virus interleukin-18 (IL-18) binding protein is secreted as a full-length form that binds cell surface glycosaminogly-cans through the C-terminal tail and a furin-cleaved form with only the IL-18 binding domain. J Virol 2003;77(4):2623–30.
122. Heng MC, Steuer ME, Levy A, et al. Lack of host cellular immune response in eruptive molluscum contagiosum. Am J Dermatopathol 1989;11(3):248–54.
123. Boguniewicz M, Nicol N, Kelsay K, et al. A multidisciplinary approach to evaluation and treatment of atopic dermatitis. Semin Cutan Med Surg 2008;27(2):115–27.
124. Cury Martins J, Martins C, Aoki V, et al. Topical tacrolimus for atopic dermatitis. Cochrane Database Syst Rev 2015;(7):CD009864.
125. Boguniewicz M, Fiedler VC, Raimer S, et al. A randomized, vehicle-controlled trial of tacrolimus ointment for treatment of atopic dermatitis in children. Pediatric Tacrolimus Study Group. J Allergy Clin Immunol 1998;102(4 Pt 1):637–44.
126. Ong PY. Recurrent MRSA skin infections in atopic dermatitis. J Allergy Clin Immunol Pract 2014;2(4):396–9.
127. Breuer K, Haussler S, Kapp A, et al. Staphylococcus aureus: colonizing features and influence of an antibacterial treatment in adults with atopic dermatitis. Br J Dermatol 2002;147:55–61.
128. Rosa JS, Ross LA, Ong PY. Emergence of multiresistant methicillin-resistant Staphylococcal aureus in two patients with atopic dermatitis requiring linezolid treatment. Pediatr Dermatol 2014;31(2):245–8.
129. Fritz SA, Hogan PG, Hayek G, et al. Household versus individual approaches to eradication of community-associated Staphylococcus aureus in children: a randomized trial. Clin Infect Dis 2012;54(6):743–51.
130. Fritz SA, Camins BC, Eisenstein KA, et al. Effectiveness of measures to eradicate Staphylococcus aureus carriage in patients with community-associated skin and soft-tissue infections: a randomized trial. Infect Control Hosp Epidemiol 2011;32(9):872–80.
131. Huang JT, Abrams M, Tlougan B, et al. Treatment of Staphylococcus aureus colonization in atopic dermatitis decreases disease severity. Pediatrics 2009;123(5):e808–14.
132. Wollenberg A, Wetzel S, Burgdorf WHC, et al. Viral infections in atopic dermatitis: pathogenic aspects and clinical management. J Allergy Clin Immunol 2003;112(4):667–74.
133. Reed JL, Scott DE, Bray M. Eczema vaccinatum. Clin Infect Dis 2012;54(6):832–40.
134. Petersen BW, Damon IK, Pertowski CA, et al. Clinical guidance for smallpox vaccine use in a postevent vaccination program. MMWR Recomm Rep 2015;64(RR-02):1–26.
135. Beck LA, Thaçi D, Hamilton JD, et al. Dupilumab treatment in adults with moderate-to-severe atopic dermatitis. N Engl J Med 2014;371(2):130–9.
136. Wang D, Beck LA. Immunologic targets in atopic dermatitis and emerging therapy: an update. Am J Clin Dermatol 2016. [Epub ahead of print].
137. Hanifin JM, Ellis CN, Frieden IJ, et al. OPA-15406, a novel, topical, nonsteroidal, selective phosphodiesterase-4 (PDE4) inhibitor, in the treatment of adult and adolescent patients with mild to moderate atopic dermatitis (AD): A phase-II randomized, double-blind, placebo-controlled study. J Am Acad Dermatol 2016;75(2):297–305.
138. Mohammedsaeed W, McBain AJ, Cruickshank SM, et al. Lactobacillus rhamnosus GG inhibits the toxic effects of Staphylococcus aureus on epidermal keratinocytes. Appl Environ Microbiol 2014;80(18):5773–81.

Biologics in Chronic Urticaria

Adeeb Bulkhi, MD[a,b], Andrew J. Cooke, MD[a], Thomas B. Casale, MD[a,*]

KEYWORDS

- Chronic urticaria • Biologics • Omalizumab • Therapy • Rituximab • TNF antagonist
- Intravenous immunoglobulin therapy

KEY POINTS

- Omalizumab is the only monoclonal antibody that is approved for chronic urticaria (CU).
- Randomized, placebo-controlled trials and extensive clinical experience show that omalizumab is both safe and efficacious for CU.
- A few reports demonstrated effectiveness of high-dose immunoglobulin therapy.
- Weak evidence supports rituximab and tumor necrosis factor antagonist efficacy in antihistamine-refractory CU.

Chronic urticaria (CU), also referred to as chronic spontaneous urticaria, is defined as wheals, angioedema, or both lasting longer than 6 weeks.[1] CU is associated with intense pruritus, disfiguring wheals, and higher odds of reporting depression, anxiety, and sleep difficulty.[2–4] Patients with CU experience a tremendous burden, with quality-of-life estimates on par with patients with coronary artery disease awaiting bypass.[5,6] Urticaria of any type is estimated to have a lifetime prevalence of 8.8%, whereas CU has an annual prevalence of 0.5% to 5.0% and a lifetime prevalence rate of 1.8%.[2,7–12] The first-line therapies for CU are second-generation H_1 antihistamines, often required at 2 to 4 times the doses approved by the Food and Drug Administration (FDA).[12] Unfortunately, many patients will fail antihistamines and will require alternative therapies to control their symptoms. For these patients, biologics have proven to be relatively safe and efficacious.

Conflicts of Interest: Dr A. Bulkhi and Dr A.J. Cooke have no conflicts of interest to disclose. Dr T.B. Casale has been an investigator on grants from Novartis and Genentech to his University and has been on advisory boards for Novartis and Genentech with all funds to his University employer.
Funding: No sources of funding were used to support the writing of this article.
[a] Division of Allergy and Immunology, Department of Internal Medicine, University of South Florida, Tampa, FL, USA; [b] Department of Internal Medicine, College of Medicine, Umm Al-Qura University, Makkah, Saudi Arabia
* Corresponding author. 12901 Bruce B. Downs Boulevard, MDC 19, Tampa, FL 33612.
E-mail address: tbcasale@health.usf.edu

The FDA defines biologics as a wide range of products, such as vaccines, blood and blood components, allergenics, somatic cells, gene therapy, tissues, and recombinant therapeutic proteins.[13] Although biologics have been used for years, the first licensed monoclonal antibody (mAb) was muromonob-CD3, an mAb directed at CD3, in 1986.[14] Since then, the use of targeted biological therapies has expanded. For the treatment of the urticarial diseases, mAb, recombinant antagonists, and donor immunoglobulin have played important roles (**Fig. 1**). The most important biologic used in CU is omalizumab.

ANTI–IMMUNOGLOBULIN E MONOCLONAL ANTIBODIES
Overview and Mechanism of Action of Omalizumab

Although the exact cause of CU is not entirely known, many patients have autoantibodies to the alpha chain of the high-affinity receptor FcεR1 or to immunoglobulin (Ig)E, with the former more specific for CU.[15] Omalizumab is a recombinant humanized monoclonal anti-IgE antibody that binds to the C epsilon 3 domain of IgE (the site of high-affinity IgE receptor binding) and inhibits it from binding to the cell receptor.[16,17] Omalizumab binds to the free IgE, leading to a reduction of free IgE levels and, consequently, decreased expression of FcεRI receptors on mast cells, basophils, and dendritic cells.[18–22] This effect may reduce mast cell numbers, as mast cell proliferation and survival are theorized to depend on IgE-FcεRI–dependent pathways.[23] It is also

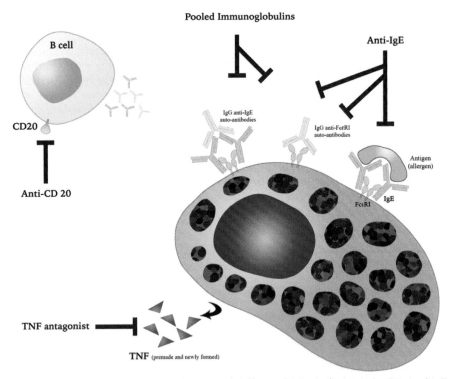

Fig. 1. The proposed mechanism of action of different biological agents in CU. Anti-IgE blocks the effect of IgE at the level of IgE-antigen cross-linking, IgE–anti-IgE IgG cross-linking, and anti-FcεRI IgG (downregulation). Anti-CD20 blocks CD20 B cells. TNF antagonist blocks both premade and newly synthesized TNF.

postulated that IgE-FcεRI interaction on mast cells lowers the threshold for degranulation to various stimuli, which would be attenuated with IgE depletion.[21] Recently, it has been proposed that omalizumab inhibits mast cell activation by dissociation of preattached IgE from its receptor.[24] This might explain the quick response (sometimes within 48 hours) seen in some patients after omalizumab initiation, which in this time frame would not be expected to decrease FcεRI expression. Omalizumab was originally approved for the treatment of moderate to severe persistent allergic asthma, but it quickly found a niche with CU.[12]

Omalizumab Proof-of-Concept and Phase 2 Studies

Early on, omalizumab was theorized to benefit patients with CU with autoantibodies.[25] Theory transitioned to practice with a few case reports showing the benefit of omalizumab.[26–32] Case reports were soon followed by small pilot studies. Kaplan and colleagues[33] performed one of the first of these studies in 2008. Twelve patients with autoimmune CU, identified by a basophil histamine release assay and/or autologous skin test, and a serum IgE of ≤700 IU/mL were randomized to 4 weeks of placebo followed by 16 weeks of omalizumab, with a dosing schedule based on the asthma package insert. All subjects had a significant reduction in hives and itch while on the omalizumab when compared with baseline and 7 of the 12 experienced complete remission.[33] A subsequent open-label prospective observational study assessed the efficacy of omalizumab on subjects with nonautoimmune CU refractory to antihistamines. The investigators included 9 subjects who were deemed nonautoimmune by negative basophil histamine release. All subjects experienced improvement in hive and itch with omalizumab with 2 experiencing complete remission.[34] A larger double-blind, placebo-controlled trial, performed by Maurer and colleagues,[35] enrolled 49 subjects with antihistamine-refractory CU with a positive IgE against thyroperoxidase. Subjects were randomized to either 24 weeks of omalizumab or placebo and dosed based on the asthma package insert using both body weight and serum IgE. The investigators showed efficacy of omalizumab in CU by a reduction in weekly urticaria activity score (UAS7) from baseline of 17.8, of a possible 42, compared with a reduction of 7.1 with placebo. Additionally, 19 subjects (70.4%) developed complete remission of wheals with the omalizumab compared with one with placebo.[35]

Saini and colleagues[36] performed a double-blind, placebo-controlled, dose-ranging study, using 90 subjects with antihistamine-refractory CU. The subjects were randomized to either 4 weeks of 75 mg, 300 mg, or 600 mg omalizumab or placebo then were followed for an additional 12 weeks after stopping omalizumab. The 300-mg and 600-mg omalizumab groups showed improvement over placebo in both itch and hive, whereas no difference from placebo was seen with the 75-mg omalizumab arm. Additionally, 36.0% of subjects in the 300-mg omalizumab group and 28.6% of subjects in the 600-mg omalizumab group achieved complete remission, whereas 0% in the placebo group achieved complete remission.[36] These data supported the doses chosen for the pivotal phase 3 studies described as follows.

Omalizumab Phase 3 Trials

The first large-scale phase 3 trial results published were from the ASTERIA II trial. This double-blinded study randomized 323 subjects with CU refractory to standard dosing of H1 antihistamines. Subjects were randomized to receive 3 subcutaneous injections of 75 mg, 150 mg, or 300 mg omalizumab or placebo, at 4-week intervals, followed by a 16-week observation period. The primary endpoint was change from baseline to week 12 in the weekly itch-severity score (of a possible 21). Weekly itch scores improved for subjects receiving 150 mg omalizumab and 300 mg omalizumab by (−8.1 ± 6.4, P = .001) and (−9.8 ± 6.0, P<.001), respectively, but not in those assigned to either placebo or 75 mg omalizumab. In addition to the weekly itch score, the UAS7 improved significantly for both the 150 mg and 300 mg omalizumab groups when compared with baseline, whereas the placebo and 75-mg omalizumab groups did not change significantly. During the follow-up observation period, the mean UAS7 for all groups increased to reach the placebo group and none returned to baseline. Complete response was seen in 44% of 300-mg omalizumab group, 22% of the 150-mg group, 16% of the 75-mg omalizumab group, and 5% of the placebo group.[37]

GLACIAL was the next large phase III double-blinded placebo-controlled trial results published. This study, unlike prior studies, required subjects with CU to fail H_1 antihistamines plus an H_2-blocker and/or leukotriene antagonist. A total of 336 subjects were randomized in a 3:1 fashion to 24 weeks of either 6 monthly injections of 300 mg omalizumab or 6 monthly injections of placebo, respectively. Throughout the study, subjects were required to maintain stable doses of the prerandomization combination of H_1-antihistamines plus H_2 antihistamines and/or leukotriene antagonists. The primary outcome for the study was safety of omalizumab when compared with placebo. The adverse events for omalizumab and placebo groups during the study were similar (65.1% and 63.9%, respectively). Headaches and upper respiratory infections were the most common adverse events noted in the omalizumab group. Serious adverse events were reported in 6.9% of subjects during the study period, 7.1% in the omalizumab group and 6.0% in the placebo group, but none were deemed related to omalizumab. To assess efficacy, investigators evaluated the weekly itch-severity score and proportion of subjects with complete response by week 12 compared with baseline. The overall improvement in weekly itch score at week 12 compared with baseline, from 0 to 21 with higher indicating more severe symptoms, was −8.6 for the omalizumab arm and −4.0 for the placebo arm. As with prior studies, once the active medication was discontinued, the weekly itch score increased to equal the placebo scores, neither of which returned to baseline. In terms of complete responders, at week 12, 33.7% of subjects in the omalizumab group were free of urticaria symptoms, whereas only 4.8% of subjects in the placebo group were free of urticaria.[38] These benefits were sustained to week 24.

ASTERIA I was also a large-scale phase 3 clinical trial. This trial was a 40-week double-blind, placebo-controlled trial that was designed similarly to ASTERIA II, but the treatment phase of the trial was twice the length. A total of 319 subjects were randomized to 24 weeks of subcutaneous omalizumab at 75 mg, 150 mg, or 300 mg or placebo every 4 weeks. The primary endpoint for the study was weekly itch-severity score at 12 weeks compared with baseline. Interestingly, subjects in all groups noticed improvements in weekly itch score as early as week 1, most significantly in the omalizumab 300-mg group. All active groups of the trial showed improvement over baseline with a reduction in weekly itchy score of 6.46 with omalizumab 75 mg, 6.66 with omalizumab 150 mg, and 9.40 with omalizumab 300 mg. Placebo showed a reduction by 3.63 over baseline at week 12. The reduction in weekly itch score was generally maintained while on the active treatment, and on cessation of medication, the weekly itch scores rose to that of the placebo. Nearly 36% of subjects in the 300-mg omalizumab group experienced complete remission of symptoms versus approximately 9% in the placebo group.[39]

The X-ACT trial was double-blind, placebo-controlled trial evaluating the efficacy of omalizumab on antihistamine-refractory CU with angioedema. A total of 91 subjects were randomized to either 28 weeks of 300 mg omalizumab or placebo given as subcutaneous injections every 4 weeks. The primary outcome for this trial was the treatment symptom score at 28 weeks when compared with baseline by using the Chronic Urticaria Quality of Life (CU-Q$_2$oL). Subjects assigned to the 300-mg omalizumab group had a threefold improvement in angioedema burden in days per week versus placebo, 0.3 and 1.1, respectively.[40]

These large clinical trials have shown that omalizumab is a safe and efficacious therapy for CU, often improving subjects' symptoms before week 4 with benefit persisting while on treatment.[41,42] In addition, the data suggest omalizumab is effective for CU despite background therapy.[39] Finally, omalizumab retreatment of patients with a recurrence of CU has been shown to be safe and effective (**Table 1**).[43]

Omalizumab and Urticaria Guidelines

The result of these large clinical trials is that the US and European guidelines for management of CU have added omalizumab as a recommended therapy following a stepwise approach. The American Academy of Allergy, Asthma, and Immunology and American College of Allergy, Asthma, and Immunology have recommended that omalizumab be added to therapy as a fourth step after failure of antihistamines at both standard and high doses, failure of the addition of an H$_2$-antihistamine and leukotriene antagonist, and failure of a high-potency antihistamine like doxepin or hydroxyzine (**Table 2**).[12] The European guidelines are slightly different, with the addition of omalizumab as the third step after the failure of nonsedating antihistamine at standard and high doses.[44]

Effectiveness of Omalizumab in Other Forms of Urticaria

Beyond CU, omalizumab has been used in urticarial vasculitis[30] and a variety of physical forms of urticaria. These include cholinergic urticaria,[29,45] cold-induced urticaria,[26,46,47] delayed pressure urticaria,[46,48,49] heat urticaria,[46,50,51] aquagenic urticaria,[52] dermatographism,[46] and solar urticaria.[31,46,53] Recently, omalizumab was investigated for the treatment of solar urticaria in a phase II trial evaluating the efficacy of 300 mg omalizumab given as 3 subcutaneous injections at 4-week intervals on 10 subjects. To qualify, subjects were required to have the appearance of wheals within 15 minutes following sun exposure and resolving in less than 2 hours in the shade. The primary outcome was the proportion of subjects who required a 10-fold increase in intensity of ultraviolet dose above baseline to trigger minimal urticarial dose at week 12 when compared with baseline. By the end of the 12 weeks, 2 of the 10 patients reached the primary endpoint. Although the trial did not reach statistical significance, it shows that omalizumab may have a role in the physical urticarias and more studies are needed.[54]

Omalizumab in Pregnancy

Although omalizumab is a safe and efficacious medication for most patients with CU, the safety in pregnancy is not completely elucidated. To assess this unique patient population, a registry was established for patients with asthma. By November 2012, 191 pregnant patients had been exposed to omalizumab during the first trimester. The outcomes of 169 of the pregnancies were known and the overall proportions of congenital anomalies, prematurity, and low birth weight were consistent with the general asthma population, without an apparent increased prevalence of major anomalies.[55] It is unlikely that this safety profile would differ in patients with CU.

Advances in Anti–immunoglobulin E Monoclonal Antibodies

New biologics targeting IgE are currently in development and will likely play an important role alongside omalizumab in the treatment of CU.[56] A second-generation anti-IgE

Table 1
Summary of the major trials involving omalizumab

Trial Name/ First Author	Number of Subjects	Study Design	Key Inclusion	Key Exclusion	Change in Weekly Itch Score
XCUISITE/Maurer et al[35]	49	RDBPC trial 3-wk screening period + 24-wk active phase Two arms: • Placebo • Omalizumab • Dosing per asthma guidelines	Uncontrolled CU ≥6 wk despite standard dosed H₁-antihistamines • Weight 20–150 kg • Serum IgE from 30–700 IU/mL • Serum IgE–anti-TPO antibody level of ≥5.0 IU/mL at most 3 mo before randomization • UAS7 ≥10	• Acute urticaria • Elevated serum IgE for reasons other than allergy or urticaria • Medications 4 wk before enrollment ○ Systemic corticosteroids ○ Methotrexate ○ Cyclosporine ○ Other immunosuppressants	Mean (SD) ΔWIS baseline to week 12 • Placebo ○ −3.57 (4.95) • 150 mg omalizumab ○ −5.9 (4.43) • 300 mg omalizumab ○ −11.19 (6.46) • 600 mg omalizumab ○ −11.19 (6.46)
MYSTIQUE/Saini et al[36]	90	RDBPC trial 1-wk screening period + 1-wk run-in + 4-wk active phase + 12-wk follow-up Four arms: • Placebo • 75 mg omalizumab • 300 mg omalizumab • 600 mg omalizumab	Uncontrolled CU ≥6 wk despite standard dosed H₁-antihistamines • UAS7 ≥12	• A cause for the CU • Routine administration of the following medications 3 mo before enrollment: ○ Dapsone ○ Hydroxychloroquine ○ Sulfasalazine ○ Methotrexate ○ Cyclophosphamide ○ Intravenous immunoglobulin ○ Plasmapheresis ○ Other monoclonal antibodies • Routine administration of the following medication 6 wk before enrollment: ○ Doxepin • Routine administration of the following medication 4 wk before enrollment: ○ Cyclosporine • Use of systemic steroids was not allowed during the trial	Mean (SD) ΔWIS baseline to wk 12 • Placebo ○ −3.5 (4.23) • 75 mg omalizumab ○ −4.5 (5.84) • 300 mg omalizumab ○ −9.2 (5.98) • 600 mg omalizumab ○ −6.5 (5.63)

ASTERIA II/Maurer et al[37]	323	RDBPC trial
		2-wk screening period + 12-wk active phase + 16-wk follow-up period
		Four arms:
		• Placebo
		• 75 mg omalizumab
		• 150 mg omalizumab
		• 300 mg omalizumab
			Uncontrolled CU for 6 mo despite use of standard dosed H_1-antihistamines
			• UAS7 ≥16
			• WIS ≥8
				• A cause for the CU
				• The use of any of the following within 7 d before the screening visit.
				  ◦ H_2 - antihistamine
				  ◦ Leukotriene antagonist
				• Routine administration of the following medications 30 d before enrollment:
				  ◦ Systemic glucocorticoids
				  ◦ Hydroxychloroquine
				  ◦ Methotrexate
				  ◦ Cyclosporine
				  ◦ Cyclophosphamide
				  ◦ Intravenous immuno globulin
					Mean (SD) ΔWIS baseline to wk 12
					• Placebo
					  ◦ −5.1 (5.6)
					• 75 mg omalizumab
					  ◦ −5.9 (6.5)
					• 150 mg omalizumab
					  ◦ −8.1 (6.4)
					• 300 mg omalizumab
					  ◦ −9.8 (6.0)

GLACIAL/Kaplan et al[38]	336	RDBPC trial
		2-wk screening period + 24-wk active phase + 16-wk follow-up period
		Two arms:
		• Placebo
		• 300 mg omalizumab
			CU despite up to 4 times approved dose of H_1-antihistamines AND H_2- antihistamines or Leukotriene antagonist, or all 3 in combination
			• UAS7 ≥16
			• WIS ≥8
				• A cause for the CU
				• Routine administration of the following medications 30 d before enrollment:
				  ◦ Systemic glucocorticoids
				  ◦ Hydroxychloroquine
				  ◦ Methotrexate
				  ◦ Cyclosporine
				  ◦ Cyclophosphamide
				  ◦ Intravenous immunoglobulin
					Mean (95% confidence interval [CI]) ΔWIS baseline to wk 12
					• Placebo
					  ◦ −4.0 (95% CI −5.3 to −2.7)
					• 300 mg omalizumab
					  ◦ −8.6 (95% CI −9.3 to −7.8)

(continued on next page)

Table 1
(continued)

Trial Name/ First Author	Number of Subjects	Study Design	Key Inclusion	Key Exclusion	Change in Weekly Itch Score

ASTERIA I/Saini et al[39]	319	RDBPC trial
		2-wk screening +
		24-wk treatment +
		16-wk follow-up
		Four arms:
		• Placebo
		• 75 mg omalizumab
		• 150 mg omalizumab
		• 300 mg omalizumab
			Uncontrolled CU for 8 mo despite use of H_1-antihistamines
			• UAS7 $\geq$16
			• WIS $\geq$8
				• A cause for the CU
				• The use of any of the following within 7 d before the screening visit:
				  ○ H_2-antihistamine
				  ○ Leukotriene antagonist
				• Routine administration of the following medications 30 d before enrollment:
				  ○ Systemic glucocorticoids
				  ○ Hydroxychloroquine
				  ○ Methotrexate
				  ○ Cyclosporine
				  ○ Cyclophosphamide
				  ○ Intravenous immunoglobulin
					Mean (SD) ΔWIS baseline to wk 12
					• Placebo
					  ○ −3.63 (5.22)
					• 75 mg omalizumab
					  ○ −6.46 (6.14)
					• 150 mg omalizumab
					  ○ −6.66 (6.28)
					• 300 mg of omalizumab
					  ○ −9.40 (5.73)

| X-ACT/Staubach et al[40] | 91 | RDBPC trial
2-wk screening +
24-wk treatment +
8-wk follow-up
Two arms:
• Placebo
• 300 mg omalizumab | Uncontrolled CU for 6 mo with 4 occurrences of angioedema despite use of 2–4 times standard dosed H₁-antihistamines
• UAS7 ≥14
• CU-Q₂oL ≥30 | • Hereditary angioedema
• Acquired angioedema
• The use of any of the following within 7 d before the screening visit:
 ○ H₂-antihistamine
 ○ Leukotriene antagonist
• Routine administration of the following medications 30 d before enrollment:
 ○ Systemic glucocorticoids
 ○ Hydroxychloroquine
 ○ Methotrexate
 ○ Cyclosporine
 ○ Cyclophosphamide
 ○ Intravenous immunoglobulin | Mean (SD)
ΔWIS baseline to wk 12
• Placebo
 ○ −2.2 (8.99)
• 300 mg omalizumab
 ○ −8.3 (7.58) |

Abbreviations: CU, chronic urticaria; CU-Q₂oL, this questionnaire measures various aspects of quality of life (scale: 0–100; high scores indicate low quality of life) that are specific to chronic urticaria; RDBPC, randomized, double-blind, placebo-controlled; UAS7, weekly urticaria score and is a scoring system based on a daily diary that uses numeric severity ratings from 0 to 3 (0, none; 3, intense) for the number of wheals over 24 hours and the intensity of pruritus, therefore the total daily score (sum of the wheal and pruritus scores) could assume any value between 0 and 6 and is summed over a week with a maximum of 42 and minimum of 0; WIS, weekly itch score: a weekly itch scale based on a 7-day sum of a daily itch diary with symptoms on a scale ranging from 0 to 3, a weekly score of 0 to 21, with higher scores indicating more severe itching; ΔUAS7, the change in UAS7; ΔWIS, change in WIS score.

Table 2
Omalizumab indications, dosage, adverse effects, contraindications, and limitations as per the package insert approved by the US Food and Drug Administration

Agent	Indications	Dosage for CU	Side Effects	Contraindications	Limitations
Omalizumab (Xolair)	• Moderate to severe persistent asthma in patients 6 y of age and older with a positive skin test or in vitro reactivity to a perennial aeroallergen and symptoms that are inadequately controlled with inhaled corticosteroids. • Chronic idiopathic urticaria in adults and adolescents 12 y of age and older who remain symptomatic despite H1 antihistamine treatment.	150 mg or 300 mg every 4 wk (dosing independent of IgE level and body weight).	The most common adverse reactions ($\geq$2% Xolair-treated patients with urticaria and more frequent than in placebo) included the following: nausea, nasopharyngitis, sinusitis, upper respiratory tract infection, viral upper respiratory tract infection, arthralgia, headache, and cough and injection site reaction. Black box warning for anaphylaxis.	Absolute: Severe hypersensitivity (previous immediate-type hypersensitivity or anaphylaxis) Relative: Malignancy, severe cardiovascular disease, active parasitic infection.	• Cost. • Insurance approval. • Reconstitution and preparation. • Lack of approval for other urticarial forms.

Abbreviation: CU, chronic urticaria.

mAb, QGE031 (ligelizumab), is now being studied for both asthma and CU. This humanized monoclonal $IgG1_K$ anti-IgE has a 40-fold to 50-fold higher affinity to the Cε3 domain of IgE compared with omalizumab.[57] An initial trial evaluating its efficacy versus placebo and omalizumab for 20 weeks in patients with CU is ongoing (clinicaltrial.gov NCT02477332). Another study is evaluating the long-term safety of QGE031 for 52 weeks in CU (clinicaltrial.gov NCT02649218).

Quilizumab is another novel humanized IgG1 mAb recently studied in asthma and CU. Unlike anti-IgE antibodies, quilizumab targets the M1-prime segment of membrane-expressed IgE on IgE-switched and memory B cells, leading to their depletion. Recently, the results of the first filed trial of quilizumab in asthma were published.[58] Total IgE was reduced by approximately 40%. However, there were no significant improvements in asthma outcomes versus placebo. The results of a recently completed trial assessing the efficacy and safety of quilizumab in CU resistant to antihistamine therapy for 20 weeks have yet to be published (clinicaltrial.gov NCT01987947).

ANTI-CD20 MONOCLONAL ANTIBODY

Rituximab is a chimeric mAb that is a cytolytic antibody that targets CD20 on B cells. CD20 is known to be expressed at high levels on B cells, including immature, mature, and memory cells. By targeting the B cells that produce IgE and functional IgG autoantibodies against FcεRI, rituximab is postulated to be an effective way to treat refractory CU. Currently, rituximab is indicated for the treatment of multiple hematology malignancies and patients with certain autoimmune diseases.[59] Given the medication's efficacy with autoimmune diseases and its potential mechanism of action, the drug has been tried on multiple occasions for patients with severe refractory CU.

One of the first reports of the use of rituximab in CU occurred in a patient with both urticaria and angioedema along with pressure-induced urticaria of the hands and feet. The patient had failed conventional and nonconventional therapy, including immunomodulators and intravenous immunoglobulin (IVIG) and became corticosteroid dependent. The patient received 4 weekly infusions of rituximab 375 mg/m². Unfortunately, the patient did not respond to the rituximab.[60] Since then, a few additional case reports have shown promising results. One case was of a 12-year-old boy with refractory CU with angioedema and immunodeficiency who was treated with 4 infusions of rituximab 375 mg/m². A week after the first infusion, the patient become asymptomatic, and the effect lasted for 12 months. Although symptoms did eventually recur, they were easily managed with antihistamines.[61] Another investigator examined the effects of rituximab in a patient with CU and an urticarial lesion biopsy showing IgG autoantibodies against FcεRI on immunohistochemistry. Four weekly intravenous infusions of rituximab at 375 mg/m² were administered. Six weeks after the last infusion, the patient achieved complete remission with evidence of basophil activation suppression.[62] More recently, a patient with refractory steroid-dependent CU received 2 infusions of rituximab 1 g 2 weeks apart, and had temporary remission lasting for 10 months. Antihistamines were restarted, and the patient was advised to undergo another cycle of rituximab.[63]

Rituximab also has been tried in urticarial vasculitis. The first was in a patient with hypocomplementemic urticarial vasculitis (HUVS) who had failed mycophenolate mofetil and corticosteroids. Rituximab was given at 375 mg/m² in 4 weekly doses. Complete remission of the HUVS was attained following rituximab therapy.[64] Another case of steroid-dependent refractory urticarial vasculitis in a patient with ulcerative colitis was treated with rituximab. Two cycles of 1 g rituximab resulted in remission for

8 months before relapse.[65] Despite these few case reports of the possible therapeutic efficacy of rituximab in CU and urticarial vasculitis, more studies are needed to support its utility in those who fail standard of care.

INTRAVENOUS IMMUNOGLOBULIN

IVIG is a purified preparation of human polyclonal IgG prepared by pooling plasma obtained from thousands of healthy donors. IVIG is used as a replacement therapy for patients with primary and secondary immunodeficiency, as well as an immunomodulator in autoimmune and inflammatory disorders at higher doses.[66] IVIG appears to work as an immune suppressant by a variety of immune effector responses, including Fc receptor blockade, enhanced autoantibody clearance, immune regulation of B-cell and T-cell functions, amelioration of regulatory T cells, and upregulation the FcγRIIB expression.[67] These immunomodulatory mechanisms are likely responsible for its effectiveness in autoimmune and inflammatory disorders, such as Kawasaki syndrome, myositis disorders, idiopathic thrombocytopenia, and myasthenia gravis.[68–71] As indicated earlier, autoantibodies to the α chain of high-affinity FcεR1 or IgE are present in approximately 30% to 40% of cases of CU, with some proposing that the vast majority of CU may have an autoimmune mechanism.[72,73] The detection of these autoantibodies can be determined by histamine-releasing activity, autologous serum skin test (ASST), Western blot, and enzyme-linked immunosorbent assay.[73,74] However, the role of these autoantibodies in CU pathogenesis has not been definitively elucidated.[72] Due to the potential role that autoimmunity plays in CU, IVIG has been evaluated by multiple therapeutic trials in CU.

Plasmapheresis was the gate that backed IVIG use as a potential therapeutic option in CU with autoantibodies based on ASST. In 1992, Grattan and colleagues[75] used plasmapheresis in subjects with CU deemed as autoimmune by ASST. Fifty percent of the patients responded at least somewhat and 25% had complete remission. This finding prompted other investigators to try IVIG in patients with CU with a positive ASST. In their trial, O'Donnell and colleagues[76] treated 10 patients with severe autoimmune CU with 0.4 g/kg per day IVIG for 5 days. They reported that 9 of 10 responded and 3 had complete remission at 3-year follow-up. Later reports examined the effectiveness of low-dose IVIG in patients with refractory CU. One report evaluated 2 doses of 0.2 g/kg given at 4 weeks apart with reporting an improvement in the urticarial score.[77] Another report evaluated the effect of monthly infusion of 0.15 g/kg IVIG on patients with CU. Subjects underwent infusions from 6 to 51 months; 90% of subjects who received IVIG had a response with 65% having complete remission.[78] More recently, a retrospective study to assess the efficacy and safety of high-dose IVIG (2 g/kg over 2 days every 4–6 weeks) on patients with refractory CU was conducted.[13] Of 6 patients, 5 had complete remission and 1 had a partial response after 1 to 11 cycles of IVIG and 11 to 24 months of follow-up. The mechanisms of IVIG therapeutic benefits in CU are not yet clear, with some reports questioning its efficacy as a true immunomodulatory therapy rather than as an anti-idiotype therapy.[79,80]

Perhaps resulting from the positive response seen in CU, IVIG has been tried in a variety of physical urticarias. Dawn and colleagues[81] examined the use of high-dose IVIG of 2 g/kg over 2 to 3 days on 8 patients with delayed pressure urticaria. Five of 8 patients responded to the infusions with 3 achieving complete remission. IVIG also has been evaluated for its utility in solar urticaria. IVIG is theorized to help by targeting the Fc receptors of specific IgE of a hypothetical provocative chromophore allergen activated by ultraviolet light in patients with solar urticaria.[82] A few case series have showed IVIG to be an efficacious therapeutic modality in solar urticaria.[83–85] In a retrospective analysis of 7 patients with solar urticaria treated with IVIG (1.4–2.5 g/kg over 2–5 days), 5 of 7 patients had complete remission.[82] Recently, Aubin and colleagues[86] evaluated IVIG in a phase II open-label trial involving 9 patients with refractory solar urticaria. The patients were treated with 2 g/kg over 2 days and then evaluated at 4 and 12 weeks. Of the 9 patients, only 2 showed remission at 4 and 12 weeks.

Although IVIG has been used for many years for a variety of conditions, it has been associated with a few adverse effects. The main adverse effects of IVIG include flushing, myalgia, headache, fever, chills, nausea or vomiting, chest tightness, wheezing, changes in blood pressure, tachycardia, and aseptic meningitis.[13,86] Before initiation of this therapy, the risks and benefits must be assessed. Available data based on several case series and small uncontrolled studies imply that IVIG may work in specific groups of patients with CU with autoantibodies. However, the lack of strong evidence, need for intravenous access, prolonged infusions, costs, and adverse effects make this medication a less favorable option.

TUMOR NECROSIS FACTOR-α ANTAGONISTS

Three biological tumor necrosis factor-α (TNF-α) antagonists, etanercept (TNF receptor fusion protein against TNF-α), infliximab (mAb against TNF-α), and adalimumab (mAb against TNF-α), have been tried as therapeutic options in different types of urticarial disorders. The rationale for using TNF-α antagonists is that there are data to suggest that CU is associated with an upregulation of TNF-α expression and increased TNF-α production in CU epidermis compared with control, thereby playing a significant role in the pathogenesis of CU.[87,88] One particular patient with a history of refractory delayed pressure urticaria and psoriasis underwent treatment with etanercept 25 mg twice per week for 8 weeks. Symptoms remitted in this patient and antihistamines were no longer needed after 5 days of starting etanercept. Later, etanercept was increased to 50 mg and then switched to infliximab because of uncontrolled psoriasis. The therapeutic effect of TNF-α antagonists on the urticaria persisted throughout the treatment period.[89] Etanercept was also reported to be effective in a patient with cold urticaria and psoriasis.[90] There was a subsequent case series of 6 patients with either CU or urticarial vasculitis who were treated successfully with TNF-α antagonists. Interestingly, all patients experienced a dramatic improvement that lasted for several years in some cases.[91] In another observational study, a total of 20 patients with urticarial disorders (CU with and without autoantibodies, physical urticaria, and neutrophilic urticaria) received either etanercept or adalimumab for periods ranging from 2 to 39 months. Sixty percent had complete to near complete remission, whereas 15% had partial response and the rest were unresponsive.[92]

Although these results are promising, the data are limited to case reports and small uncontrolled studies. Additionally, in many cases, physical urticarias and urticarial vasculitis was the primary problem. Therefore, it is difficult to recommend these agents until better, well-controlled trials are done with close comparison to safer alternatives, including other biologics such as omalizumab.

INTERLEUKIN-1 ANTAGONISTS

CU is a heterogeneous disease with distinct inflammatory processes key in some forms, but not others. IL-1 inhibitors (eg, canakinumab, anakinra) have been studied in distinct subsets of urticarial disease (urticarial vasculitis) with some effectiveness, and this has led to their evaluation in CU.[93] Canakinumab is a human anti–IL-1β mAb that is currently under investigation for CU (clinicaltrial.gov NCT01635127).

SUMMARY

Years of clinical experience and multiple studies suggest that certain biological agents may have an important role in the treatment of antihistamine-refractory CU. Of these biological agents evaluated, omalizumab is the first approved by the FDA for the treatment of CU. The medication is both safe and efficacious for patients with antihistamine-refractory CU. Due to the success of omalizumab, other anti-IgE agents are currently under investigation for use in antihistamine-refractory CU. Although less well studied, other biologics like rituximab, IVIG and TNF-α antagonists may be considered as an alternative option to resistant cases. The success of these biological agents are a benefit to the patients and may help with the understanding of the pathogenesis of CU and further classification of CU endotypes.

REFERENCES

1. Powell RJ, Leech SC, Till S, et al. BSACI guideline for the management of chronic urticaria and angioedema. Clin Exp Allergy 2015;45(3):547–65.
2. Balp MM, Vietri J, Tian H, et al. The impact of chronic urticaria from the patient's perspective: a survey in five European countries. Patient 2015;8(6):551–8.
3. Vietri J, Turner SJ, Tian H, et al. Effect of chronic urticaria on US patients: analysis of the National Health and Wellness Survey. Ann Allergy Asthma Immunol 2015; 115(4):306–11.
4. Staubach P, Dechene M, Metz M, et al. High prevalence of mental disorders and emotional distress in patients with chronic spontaneous urticaria. Acta Derm Venereol 2011;91(5):557–61.
5. O'Donnell BF. Urticaria: impact on quality of life and economic cost. Immunol Allergy Clin North Am 2014;34(1):89–104.
6. O'Donnell BF, Lawlor F, Simpson J, et al. The impact of chronic urticaria on the quality of life. Br J Dermatol 1997;136(2):197–201.
7. Broder MS, Raimundo K, Antonova E, et al. Resource use and costs in an insured population of patients with chronic idiopathic/spontaneous urticaria. Am J Clin Dermatol 2015;16(4):313–21.
8. Zuberbier T, Balke M, Worm M, et al. Epidemiology of urticaria: a representative cross-sectional population survey. Clin Exp Dermatol 2010;35(8):869–73.
9. Sanchez-Borges M, Asero R, Ansotegui IJ, et al. Diagnosis and treatment of urticaria and angioedema: a worldwide perspective. World Allergy Organ J 2012; 5(11):125–47.
10. Gaig P, Olona M, Munoz Lejarazu D, et al. Epidemiology of urticaria in Spain. J Investig Allergol Clin Immunol 2004;14(3):214–20.
11. Lapi F, Cassano N, Pegoraro V, et al. Epidemiology of chronic spontaneous urticaria: results from a nationwide, population-based study in Italy. Br J Dermatol 2016;174(5):996–1004.
12. Bernstein JA, Lang DM, Khan DA, et al. The diagnosis and management of acute and chronic urticaria: 2014 update. J Allergy Clin Immunol 2014;133(5):1270–7.
13. Mitzel-Kaoukhov H, Staubach P, Muller-Brenne T. Effect of high-dose intravenous immunoglobulin treatment in therapy-resistant chronic spontaneous urticaria. Ann Allergy Asthma Immunol 2010;104(3):253–8.
14. Liu JK. The history of monoclonal antibody development—progress, remaining challenges and future innovations. Ann Med Surg (Lond) 2014;3(4):113–6.
15. Kaplan AP. Therapy of chronic urticaria: a simple, modern approach. Ann Allergy Asthma Immunol 2014;112(5):419–25.

16. Normansell R, Walker S, Milan SJ, et al. Omalizumab for asthma in adults and children. Cochrane Database Syst Rev 2014;(1):CD003559.
17. Easthope S, Jarvis B. Omalizumab. Drugs 2001;61(2):253–60 [discussion: 61].
18. Niimi N, Francis DM, Kermani F, et al. Dermal mast cell activation by autoantibodies against the high affinity IgE receptor in chronic urticaria. J Invest Dermatol 1996;106(5):1001–6.
19. Holgate ST, Djukanovic R, Casale T, et al. Anti-immunoglobulin E treatment with omalizumab in allergic diseases: an update on anti-inflammatory activity and clinical efficacy. Clin Exp Allergy 2005;35(4):408–16.
20. Saavedra MC, Sur S. Down regulation of the high-affinity IgE receptor associated with successful treatment of chronic idiopathic urticaria with omalizumab. Clin Mol Allergy 2011;9(1):2.
21. Chang TW, Chen C, Lin CJ, et al. The potential pharmacologic mechanisms of omalizumab in patients with chronic spontaneous urticaria. J Allergy Clin Immunol 2015;135(2):337–42.
22. Beck LA, Marcotte GV, MacGlashan D, et al. Omalizumab-induced reductions in mast cell Fc epsilon RI expression and function. J Allergy Clin Immunol 2004; 114(3):527–30.
23. Kawakami T, Galli SJ. Regulation of mast-cell and basophil function and survival by IgE. Nat Rev Immunol 2002;2(10):773–86.
24. Serrano-Candelas E, Martinez-Aranguren R, Valero A, et al. Comparable actions of omalizumab on mast cells and basophils. Clin Exp Allergy 2016;46(1):92–102.
25. Mankad VS, Burks AW. Omalizumab: other indications and unanswered questions. Clin Rev Allergy Immunol 2005;29(1):17–30.
26. Boyce JA. Successful treatment of cold-induced urticaria/anaphylaxis with anti-IgE. J Allergy Clin Immunol 2006;117(6):1415–8.
27. Spector SL, Tan RA. Effect of omalizumab on patients with chronic urticaria. Ann Allergy Asthma Immunol 2007;99(2):190–3.
28. Sands MF, Blume JW, Schwartz SA. Successful treatment of 3 patients with recurrent idiopathic angioedema with omalizumab. J Allergy Clin Immunol 2007; 120(4):979–81.
29. Metz M, Bergmann P, Zuberbier T, et al. Successful treatment of cholinergic urticaria with anti-immunoglobulin E therapy. Allergy 2008;63(2):247–9.
30. Dreyfus DH. Observations on the mechanism of omalizumab as a steroid-sparing agent in autoimmune or chronic idiopathic urticaria and angioedema. Ann Allergy Asthma Immunol 2008;100(6):624–5.
31. Guzelbey O, Ardelean E, Magerl M, et al. Successful treatment of solar urticaria with anti-immunoglobulin E therapy. Allergy 2008;63(11):1563–5.
32. Callejas-Rubio JL, Sanchez-Cano D, Lara MA, et al. Omalizumab as a therapeutic alternative for chronic urticaria. Ann Allergy Asthma Immunol 2008;101(5):556.
33. Kaplan AP, Joseph K, Maykut RJ, et al. Treatment of chronic autoimmune urticaria with omalizumab. J Allergy Clin Immunol 2008;122(3):569–73.
34. Ferrer M, Gamboa P, Sanz ML, et al. Omalizumab is effective in nonautoimmune urticaria. J Allergy Clin Immunol 2011;127(5):1300–2.
35. Maurer M, Altrichter S, Bieber T, et al. Efficacy and safety of omalizumab in patients with chronic urticaria who exhibit IgE against thyroperoxidase. J Allergy Clin Immunol 2011;128(1):202–9.e5.
36. Saini S, Rosen KE, Hsieh HJ, et al. A randomized, placebo-controlled, dose-ranging study of single-dose omalizumab in patients with H1-antihistamine-refractory chronic idiopathic urticaria. J Allergy Clin Immunol 2011;128(3): 567–73.e1.

37. Maurer M, Rosen K, Hsieh HJ, et al. Omalizumab for the treatment of chronic idiopathic or spontaneous urticaria. N Engl J Med 2013;368(10):924–35.

38. Kaplan A, Ledford D, Ashby M, et al. Omalizumab in patients with symptomatic chronic idiopathic/spontaneous urticaria despite standard combination therapy. J Allergy Clin Immunol 2013;132(1):101–9.

39. Saini SS, Bindslev-Jensen C, Maurer M, et al. Efficacy and safety of omalizumab in patients with chronic idiopathic/spontaneous urticaria who remain symptomatic on H antihistamines: a randomized, placebo-controlled study. J Invest Dermatol 2015;135(3):925.

40. Staubach P, Metz M, Chapman-Rothe N, et al. Effect of omalizumab on angioedema in H -antihistamine resistant chronic spontaneous urticaria patients: results from X-ACT, a randomised controlled trial. Allergy 2016;71(8):1135–44.

41. Kaplan A, Ferrer M, Bernstein JA, et al. Timing and duration of omalizumab response in patients with chronic idiopathic/spontaneous urticaria. J Allergy Clin Immunol 2016;137(2):474–81.

42. Casale TB, Bernstein JA, Maurer M, et al. Similar efficacy with omalizumab in chronic idiopathic/spontaneous urticaria despite different background therapy. J Allergy Clin Immunol Pract 2015;3(5):743–50.e1.

43. Metz M, Ohanyan T, Church MK, et al. Retreatment with omalizumab results in rapid remission in chronic spontaneous and inducible urticaria. JAMA Dermatol 2014;150(3):288–90.

44. Zuberbier T, Aberer W, Asero R, et al. The EAACI/GA(2) LEN/EDF/WAO guideline for the definition, classification, diagnosis, and management of urticaria: the 2013 revision and update. Allergy 2014;69(7):868–87.

45. Otto HF, Calabria CW. A case of severe refractory chronic urticaria: a novel method for evaluation and treatment. Allergy Asthma Proc 2009;30(3):333–7.

46. Metz M, Altrichter S, Ardelean E, et al. Anti-immunoglobulin E treatment of patients with recalcitrant physical urticaria. Int Arch Allergy Immunol 2011;154(2):177–80.

47. Brodska P, Schmid-Grendelmeier P. Treatment of severe cold contact urticaria with omalizumab: case reports. Case Rep Dermatol 2012;4(3):275–80.

48. Bindslev-Jensen C, Skov PS. Efficacy of omalizumab in delayed pressure urticaria: a case report. Allergy 2010;65(1):138–9.

49. Rodriguez-Rodriguez M, Antolin-Amerigo D, Barbarroja-Escudero J, et al. Successful treatment of severe delayed pressure angio-oedema with omalizumab. Allergol Immunopathol (Madr) 2014;42(1):78–80.

50. Bullerkotte U, Wieczorek D, Kapp A, et al. Effective treatment of refractory severe heat urticaria with omalizumab. Allergy 2010;65(7):931–2.

51. Carballada F, Nunez R, Martin-Lazaro J, et al. Omalizumab treatment in 2 cases of refractory heat urticaria. J Investig Allergol Clin Immunol 2013;23(7):519–21.

52. Rorie A, Gierer S. A case of aquagenic urticaria successfully treated with omalizumab. J Allergy Clin Immunol Pract 2016;4(3):547–8.

53. Waibel KH, Reese DA, Hamilton RG, et al. Partial improvement of solar urticaria after omalizumab. J Allergy Clin Immunol 2010;125(2):490–1.

54. Aubin F, Avenel-Audran M, Jeanmougin M, et al. Omalizumab in patients with severe and refractory solar urticaria: a phase II multicentric study. J Am Acad Dermatol 2016;74(3):574–5.

55. Namazy J, Cabana MD, Scheuerle AE, et al. The Xolair Pregnancy Registry (EXPECT): the safety of omalizumab use during pregnancy. J Allergy Clin Immunol 2015;135(2):407–12.

56. Liour SS, Tom A, Chan YH, et al. Treating IgE-mediated diseases via targeting IgE-expressing B cells using an anti-CepsilonmX antibody. Pediatr Allergy Immunol 2016;27(5):446–51.
57. Arm JP, Bottoli I, Skerjanec A, et al. Pharmacokinetics, pharmacodynamics and safety of QGE031 (ligelizumab), a novel high-affinity anti-IgE antibody, in atopic subjects. Clin Exp Allergy 2014;44(11):1371–85.
58. Harris JM, Maciuca R, Bradley MS, et al. A randomized trial of the efficacy and safety of quilizumab in adults with inadequately controlled allergic asthma. Respir Res 2016;17:29.
59. Townsend MJ, Monroe JG, Chan AC. B-cell targeted therapies in human autoimmune diseases: an updated perspective. Immunol Rev 2010;237(1):264–83.
60. Mallipeddi R, Grattan CE. Lack of response of severe steroid-dependent chronic urticaria to rituximab. Clin Exp Dermatol 2007;32(3):333–4.
61. Arkwright PD. Anti-CD20 or anti-IgE therapy for severe chronic autoimmune urticaria. J Allergy Clin Immunol 2009;123(2):510–1 [author reply: 511].
62. Chakravarty SD, Yee AF, Paget SA. Rituximab successfully treats refractory chronic autoimmune urticaria caused by IgE receptor autoantibodies. J Allergy Clin Immunol 2011;128(6):1354–5.
63. Steinweg SA, Gaspari AA. Rituximab for the treatment of recalcitrant chronic autoimmune urticaria. J Drugs Dermatol 2015;14(12):1387.
64. Saigal K, Valencia IC, Cohen J, et al. Hypocomplementemic urticarial vasculitis with angioedema, a rare presentation of systemic lupus erythematosus: rapid response to rituximab. J Am Acad Dermatol 2003;49(5 Suppl):S283–5.
65. Swaminath A, Magro CM, Dwyer E. Refractory urticarial vasculitis as a complication of ulcerative colitis successfully treated with rituximab. J Clin Rheumatol 2011;17(5):281–3.
66. Negi VS, Elluru S, Siberil S, et al. Intravenous immunoglobulin: an update on the clinical use and mechanisms of action. J Clin Immunol 2007;27(3):233–45.
67. Ballow M. The IgG molecule as a biological immune response modifier: mechanisms of action of intravenous immune serum globulin in autoimmune and inflammatory disorders. J Allergy Clin Immunol 2011;127(2):315–23 [quiz: 24–5].
68. Leung DY, Schlievert PM, Meissner HC. The immunopathogenesis and management of Kawasaki syndrome. Arthritis Rheum 1998;41(9):1538–47.
69. Dalakas MC. Polymyositis, dermatomyositis and inclusion-body myositis. N Engl J Med 1991;325(21):1487–98.
70. Neunert C, Lim W, Crowther M, et al. The American Society of Hematology 2011 evidence-based practice guideline for immune thrombocytopenia. Blood 2011;117(16):4190–207.
71. Donofrio PD, Berger A, Brannagan TH 3rd, et al. Consensus statement: the use of intravenous immunoglobulin in the treatment of neuromuscular conditions report of the AANEM ad hoc committee. Muscle Nerve 2009;40(5):890–900.
72. Saini SS. Chronic spontaneous urticaria: etiology and pathogenesis. Immunol Allergy Clin North Am 2014;34(1):33–52.
73. Kaplan AP, Greaves M. Pathogenesis of chronic urticaria. Clin Exp Allergy 2009;39(6):777–87.
74. Hide M, Francis DM, Grattan CE, et al. Autoantibodies against the high-affinity IgE receptor as a cause of histamine release in chronic urticaria. N Engl J Med 1993;328(22):1599–604.
75. Grattan CE, Francis DM, Slater NG, et al. Plasmapheresis for severe, unremitting, chronic urticaria. Lancet 1992;339(8801):1078–80.

76. O'Donnell BF, Barr RM, Black AK, et al. Intravenous immunoglobulin in autoimmune chronic urticaria. Br J Dermatol 1998;138(1):101–6.
77. Kroiss M, Vogt T, Landthaler M, et al. The effectiveness of low-dose intravenous immunoglobulin in chronic urticaria. Acta Derm Venereol 2000;80(3):225.
78. Pereira C, Tavares B, Carrapatoso I, et al. Low-dose intravenous gammaglobulin in the treatment of severe autoimmune urticaria. Eur Ann Allergy Clin Immunol 2007;39(7):237–42.
79. Asero R. Are IVIG for chronic unremitting urticaria effective? Allergy 2000;55(11):1099–101.
80. Hrabak T, Calabria CW. Multiple treatment cycles of high-dose intravenous immunoglobulin for chronic spontaneous urticaria. Ann Allergy Asthma Immunol 2010;105(3):245 [author reply: 245–6].
81. Dawn G, Urcelay M, Ah-Weng A, et al. Effect of high-dose intravenous immunoglobulin in delayed pressure urticaria. Br J Dermatol 2003;149(4):836–40.
82. Adamski H, Bedane C, Bonnevalle A, et al. Solar urticaria treated with intravenous immunoglobulins. J Am Acad Dermatol 2011;65(2):336–40.
83. Correia I, Silva J, Filipe P, et al. Solar urticaria treated successfully with intravenous high-dose immunoglobulin: a case report. Photodermatol Photoimmunol Photomed 2008;24(6):330–1.
84. Hughes R, Cusack C, Murphy GM, et al. Solar urticaria successfully treated with intravenous immunoglobulin. Clin Exp Dermatol 2009;34(8):e660–2.
85. Maksimovic L, Fremont G, Jeanmougin M, et al. Solar urticaria successfully treated with intravenous immunoglobulins. Dermatology 2009;218(3):252–4.
86. Aubin F, Porcher R, Jeanmougin M, et al. Severe and refractory solar urticaria treated with intravenous immunoglobulins: a phase II multicenter study. J Am Acad Dermatol 2014;71(5):948–53.e1.
87. Hermes B, Prochazka AK, Haas N, et al. Upregulation of TNF-alpha and IL-3 expression in lesional and uninvolved skin in different types of urticaria. J Allergy Clin Immunol 1999;103(2 Pt 1):307–14.
88. Piconi S, Trabattoni D, Iemoli E, et al. Immune profiles of patients with chronic idiopathic urticaria. Int Arch Allergy Immunol 2002;128(1):59–66.
89. Magerl M, Philipp S, Manasterski M, et al. Successful treatment of delayed pressure urticaria with anti-TNF-alpha. J Allergy Clin Immunol 2007;119(3):752–4.
90. Gualdi G, Monari P, Rossi MT, et al. Successful treatment of systemic cold contact urticaria with etanercept in a patient with psoriasis. Br J Dermatol 2012;166(6):1373–4.
91. Wilson LH, Eliason MJ, Leiferman KM, et al. Treatment of refractory chronic urticaria with tumor necrosis factor-alfa inhibitors. J Am Acad Dermatol 2011;64(6):1221–2.
92. Sand FL, Thomsen SF. TNF-alpha inhibitors for chronic urticaria: experience in 20 patients. J Allergy (Cairo) 2013;2013:130905.
93. Krause K, Mahamed A, Weller K, et al. Efficacy and safety of canakinumab in urticarial vasculitis: an open-label study. J Allergy Clin Immunol 2013;132(3):751–4.e5.

Itch in Atopic Dermatitis

Makiko Kido-Nakahara, MD, PhD[a],*, Masutaka Furue, MD, PhD[a],
Dugarmaa Ulzii, MD[a], Takeshi Nakahara, MD, PhD[b]

KEYWORDS

- Atopic dermatitis • Pruritus • Pruritogen • Hypersensitivity of pruritus • New therapy

KEY POINTS

- Numerous types of pruritogens produced with inflammation are involved in atopic itch.
- Hypersensitivity of pruritus occurs in the peripheral and central nervous system in atopic dermatitis.
- The appropriate conventional treatment of atopic dermatitis should generally lead to the reduction of itch sensation.
- The future development of new therapeutic drugs for itch is expected.

INTRODUCTION

Atopic dermatitis (AD) is characterized by chronic cutaneous inflammation and dry skin. Intense pruritus is the major and most burdensome symptom of AD.[1] Itch is a specialized perception of skin leading to a scratching behavior that is often recognized in terrestrial mammals. Itch-induced scratching appears to exacerbate skin lesions in clinical and experimental settings.[2] Itching and scratching cause sleep loss and severely disturb the quality of life of affected individuals.

PERIPHERAL ITCH
Transmission of Peripheral Itch

Itch is mediated by unmyelinated C-fiber afferents and thinly myelinated Aδ fiber afferents, and these cutaneous sensory nerve fibers originate from cell bodies in the dorsal root ganglion (DRG).[3–5] The free nerve endings exist in the epidermis and papillary dermis and around skin appendages and are activated by endogenous and exogenous pruritogens through relevant receptors. The electrical signals generated by sensory nerve stimulation are sent to the central nervous system. Itch-specific peripheral neurons are positive for Mas-related G-protein-coupled receptor (GPCR) A3

Conflict of Interest: The authors declare no conflicts of interest.
[a] Department of Dermatology, Kyushu University, Maidashi 3-1-1, Higashiku, Fukuoka 812-8582, Japan; [b] Division of Skin Surface Sensing, Kyushu University, Maidashi 3-1-1, Higashiku, Fukuoka 812-8582, Japan
* Corresponding author.
E-mail address: macky@dermatol.med.kyushu-u.ac.jp

(MargprA3) because genetic ablation of MargprA3 expression neurons attenuated scratch responses to chloroquine and histamine without affecting pain behaviors.[6] At least 2 types of pruriceptive neurons have been identified in the murine DRG, namely, histamine-dependent and histamine-independent afferents, with substantial overlap (**Fig. 1**).[7] These 2 systems, although closely related, seem to exist separately and independently from one another. The histaminergic itch pathway uses transient receptor potential channel V1 (TRPV1) as a direct downstream target. In nonhistaminergic itch, some pruritogens (eg, chloroquine) use TRPA1, whereas others are not necessary for TRPV1 or TRPA1.[8] Antipruritic effects of antihistamines are limited in the treatment of AD. This clinical observation implies that atopic itch is induced mainly by the nonhistaminergic pathway.

Hyperinnervation in Epidermis

Another intriguing finding is that epidermal hyperinnervation or elongation of sensory nerve fibers in AD may cause itchy and sensitive skin.[5] The hyperinnervation is mainly caused by an imbalance between nerve elongation factors (eg, nerve growth factor [NGF]) and nerve repulsion factors (eg, semaphorin 3A [Sema3A]) that are produced by keratinocytes. In fact, the expression of NGF is upregulated in the lesional skin of patients with AD with reciprocal downregulation of Sema3A expression. The imbalance of NGF/Sema3A in the epidermis is normalized in the improved skin lesions treated with ultraviolet radiation.

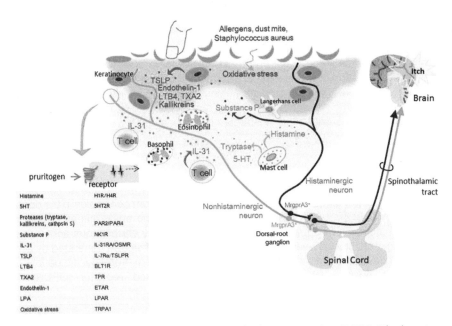

Fig. 1. Pathophysiology of pruritus in AD. 5HT, 5 hydroxytryptamine; 5HT2R, 5 hydroxytryptamine 2 receptor; BLT1R, leukotriene B4 receptor 1; ETAR, endothelin receptor type A; H1R, histamine H1 receptor; H4R, histamine H4 receptor; IL-31RA, interleukin-31 receptor A; IL-7Rα, interleukin-7 receptor alpha; LPA, lysophosphatidic acid; LPAR, lysophosphatidic acid receptor; LTB4, leukotriene B4; Mrgpr, Mas-related G-protein-coupled receptor; NK1R, neurokinin 1 receptor; OSMR, oncostatin M receptor; TPR, thromboxane prostanoid receptor; TRPA1, transient receptor potential cation channel subfamily A member 1; TSLPR, thymic stromal lymphopoietin receptor; TXA2, thromboxane A2.

Thermal Hyperalgesia by Artemin

Patients with AD suffer from abnormal itching that develops from a normally nonitchy stimulus, such as thermal stimuli,[9] which is called alloknesis. Murota and Katayama[9] first proposed a possible involvement of artemin, a member of the glial cell–derived neurotrophic factor-related family, in warmth-provoked itching. Artemin accumulates in the upper dermis of lesional skin in patients with AD. Intradermal injection of artemin in mice increased the number of peripheral nerve fibers, and mice exhibited grooming of the entire body beyond the injection site, suggesting that artemin may cause thermal alloknesis.

PRURITOGENS

Various pruritogens and their specific receptors evoke itch signaling in the skin of patients with AD, as shown in **Fig. 1**.[3,4] Many endogenous and exogenous pruritogens produced from inflammation are involved, including histamine, tryptase, substance P, interleukin-31 (IL-31), thymic stromal lymphopoietin (TSLP), leukotrienes, and endothelin-1 (ET-1). Some of the important mediators in atopic itch are mentioned in the following sections.

Histamine

Histamine is one of the major itch mediators that has been well evaluated. Direct application of histamine to human skin induces itching and a subsequent axonal reflective vasodilation or flare. Of the 4 histamine receptors, 2 (H1R and H4R) have been identified as potential pruritoception.[10] Cowden and colleagues[11] showed that inhibitors of H4R have dual effects on pruritus and Th2-mediated inflammation, resulting in significant reductions in both. Furthermore, simultaneous blockade of H1R and H4R was more effective in reducing itch and inflammation than either alone. However, it is not clear how much of a role histamine plays as the cause of itching in AD.

Protease and Protease-Activated Receptors and Their Agonists

Protease-activated receptors (PARs) belong to the GPCR family, which is activated by various endogenous and exogenous proteases, including tryptase, dust mites, and *Staphylococcus aureus*, resulting in the induction of nonhistaminergic itch.[12] Tryptase and its receptor, PAR2, were significantly increased in the lesional skin of patients with AD. Both PAR2 and PAR4 are expressed on several cell types, including keratinocytes and pruriceptive neurons in the DRGs. The expression of PAR2 on keratinocytes was upregulated in both the lesional and nonlesional skin of patients with AD, with the highest level of expression occurring in the lesional skin.[13] Application of intralesional PAR2 agonist induced a prolonged itch sensation in patients with AD.[14]

Interleukin-31

IL-31, which is produced primarily by Th2 cells, has attracted attention as a pruritogen in patients with AD. Its receptor, which is a complex composed of IL-31 receptor A and oncostatin M receptor, is expressed on peripheral nerve fibers, DRGs, and keratinocytes.[10] Serum IL-31 levels are elevated in patients with AD, and activated leukocytes in patients with AD expressed higher levels of IL-31 compared with healthy individuals. Administration of anti–IL-31 receptor antibodies in AD model mice significantly suppressed scratching behavior and skin inflammation. In a recent study, IL-31 did not induce an immediate itch response but did induce late-onset pruritus in humans, indicating that IL-31 exerts its pruritic action via an indirect mechanism that may involve keratinocytes.[15] Nevertheless, the first clinical trial of an anti–IL-31 receptor A antibody against AD was successful in significantly reducing atopic itch.[16]

Thymic Stromal Lymphopoietin

TSLP is an epithelial-derived cytokine that is implicated in the pathogenesis of AD,[17] and TSLP serum levels are a sensitive biomarker for evaluating the severity of AD.[18] TSLP acts as a potent stimulator of Th2 cytokines, including IL-4, IL-5, and IL-13, with subsequent immunoglobulin E production. Wilson and colleagues[19] discovered that TSLP acts as a primary pruritogen, whereby calcium-dependent TSLP release by keratinocytes directly activates primary afferent sensory neurons through the TSLP receptors expressed on them and stimulates immune cells to induce itch and promote inflammatory responses in the skin.

Endothelin-1

ET-1 is a 21-amino-acid peptide that is expressed by a variety of cell types, including immune cells, endothelial cells, neurons, and glial cells of the central and peripheral nervous system.[20] ET-1 is a potent vasoconstrictor that can also evoke pain and itch sensations in rodents and humans. Using iontophoresis, we demonstrated that ET-1 causes a potent, partially histamine-independent pruritus in humans.[20] Immunohistochemically, ET-1 was upregulated in the lesional epidermis of mice and humans with AD[21]; therefore, ET-1 could play a role in atopic itch.

CENTRAL ITCH
Transmission of Itch from the Spinal Cord to the Brain

Mice deficient in gastrin-releasing peptide receptor (GRPR) or natriuretic polypeptide B (NPPB) exhibited a profound scratching deficit to all of the pruritogenic stimuli, whereas pain behaviors were unaffected.[22,23] Intrathecal injection of NPPB elicited scratching behaviors. Natriuretic peptide receptor A (NPRA) is a specific receptor for NPPB. Mice in which NPRA was ablated exhibited impaired scratching responses to histamine and NPPB but not gastrin-releasing peptide (GRP), indicating that GRP is downstream of NPPB.[24] NPPB and glutamate released from primary pruriceptive afferent neurons seem to mediate the itch signal to NPRA + interneurons, which were positive for GRP (see **Fig. 1**). Then, GRP activates tertiary neurons that express the GRP receptor. The transmitter used by GRPR-expressing neurons has not yet been identified, but substance P is believed to play a role in the activation of the last step transmitter in the spinal cord and the stimulation of spinothalamic projection interneurons (**Fig. 2**).[23]

Inhibitory Nerve for Itch

Painful nociceptive neural input inhibits pruritus. It is now hypothesized that noxious stimuli through glutamatergic afferents of nociceptors activate Bhlhb5-expressing inhibitory interneurons in the spinal cord.[25] Bhlhb5 inhibitory interneurons mediate their signal by releasing dynorphin, which activates kappa-opioid receptors.[26] Glycine and γ-aminobutyric acid (GABA) also are inhibitory transmitters in the spinal cord, but the exact source and cellular substrates of these molecules remain unknown.[27] Inhibitory interneurons may be positively regulated by the descending pathway from the brain (see **Fig. 2**).

Involvement of Astrocytes in Atopic Itch

In addition to the sensory nerve itself, astrocytes, which are a subtype of glial cells, also are involved in chronic itch in AD. Shiratori-Hayashi and colleagues[28] first discovered that signal transducer and activator of transcription 3 (STAT3) is activated in astrocytes of the dorsal horn of spinal segments, corresponding to the itchy area of a

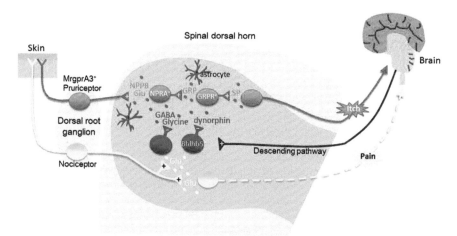

Fig. 2. Schematic of an itch circuit in the dorsal horn of the spinal cord. Glu, glutamate; GRP, gastrin-releasing peptide; Mrgpr, Mas-related G-protein-coupled receptor; SP, substance P. (*Adapted from* Mishra SK, Hoon MA. Transmission of pruriceptive signals. Handb Exp Pharmacol 2015;226:156; with permission.)

lesion, and conditional disruption of astrocytic STAT3 alleviates chronic itch. Moreover, lipocalin-2, which is produced by astrocytes in a STAT3-dependent manner, acts as a critical amplifier of itching, thereby providing a previously unrecognized target for treating chronic itch.

Itch and the Brain

Recent neuroimaging studies have focused on brain imaging of histamine-induced itch in humans. In healthy humans, acute histamine-induced itch captivates the anterior cingulate cortex, insular and primary somatosensory cortex, premotor and supplementary motor areas, prefrontal cortex, and thalamus. In contrast, patients with AD exhibit excitation of broader areas of the brain compared with healthy subjects. These results suggest the strong itch intensity or central sensitization of itch in patients with AD.[29]

Mochizuki and colleagues[30] reported that brain regions known as the reward system, such as the midbrain and striatum, react strongly when itchy lesions are scratched compared with nonitchy lesions. Reward system activation may cause excessive and repetitive scratching behavior, resulting in the scratching-mediated exacerbation of AD.

The central sensitization of pruritus occurred in patients with AD, and the perception and interpretation of pruritus are very much influenced by cognitive and affective process.[31] Therefore, the drugs that modulate the central nervous system might work well for reducing pruritus. Several psychotropic drugs were reported to show an antipruritic effect in patients with AD, including antidepressants (tricyclic antidepressants and selective serotonin reuptake inhibitors) and structural analogs of the inhibitory neurotransmitter, GABA, but the precise mechanisms of antipruritic effect of these drugs are still unclear.[32,33]

ASSESSMENT OF CHRONIC ITCH

As a subjective symptom, pruritus is difficult to measure precisely in an objective manner. Evaluating the intensity of pruritus is necessary to determine disease severity and treatment effectiveness. There are several established subjective evaluation methods to quantitatively estimate the intensity of pruritus, including the visual analog scale (VAS), which is one of the most widely distributed methods used to estimate the intensity of pruritus. Recently, the following 10-point maximum VAS categories were proposed: 0 = no pruritus, >0 to <3 points = mild pruritus, $\geq$3 to <7 points = moderate pruritus, $\geq$7 to <9 points = severe pruritus, and $\geq$9 points = very severe pruritus in Caucasian and Japanese populations.[34,35]

ANTIPRURITIC EFFECTS OF CONVENTIONAL TREATMENTS

First-line treatments for AD include the application of emollients for dry skin, topical steroids, and tacrolimus for skin inflammation and oral antihistamines for pruritus, followed by second-line adjunct therapies, such as systemic cyclosporine, short-term oral steroids, and ultraviolet radiation.[1] A questionnaire survey revealed that 81 (82.7%) of 98 patients with AD reported that the emollient was effective or somewhat effective in treating their pruritus,[36] consistent with the fact that emollients prevent dry skin–inducible intraepidermal hyperinnervation.[37] Topical application of 0.1% fluocinonide for 2 weeks significantly reduced pruritus by 3.5 $\pm$ 3.4 points according to a 10-point maximum VAS.[38] Topical tacrolimus significantly inhibited pruritus flare-ups compared with emollient application in maintenance therapy.[39] Fexofenadine, a nonsedating H1R antagonist, significantly decreased the severity of pruritus compared with placebo in patients with AD.[40] This improvement was observed after 1 day of treatment and was maintained throughout the treatment period. However, nonsedating antihistamines have not been helpful as antipruritic agents in clinical experience. Cyclosporine significantly inhibited pruritus in patients with AD in association with decreased IL-31 serum levels.[41] Although numerous reports confirmed the itch-relieving effects of conventional treatments, the satisfaction of most patients with moderate and severe pruritus remains very limited.

RECENT REPORTS ON NEW ANTIPRURITIC DRUGS
Dupilumab

Dupilumab is a fully human monoclonal antibody directed against the alpha subunit of the IL-4 receptors that block signaling from both IL-4 and IL-13. In phase I and II studies of adults with moderate to severe AD, administration of dupilumab resulted in rapid, significant improvements in inflammation and pruritus and decreases in Th2-related biomarkers with no dose-limiting toxicity.[42,43] These findings indicate that dupilumab is a promising new anti-inflammatory and antipruritic treatment for AD.

Histamine H4 Receptor Antagonist

Based on its antipruritic and anti-inflammatory effects in experimental animals, a clinical trial of the oral administration of H4R antagonist (JNJ-39758979) was conducted in Japanese patients with AD.[44] Although the H4R antagonist significantly reduced daytime and nighttime pruritus in patients with AD, the clinical study was terminated because of the severe adverse effects of agranulocytosis. In addition to its neural expression,[4] H4R may be a prerequisite molecule for bone marrow maturation.

Phosphodiesterase 4 Inhibitors

Phosphodiesterase 4 inhibitors exhibit immunosuppressive activity and inhibit IL-4 in the mononuclear cells of patients with AD. In clinical trials to date, several topical phosphodiesterase 4 inhibitors, including E6005[45] and OPA-15406,[46] demonstrated effectiveness against inflammation and pruritus in AD. Phosphodiesterase 4 inhibitors constitute one set of drugs expected to be administered for atopic itch.

Anti–Interleukin-31 Receptor Antibody

Anti–IL-31 receptor antibody may be another promising agent with which to inhibit atopic itch. In humans and mice, IL-31 is predominantly produced by T-helper 2 cells, and its cutaneous injection induces pruritus.[47] A recent clinical trial in Japan revealed that a single injection of anti–IL-31 receptor antibody (CIM331) significantly inhibited pruritus in patients with moderate to severe AD for up to 4 weeks after administration.[16]

The Kappa-Opioid Agonist Nalfurafine

The kappa-opioid agonist nalfurafine was approved in Japan for the treatment of itching in patients with chronic kidney and liver diseases.[48] In an experimental model, a recent study showed that nalfurafine reduced scratching evoked by histamine and chloroquine. Nalfurafine also abolished spontaneous scratching induced by dry skin.[49] These data suggest that nalfurafine may be a potential antipruritic drug for AD.

Topical Tropomyosin Receptor Kinase A Inhibitor

Tropomyosin receptor kinase A (TrkA) is a high-affinity NGF receptor. Nerve fibers positive for TrkA were detected in human epidermis, dermis, and DRG.[50] A recent clinical trial by Roblin and colleagues[50] demonstrated that the topical TrkA kinase inhibitor CT327 is an effective treatment for pruritus due to psoriasis. Further trials of topical CT327 are expected for atopic itch.

SUMMARY

Many types of pruritogens derived from local and systemic inflammation are likely to be involved in atopic itch. Hypersensitivity and chronicity of pruritus in the peripheral and central nervous systems may be other important concerns. Biological treatments using anti–IL-31 receptor A or anti–IL-4 receptor alpha appear to be beneficial in reducing atopic itch. Combined therapy with conventional topical remedies and these biologics may provide new treatment strategies for atopic patients. Recent genome-wide association studies and immunochip analysis indicated at least 19 significant susceptibility loci for AD.[51] These loci contain chromosomes 5q31 and 17q21.32, where IL-4/IL-3 and the NGF receptor are, respectively, located. Considering the favorable antipruritic effects of new remedies targeting IL-4/IL-3 and the NGF receptor, gene products of other susceptible loci may be possible targets in the development of new agents that control atopic itch.

REFERENCES

1. Saeki H, Furue M, Furukawa F, et al. Guidelines for management of atopic dermatitis. J Dermatol 2009;36:563–77.
2. Takeuchi S, Yasukawa F, Furue M, et al. Collared mice: a model to assess the effects of scratching. J Dermatol Sci 2010;57:44–50.
3. Furue M, Kadono T. New therapies for controlling atopic itch. J Dermatol 2015;42: 847–50.
4. Akiyama T, Carstens E. Neural processing of itch. Neuroscience 2013;250: 697–714.
5. Tominaga M, Takamori K. Itch and nerve fibers with special reference to atopic dermatitis: therapeutic implications. J Dermatol 2014;41:205–12.

6. Han L, Ma C, Liu Q, et al. A subpopulation of nociceptors specifically linked to itch. Nat Neurosci 2012;16:174–82.
7. Schmelz M. Neurophysiology and itch pathways. Handb Exp Pharmacol 2015; 226:39–55.
8. Imamachi N, Park GH, Lee H, et al. TRPV1-expressing primary afferents generate behavioral responses to pruritogens via multiple mechanisms. Proc Natl Acad Sci U S A 2009;106:11330–5.
9. Murota H, Katayama I. Evolving understanding on the aetiology of thermally provoked itch. Eur J Pain 2016;20:47–50.
10. Mollanazar NK, Smith PK, Yosipovitch G, et al. Mediators of chronic pruritus in atopic dermatitis: getting the itch out? Clin Rev Allergy Immunol 2015. http://dx.doi.org/10.1007/s12016-015-8488-5.
11. Cowden JM, Zhang M, Dunford PJ, et al. The histamine H4 receptor mediates inflammation and pruritus in Th2-dependent dermal inflammation. J Invest Dermatol 2010;130:1023–33.
12. Kempkes C, Buddenkotte J, Cevikbas F, et al. Role of PAR-2 in neuroimmune communication and itch. In: Carstens E, Akiyama T, editors. Itch: mechanisms and treatment. Boca Raton (FL): CRC Press/Taylor & Francis; 2014 [Chapter 11. Frontiers in Neuroscience]. p. 193–212.
13. Buddenkotte J, Stroh C, Engels IH, et al. Agonists of proteinase-activated receptor-2 stimulate upregulation of intercellular cell adhesion molecule-1 in primary human keratinocytes via activation of NF-kappa B. J Invest Dermatol 2005;124:38–45.
14. Steinhoff M, Neisius U, Ikoma A, et al. Proteinase-activated receptor-2 mediates itch: a novel pathway for pruritus in human skin. J Neurosci 2003;23:6176–80.
15. Hawro T, Saluja R, Weller K, et al. Interleukin-31 does not induce immediate itch in atopic dermatitis patients and healthy controls after skin challenge. Allergy 2014; 69:113–7.
16. Nemoto O, Furue M, Nakagawa H, et al. The first trial of CIM331, a humanized antihuman interleukin-31 receptor A antibody, in healthy volunteers and patients with atopic dermatitis to evaluate safety, tolerability and pharmacokinetics of a single dose in a randomized, double-blind, placebo-controlled study. Br J Dermatol 2016;174:296–304.
17. Leyva-Castillo JM, Hener P, Michea P, et al. Skin thymic stromal lymphopoietin initiates Th2 responses through an orchestrated immune cascade. Nat Commun 2013;4:2847.
18. Kataoka Y. Thymus and activation-regulated chemokine as a clinical biomarker in atopic dermatitis. J Dermatol 2014;41:221–9.
19. Wilson SR, Thé L, Batia LM. The epithelial cell-derived atopic dermatitis cytokine TSLP activates neurons to induce itch. Cell 2013;155:285–95.
20. Kido-Nakahara M, Buddenkotte J, Kempkes C, et al. Neural peptidase endothelin-converting enzyme 1 regulates endothelin 1-induced pruritus. J Clin Invest 2014;124:2683–95.
21. Aktar MK, Kido-Nakahara M, Furue M, et al. Mutual upregulation of endothelin-1 and IL-25 in atopic dermatitis. Allergy 2015;70:846–54.
22. Sun YG, Zhao ZQ, Meng XL, et al. Cellular basis of itch sensation. Science 2009; 325:1531–4.
23. Mishra SK, Hoon MA. Transmission of pruriceptive signals. Handb Exp Pharmacol 2015;226:151–62.
24. Mishra SK, Hoon MA. The cells and circuitry for itch responses in mice. Science 2013;340:968–71.

25. Ross SE, Mardinly AR, McCord AE, et al. Loss of inhibitory interneurons in the dorsal spinal cord and elevated itch in Bhlhb5 mutant mice. Neuron 2010;65: 886–98.
26. Kardon AP, Polgár E, Hachisuka J, et al. Dynorphin acts as a neuromodulator to inhibit itch in the dorsal horn of the spinal cord. Neuron 2014;82:573–86.
27. Akiyama T, Iodi Carstens M, Carstens E. Transmitters and pathways mediating in-hibition of spinal itch-signaling neurons by scratching and other counterstimuli. PLoS One 2011;6:e22665.
28. Shiratori-Hayashi M, Koga K, Tozaki-Saitoh H, et al. STAT3-dependent reactive astrogliosis in the spinal dorsal horn underlies chronic itch. Nat Med 2015;21: 927–31.
29. Ishiuji Y, Coghill RC, Patel TS, et al. Distinct patterns of brain activity evoked by histamine-induced itch reveal an association with itch intensity and disease severity in atopic dermatitis. Br J Dermatol 2009;161:1072–80.
30. Mochizuki H, Kakigi R. Itch and brain. J Dermatol 2015;42:761–7.
31. Mochizuki H, Papoiu ADP, Yosipovitch G. Brain processing of itch and scratching. In: Carstens E, Akiyama T, editors. Itch: mechanisms and treatment. Boca Raton (FL): CRC Press; 2014. p. 391–407.
32. Leslie TA, Greaves MW, Yosipovitch G. Current topical and systemic therapies for itch. Handb Exp Pharmacol 2015;226:337–56.
33. Kim K. Neuroimmunological mechanism of pruritus in atopic dermatitis focused on the role of serotonin. Biomol Ther 2012;20(6):506–12.
34. Reich A, Heisig M, Phan NQ, et al. Visual analogue scale: evaluation of the instru-ment for the assessment of pruritus. Acta Derm Venereol 2012;92:497–501.
35. Kido-Nakahara M, Katoh N, Saeki H, et al. Comparative cut-off value setting of pruritus intensity in visual analogue scale and verbal rating scale. Acta Derm Ve-nereol 2015;95:345–6.
36. Kawakami T, Soma Y. Questionnaire survey of the efficacy of emollients for adult patients with atopic dermatitis. J Dermatol 2011;38:531–5.
37. Kamo A, Tominaga M, Negi O, et al. Topical application of emollients prevents dry skin-inducible intraepidermal nerve growth in acetone-treated mice. J Dermatol Sci 2011;62:64–6.
38. Woods MT, Brown PA, Baig-Lewis SF, et al. Effects of a novel formulation of fluo-cinonide 0.1% cream on skin barrier function in atopic dermatitis. J Drugs Derma-tol 2011;10:171–6.
39. Takeuchi S, Saeki H, Tokunaga S, et al. A randomized, open-label, multicenter trial of topical tacrolimus for the treatment of pruritis in patients with atopic derma-titis. Ann Dermatol 2012;24:144–50.
40. Kawashima M, Tango T, Noguchi T, et al. Addition of fexofenadine to a topical corticosteroid reduces the pruritus associated with atopic dermatitis in a 1-week randomized, multicentre, double-blind, placebo-controlled, parallel-group study. Br J Dermatol 2003;148:1212–21.
41. Otsuka A, Tanioka M, Nakagawa Y, et al. Effects of cyclosporine on pruritus and serum IL-31 levels in patients with atopic dermatitis. Eur J Dermatol 2011;21: 816–7.
42. Thaçi D, Simpson EL, Beck LA, et al. Efficacy and safety of dupilumab in adults with moderate-to-severe atopic dermatitis inadequately controlled by topical treatments: a randomised, placebo-controlled, dose-ranging phase 2b trial. Lan-cet 2016;387:40–52.
43. Hamilton JD, Ungar B, Guttman-Yassky E. Drug evaluation review: dupilumab in atopic dermatitis. Immunotherapy 2015;7:1043–58.

44. Murata Y, Song M, Kikuchi H, et al. Phase 2a, randomized, double-blind, placebo-controlled, multicenter, parallel-group study of a H4R-antagonist (JNJ-39758979) in Japanese adults with moderate atopic dermatitis. J Dermatol 2015;42:129–39.

45. Furue M, Kitahara Y, Akama H, et al. Safety and efficacy of topical E6005, a phosphodiesterase 4 inhibitor, in Japanese adult patients with atopic dermatitis: results of a randomized, vehicle-controlled, multicenter clinical trial. J Dermatol 2014;41:577–85.

46. Hanifin JM, Ellis CN, Frieden IJ, et al. OPA-15406, a novel, topical, nonsteroidal, selective phosphodiesterase-4 (PDE4) inhibitor, in the treatment of adult and adolescent patients with mild to moderate atopic dermatitis (AD): a phase-II randomized, double-blind, placebo-controlled study. J Am Acad Dermatol 2016; 75(2):297–305.

47. Cevikbas F, Wang X, Akiyama T, et al. A sensory neuron-expressed IL-31 receptor mediates T helper cell-dependent itch: involvement of TRPV1 and TRPA1. J Allergy Clin Immunol 2014;133:448–60.

48. Kumagai H, Ebata T, Takamori K, et al. Effect of a novel kappa-receptor agonist, nalfurafine hydrochloride, on severe itch in 337 haemodialysis patients: a Phase III, randomized, double-blind, placebo-controlled study. Nephrol Dial Transplant 2010;25:1251–7.

49. Akiyama T, Carstens MI, Piecha D, et al. Nalfurafine suppresses pruritogen- and touch-evoked scratching behavior in models of acute and chronic itch in mice. Acta Derm Venereol 2015;95:147–50.

50. Roblin D, Yosipovitch G, Boyce B, et al. Topical TrkA kinase inhibitor CT327 is an effective, novel therapy for the treatment of pruritus due to psoriasis: results from experimental studies, and efficacy and safety of CT327 in a phase 2b clinical trial in patients with psoriasis. Acta Derm Venereol 2015;95:542–8.

51. Tamari M, Hirota T. Genome-wide association studies of atopic dermatitis. J Dermatol 2014;41:213–20.

Wet Wrap Therapy in Moderate to Severe Atopic Dermatitis

Noreen Heer Nicol, PhD, RN, FNP[a],*, Mark Boguniewicz, MD[b]

KEYWORDS

- Wet wrap therapy • Wet wrap • Wet dressings • Occlusive dressings
- Occlusion therapy • Atopic dermatitis • Atopic eczema

KEY POINTS

- Atopic dermatitis (AD) remains a complex, common, chronic, and relapsing skin disorder, and a global public health problem.
- National and international guidelines address AD care in a stepwise fashion. Wet wrap therapy (WWT) is a therapeutic intervention for moderate to severe AD.
- WWT plays an important role as an acute therapeutic intervention for management of moderate to severe AD used with undiluted topical corticosteroids of appropriate potency.
- WWT should not be used for mild AD or as a chronic or maintenance therapy.
- WWT should be considered as a treatment option ahead of the systemic therapies for patients failing conventional topical therapy.

INTRODUCTION

Atopic dermatitis (AD) remains a complex, common, chronic, and relapsing skin disorder of infants and children but can affect patients of any age. In the United States, prevalence in school-aged children has been found to be up to 18%.[1] In addition, recent data from the National Health Interview Survey show that up to 10% of adults in the United States report having eczema and the prevalence is higher in those with concomitant allergies or asthma.[2] In other industrialized countries, prevalence greater than 20% has been reported.[3] Of note, in a large cohort of subjects with mild to moderate AD, it was not until age 20 that 50% had at least 1 lifetime 6-month period free of symptoms and treatment.[4] More than half of these patients will develop asthma and allergies suggesting an atopic march in a significant number of patients with AD.[5]

[a] College of Nursing, University of Colorado, 13120 East 19th Avenue, Mail Stop C288-18, Aurora, CO 80045, USA; [b] Department of Pediatrics, National Jewish Health, University of Colorado School of Medicine, Denver, CO 80206, USA
* Corresponding author.
E-mail address: Noreen.nicol@ucdenver.edu

Immunol Allergy Clin N Am 37 (2017) 123–139
http://dx.doi.org/10.1016/j.iac.2016.08.003
0889-8561/17/© 2016 Elsevier Inc. All rights reserved.

immunology.theclinics.com

AD occurs in genetically predisposed individuals with a defective skin barrier and abnormal immune responses to irritants, allergens, and microbial organisms.[6] AD is characterized by abnormal skin barrier function associated with abnormalities in cornified envelope genes, reduced ceramide levels, increased levels of endogenous proteolytic enzymes, and enhanced transepidermal water loss (TEWL).[7] Skin barrier may also be damaged by exposure to exogenous proteases from *Staphylococcus aureus*.[8] Skin barrier abnormalities contribute to increased allergen absorption and microbial colonization. Exposing the immune system of the skin to allergen compared with systemic or airway sensitization results in a higher allergic antibody response and could predispose susceptible children to developing asthma and allergic rhinitis later in life.[9] Patients with AD typically have severe pruritus and disrupted sleep that affects their quality of life, as well as that of family members.[10] When AD remains in poor control, patients and caregivers can experience multiple medical and psychosocial issues. Associated with this, AD imposes a significant economic burden on the patient, family, and society.[11]

ROLE OF MULTIDISCIPLINARY CARE

A multidisciplinary care model that incorporates a stepwise approach to the management of moderate to severe AD has been used by the authors for almost 3 decades.[12,13] In this approach, the importance of teaching patients or caregivers skills to self-monitor and manage disease with the help of an individualized plan is a key component.[14] In the authors' center, the multidisciplinary team is composed of pediatric allergist-immunologists with extensive experience in basic and clinical research in AD, pediatric nurse specialists, behavioral clinicians, fellows-in-training, physician assistants, nurse educators, child-life specialists, art therapists, social workers, dietitians, and rehabilitation therapists. Dermatologists are available for consultation if the diagnosis of AD is in question or alternative therapies, such as phototherapy, are being considered. The philosophy of care is based on a personalized approach with comprehensive evaluation and treatment tailored to the needs and goals of the patient and caregiver.

In this treatment model, all members of the multidisciplinary team teach the same key concepts and reinforce the messages being delivered to the patients and caregivers regardless of which educational strategy is incorporated. Educational strategies include one-on-one communication, direct demonstration with reinforcement, group discussions, classroom teaching, written materials, and AD Home Care Plan or AD Action Plan. AD Home Care Plans or AD Action Plans are integral to the management of the AD patient[15–17] (**Box 1**). Development of a skin care regimen that is agreed on by the clinician, patient, and caregivers requires open communication. Patients or caregivers, especially given the degree of sleep disruption associated with AD,[18] may forget or confuse skin care recommendations given to them without a written plan. This plan should be reviewed and modified at follow-up visits.

STEPWISE MANAGEMENT OF ATOPIC DERMATITIS

National and international AD guidelines outline basic treatment of AD to establish the foundation of AD management.[9,19,20] These guidelines recommend 3 basic components of optimal skin care. First and foremost, the regular use of moisturizers[21] or emollients in conjunction with skin hydration is essential to address the skin barrier defect. Second, identification and avoidance of specific and nonspecific triggers is critical in reducing symptoms. Third, depending on the severity of AD, topical therapeutic agents may be initiated in a stepwise fashion. Topical corticosteroids are often the standard of care to which other treatments are compared.

Box 1
National Jewish Atopic Dermatitis Program step-care "AD action" plan

Maintenance or daily care

1. Take at least 1 bath or shower per day; use warm water, for 10 to 15 minutes.

2. Use a gentle cleansing bar or wash in the sensitive skin formulation as needed.

3. Pat away excess water and immediately (within 3 minutes) apply moisturizer, sealer, or maintenance medication if directed. Fragrance-free moisturizers are available in 1 pound jars include Aquaphor Ointment (Beiersdorf, Wilton, CT), Eucerin Crème (Beiersdorf, Wilton, CT), Vanicream (Pharmaceutical Specialities, Rochester, MN), CeraVe Cream (Valeant, Bridgewater, NJ), or Cetaphil Cream (Galderma, Fort Worth, TX). Vaseline is a good occlusive preparation to seal in the water; however, it contains no water so it only works effectively after a bathing. Use moisturizers liberally throughout the day. Moisturizers and sealers should not be applied over any topical medication.

4. Avoid skin irritants and proven allergens.

Mild to moderate AD

1. Bathe as above for 10 to 15 minutes, in comfortably warm water, 2 times a day, in the morning and before bedtime.

2. Use a gentle cleansing bar or wash in the sensitive skin formulation as needed.

3. Use moisturizers, as above, on healed and unaffected skin, twice daily, especially after baths, and on total body at midday.

4. Apply to affected areas of face, groin, and underarms twice daily especially after baths _____ (low potency topical corticosteroid), or_____ (topical calcineurin inhibitors), or other topical preparation as directed _____ (topical barrier repair cream; eg, Atopiclair 3 times daily).

5. Apply to other affected areas of the body twice daily, especially after baths, _____ (low to mid potency topical corticosteroid), or _____ (topical calcineurin inhibitors), or other topical preparation as directed _____.

6. Add other medications as directed: _____ (eg, oral sedating antihistamines, topical or oral antimicrobial therapy).

7. Pay close attention to things that seem to irritate the skin or make condition worse.

Moderate to severe AD

1. Bathe as above for 10 to 15 minutes, in comfortably warm water, 2 times a day, in the morning and before bedtime, or a third time midday if WWT is applied 3 times. Put no additives in bath water.

2. Use a gentle cleansing bar or wash in the sensitive skin formulation as needed. An antibacterial cleanser may be considered.

3. Use moisturizers as above on healed and unaffected skin, twice daily, especially after baths, and on total body at midday.

4. Apply to affected areas of face, groin, and underarms twice daily, especially after baths _____(low potency topical corticosteroid), or_____ (topical calcineurin inhibitors), or other topical preparation as directed _____ (topical barrier repair cream, eg, Atopiclair 3 times daily).

5. Apply to other affected areas of the body twice daily, especially after baths, _____(mid to high potency topical corticosteroid), or _____(topical calcineurin inhibitors), or other topical preparation as directed _____.

6. Use wet wraps on involved areas selectively as directed per policy and procedure. Wet wraps are left in place a minimum of 2 hours. If left in place, need to be rewet every 2 to 3 hours. In

general, wet wraps are removed after 4 hours. If patient falls asleep with wet wraps in place, they may be left on overnight. Stop rewetting during the night. Apply moisturizer total body after wet wraps are removed.

7. Add other medications as directed: _____(eg, oral sedating antihistamines, topical or oral antimicrobial therapy).

8. Pay close attention to things that irritate skin or make condition worse.

9. Step down to moderate plan above as the skin heals.

Reduce skin irritation

1. Wash all new clothes before wearing them. This removes formaldehyde and other irritating chemicals.

2. Add a second rinse cycle to ensure removal of detergent. Residual laundry detergent, particularly perfume or dye, may be irritating when it remains in the clothing. Changing to a liquid and fragrance-free, dye-free detergent may be helpful.

3. Wear garments that allow air to pass freely to skin. Open weave, loose-fitting, cotton-blend clothing may be most comfortable.

4. Work and sleep in comfortable surroundings with a fairly constant temperature and humidity level.

5. Keep fingernails very short and smooth to help prevent damage due to scratching.

6. Carry a small tube of moisturizer or sunscreen at all times. Daycare, school, or work should have a separate supply of moisturizer.

7. After swimming in chlorinated pool or using hot tub, shower or bathe using a gentle cleanser to remove chemicals, then apply moisturizer.

Courtesy of Noreen Nicol, PhD, RN, FNP, Mark Boguniewicz, MD, and Donald Leung MD, PhD, Atopic Dermatitis Program, National Jewish Health, Denver, CO. This may be modified and used for patient care citing National Jewish Health Atopic Dermatitis Program as source. (Nicol and Boguniewicz, 2008); with permission.

In severe cases that cannot be controlled with topical treatment, guidelines suggest systemic treatment options.[9,20,22] These include cyclosporine A and ultraviolet light therapy. Systemic corticosteroids are known to be effective in short-term treatment of AD but evidence is limited to support their use due to long-term side effects and rebound flaring. Systemic steroids are discouraged for continuous or chronic intermittent use in AD but may be considered for transitional therapy to nonsteroidal therapies, including phototherapy, and in acute, severe, rapidly progressive, or debilitating cases in adults or children. Use of other immunosuppressives, including cyclosporine A, methotrexate, azathioprine, or mycophenolate mofetil, is problematic because such therapy is off-label for AD in most countries and can be associated with serious side effects. A different approach in the patients with difficult to manage moderate to severe AD is acute intervention with wet wrap therapy (WWT). **Fig. 1** is a flowchart highlighting AD diagnosis and management developed by the Joint Task Force on Practice Parameters, representing the American Academy of Allergy, Asthma & Immunology; the American College of Allergy, Asthma & Immunology; and the Joint Council of Allergy, Asthma and Immunology.[9]

ROLE OF WET WRAP THERAPY IN ATOPIC DERMATITIS
Overview of Wet Wrap Treatment

Dampened bandages or water dressings are an ancient remedy described by the Babylonians and Egyptians. Their use is described in historical surgical and nursing

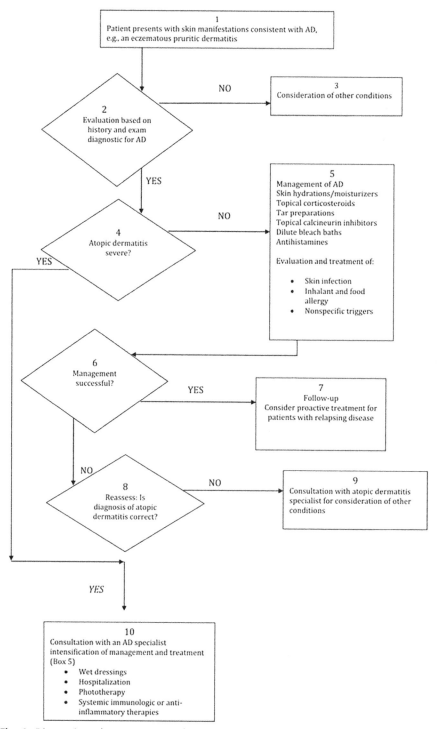

Fig. 1. Diagnosis and management of AD. (*From* Schneider L, Tilles S, Lio P, et al. Atopic dermatitis: a practice parameter update 2012. J Allergy Clin Immunol 2013;131(2):297; with permission.)

textbooks to reduce inflammation. The use of dampened bandages is still commonly used throughout the world and these treatments are often referred to as wet dressings.

Dampened bandages or moist dressings are used in for a variety of acute inflammatory states, ulcers, and other skin disorders. The simple wet dressing is used for cooling, antiinflammatory, and itch-reducing properties; it was often a cloth or dressing soaked in cool water and applied directly to the affected skin for everything from bug bites and wounds to a variety of skin disorders. Single or multiple layers of wet dressings were also used historically over a variety of topical preparations to assist in absorption. They also act as a protective barrier from the trauma associated with scratching in pruritic skin disorders.

Definition of Wet Wrap Therapy

WWT is generally defined as a treatment modality using layers of bandages, cotton clothing, or gauze over or together with topical medication. Specialized nursing care and education is important to ensure proper use of WWT. Nicol[13] published a detailed description of WWT in AD in 1987. This article described the technique using illustrative photos. The investigator also clarified the concept of simplifying wet wraps by using wet clothing in place of bandages to make this treatment simpler, less time intensive, and less expensive. This article is cited in the *Annotated Bibliography of the Dermatologic Nursing Literature* done at Oxford as the first nursing paper in the literature on the wet wrap technique specifically in AD.[23]

Over the past 3 decades, the term WWT has been used as a treatment for severe and/or refractory AD. Current reviews on the efficacy and safety of occlusive therapy, including WWT, state that this therapy is advocated as a relatively safe and effective treatment modality in moderate to severe AD when used appropriately and may be underused.[24–26]

Mechanism of Wet Wrap Therapy

WWT is well tolerated in eczema treatment due to the cooling, antiinflammatory, and antipruritic properties on the skin. Itch is reduced by cooling through vasoconstriction. WWT increases skin hydration and decreases TEWL. WWT protects the skin as a barrier against external irritants and allergens. Additional work has pointed to a beneficial effect of WWT on the skin barrier that persists even after discontinuation of this treatment modality.[27]

Reported side effects and contraindications of WWT vary greatly depending on study methodology; WWT technique, including topicals used; and time devoted to WWT oversight and patient education (**Table 1**). The biggest barrier is the time that it takes to properly teach the patient and family to avoid discomfort and poor acceptance. WWT can be a time-consuming treatment depending on methodology of application. Other complications reported in varying degrees include potential local and systemic corticosteroid side effects, allergic sensitization, skin maceration, and possible increased infectious complications, including folliculitis, impetigo, and herpes. Occlusion alone results in increased density of bacteria of both normal and lesional eczematous skin.[28] Paradoxically, WWT can promote skin dryness if sufficient emollients are not used after wet wraps are removed.

Methodology of Wet Wrap Therapy

There are 2 primary methods of WWT used in the treatment of AD:

1. Double-layer wet wrap (inner wet layer and outer dry layer) over ointment or cream applied directly to skin

Table 1
Reported complications, besides temporary systemic bioactivity, during an intervention treatment with wet-wrap dressings and (diluted) topical corticosteroids for a maximum period of 14 days

Adverse Event	Occurrence
Discomfort, including chills and poor acceptance	Frequent
Folliculitis	Common
Refractory skin lesions on the areas not covered by bandages	Common
Impetigo	Rare
Cutaneous *Pseudomonas aeruginosa* infection	Rare
Herpetic infections	Rare

From Devillers AC, Oranje AP. Efficacy and safety of 'wet-wrap' dressings as an intervention treatment in children with severe and/or refractory atopic dermatitis: a critical review of the literature. Br J Dermatol 2006;154(4):579–85; with permission.

2. Double layer wrap (1 layer impregnated with diluted steroids, rather than water, and 1 outer dry layer) applied directly to the involved skin.

In both methods, the use of an outer layer results in decreased evaporation of water from inner layer and, therefore, in prolonged moisturization and cooling.[29]

The first method has been standardized for years at the authors' AD treatment program.[12,16,30] Step care for AD as done in the National Jewish AD Program is outlined in **Box 1**.[15] This step care is the basis for the recommended AD therapies and protocol for daily provider orders, as well as patient discharge orders and instructions. As used by the authors, WWT is reserved for patients with moderate to severe AD as an acute intervention.

The typical standard for this method of care includes a 10 to 15 minute bath in warm water, immediately followed by application of a topical medication (appropriate full-strength topical steroid because topical calcineurin inhibitors in the United States carry a warning not to use with occlusive dressings) to eczematous lesions and moisturizers to clear areas. Based on clinical severity as assessed with a validated outcomes tool (eg, SCORing atopic dermatitis [SCORAD]) by the attending team, patients are prescribed 2 to 3 supervised baths per day; topical and/or oral medications; moisturizer applications, usually 2 to 3 times per day; and WWT applied up to 3 times a day, tapering all therapy with improvement. WWT is done using children's normal cotton-blend clothing and detailed in **Box 2**. This is followed by applying the water-dampened wet cotton pajamas, socks, or gauze dressings covered by a dry second outer layer (**Fig. 2**). The area requiring skilled nursing technique is the face. When the face has moderate to severe AD, a low potency topical steroid is applied and wrapped with 2 layers of wet gauze followed by 2 layers of dry gauze held in place by a tubular bandage retainer. Wet wraps are left in place for approximately 2 hours. At bedtime, they may be left on overnight and, in fact, this may be beneficial in preventing trauma from patient scratching at night. Moisturizer should be applied to total body after wet wraps are removed. Significant healing of severely excoriated eczema lesions is seen after 3 to 4 days of WWT (**Fig. 3**).

In the second method, Goodyear and colleagues[31] demonstrated efficacy of wet-wraps in a study of erythrodermic children with AD using diluted topical corticosteroids. The difference between this WWT method and the method prescribed by the investigators is that no water is applied to the bandages. The wetness results from Tubegauz impregnated with diluted topical steroids applied directly as the first layer

Box 2
Wet wrap therapy procedure

WWT will be used to relieve inflammation, itching, and burning of AD. Wet wraps facilitate the removal of scale and increase penetration of topical medications in the stratum corneum. Skin protection provided by the wraps allows healing to take place. WWT should only be used during flares of AD under the supervision of a health care provider. They should not be used as routine maintenance therapy.

Supplies:

1. Topical medications and moisturizers

2. Tap water at comfortably warm temperature

3. Basin for dampening of dressings

4. Clean dressings of approximate size to cover involved area:
   a. Face: 2 to 3 layers of wet Kerlix gauze held in place with Surginet.
   b. Arms, legs, hands, and feet: 2 to 3 layers of wet Kerlix gauze held in place with Ace bandages or tube socks, or cotton gloves, or wet tube socks followed by dry tube socks. Tube socks may be used for wraps for hands and feet, and larger ones work as leg or arm covers.
   c. Total body: combination of above, or wet pajamas or long underwear and turtleneck shirts covered by dry pajamas or sweatsuit. Pajamas with feet work well for the outer layer.

5. Blankets to prevent chilling.

6. Nonsterile gloves if desired.

Procedure:

1. Be certain that the patient's room is warm and insure privacy. Gather supplies appropriate to the individual.

2. If wraps are to be applied to a large portion of the body, work with 2 people if possible. It is necessary to work rapidly to prevent chilling.

3. Explain the procedure to the patient and parent.

4. Fill the basin with warm tap water.

5. The patient will have had a 15 to 20 minute soaking bath, in warm water without additional additives, before this procedure. Pat skin dry with a towel.

6. Apply the appropriate topical medications to affected areas and moisturizer to nonaffected areas immediately after pat drying the skin. Use clean plastic spoons or tongue depressor to avoid contamination of products in jars. This allows large areas to be covered quickly and prevent caregivers from unnecessary exposure to topical medications.

7. Soak the dressings in very warm water because they cool quickly in this process. Squeeze out excess water. Dressings should be wet, not dripping.

8. Cover an area with wet dressing chosen for the area and the patient. Immediately after wrapping, cover with appropriate dry material such as an Ace bandage, socks, or pajamas. Start at the feet and move upward. Use wet, long underwear or wet pajamas covered by dry pajamas or sweatsuit with total body involvement in place of wet gauze.

9. Take steps to avoid chilling. Blanket can be put in a dryer to warm up and cover patient but do not overheat the patient. Wraps can be removed after 2 to 4 hours or can be rewet. A warm blanket and snuggling help pass the time.

10. If patient is known or suspected to have an infection of the involved areas, place dressings in appropriate bag, and dispose according to infection control procedure.

11. After all dressings are removed, moisturizers may be applied to the entire body.

Courtesy of Noreen Nicol, PhD, RN, FNP, Mark Boguniewicz, MD, and Donald Leung MD, PhD, Atopic Dermatitis Program, National Jewish Health, Denver, CO. This may be modified and used for patient care citing National Jewish Health Atopic Dermatitis Program as source. (Nicol and Boguniewicz, 2008); with permission.

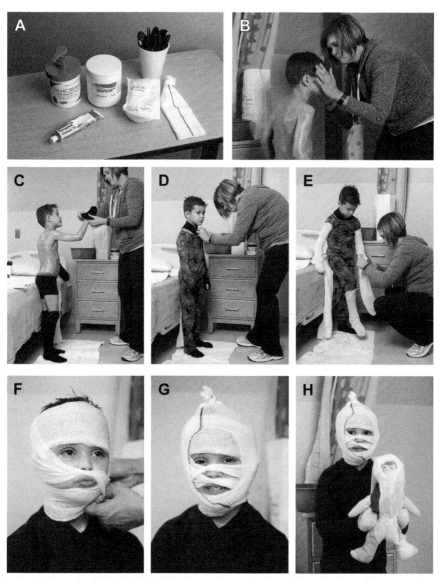

Fig. 2. (*A*) Supplies for WWT. (*B*) Topical steroids applied to affected lesions. (*C*) Wet socks to eczema of extremities. (*D*) Wet pajamas to eczema of trunk. (*E*) Dry layer applied over wet layer. (*F*) Wet Kerlix bandage (Molnlycke Healthcare, Norcross, GA) applied to facial eczema. (*G*) Face wrap held in place by burn netting. (*H*) Completed wrap (with patient's doll also wrapped!).

and covered by an outer dry layer. It is worth noting that, outside the United States, WWT is often done using a variety of expensive dressings. Some tubular bandages, such as Tubifast (Molnlycke Healthcare, Norcross, GA), are available only by prescription. The ability to wash and reuse these expensive bandages appears to range from none to up to 20. Disadvantages reported with these tubular bandages include high cost, difficulty applying, intolerance of use, increased risk of cutaneous infections, and systemic

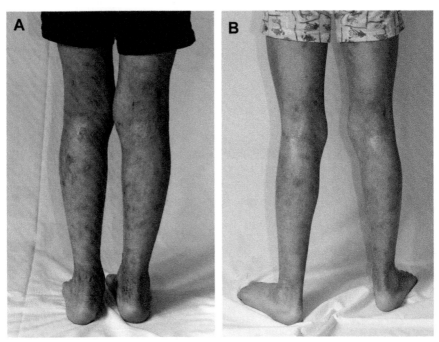

Fig. 3. (*A*) Severe excoriated eczema lesions on lower extremities before WWT. (*B*) Significant healing of severe eczema of lower extremities after 3 to 4 days of WWT.

absorption of steroid.[29] Of note, some investigators advocate use of WWT as part of a maintenance skin care regimen versus using as an acute intervention.[32]

Wide variations in WWT methodology exist from center to center and country to country. These include lack of clarity regarding use of water (or not), use with nonsteroidal topical preparations (eg, topical calcineurin inhibitors), use with only emollients, or use of only a wrap without topical medication or moisturizer. When topical corticosteroids are used in WWT, it is often unclear if they were used full-strength, as a pharmacy-diluted solution, or in some self-compounded manner. There is also lack of clarity regarding the types of dressings and bandages used, what they were soaked in, how they were applied, how long they were applied, and skin care before and after application of the WWT.

In 2006, Devillers and Oranje[26] published a critical review of the literature related to the efficacy and safety of wet-wrap dressings as interventions in children with severe and/or refractory AD. The study did an inventory of methodologies to evaluate the currently available use of WWT. These investigators summarized 9 possible differences in the methodology of WWT in AD literature: topical product, type of bandages, application technique of topical product, application frequency, rewetting of the first layer of bandages, bandages left in situ, area treated, duration of treatment, and location of treatment. These 9 differences remain as critical variables in WWT today. The investigators suggest 2 additional variables: skin care immediately before application and immediately after removal of WWT. Important details in the skin care before WWT application include noting whether and how the patient is instructed to hydrate the skin and specifying whether a local soak, shower, or bath is used. When bathing is recommended, clarify length of bathing and whether a bath additive is used (eg, oils, bleach, or other). The aftercare detail should include if or what topical is to be applied (eg, specific moisturizer or other).

Devillers and Oranje[26] concluded that large prospective studies evaluating the efficacy and safety profile of WWT are lacking. Their conclusions with a grade C of strength of recommendation included:

1. WWT using cream or ointment and a double layer of cotton bandages, with a moist first layer and a dry second layer, is an efficacious short-term intervention treatment in children with severe and/or refractory AD.
2. The use of wet-wrap dressings with diluted topical corticosteroids is a more efficacious short-term intervention treatment in children with severe and/or refractory AD than wet-wrap dressings with emollients only.
3. The use of wet-wrap dressings with diluted topical corticosteroids for up to 14 days is a safe intervention treatment in children with severe and/or refractory AD, with temporary systemic bioactivity of the corticosteroids as the only reported serious side-effect.
4. Lowering the absolute amount of applied topical corticosteroid to once daily application and further dilution of the product can reduce the risk of systemic bioactivity.

Evaluating Studies Using Wet Wrap Therapy

Several variables and unresolved issues are apparent when one examines the published reviews and clinical studies that incorporate WWT in the treatment of AD. Clinical studies on the efficacy of WWT published between 1991 and 2015 are listed in **Table 2**. Of the 18 studies examined,[30–47] only 12 studies used a validated AD severity outcomes tool and only 6 were randomized controlled trials. The total number of subjects included in these studies was small. All WWT studies demonstrated efficacy of this treatment or no worsening in the WWT treatment arms. One of the 18 WWT studies had a follow-up assessment after stopping WWT as part of the study.[30]

The largest study to date in moderate to severe AD subjects treated with WWT under direct nursing supervision and using a validated outcomes tool was done at the authors' institution.[30] This was a retrospective observational cohort study in a multidisciplinary AD treatment program. The study population consisted of 72 children with AD, mean age 4.6 years (SD = 3.12) ranging from 6 months to 12.8 years. Significant differences between SCORAD index means at admission 49.68 (SD = 17.72) and discharge 14.83 (SD = 7.45) demonstrate significant clinical improvement as a result of participation in this treatment program using WWT ($P \leq .0001$). The average number of days of receiving WWT was 7.5 (range 2–16 days); WWT was discontinued on all subjects before discharge. Of note, none of the subjects required systemic immunosuppressive therapy during this treatment program. Only 4 of the 72 subjects experienced mild folliculitis while using WWT. The AD Quickscore (ADQ)[48] is a parent administered questionnaire that correlated with SCORAD while the subjects were in the AD treatment program and 1 month after discharge. The results also suggest that these subjects were able to maintain improvement of their AD despite stopping WWT before discharge[30] (**Fig. 4**). This study demonstrates the benefit of an intensive multidisciplinary AD treatment program consisting of supervised skin care incorporating WWT in improving AD severity. Subjects treated in this unique outpatient AD program had moderate to severe AD and were failing outpatient therapy. This study showed that these subjects could be managed without systemic immunosuppressive therapy and were able to transition off of WWT before discharge from the program.

Table 2
Clinical studies on the efficacy of wet-wrap treatment

Investigators, Year	Study Design	Subjects	Validated AD Severity Yes/No, Measure Result
Abeck et al,[33] 1999	Prospective observational	N = 6 3 children (3–12 y) and 3 adults	Yes, SCORAD Improved SCORAD index in WWT
Beattie & Lewis-Jones,[34] 2004	Prospective randomized controlled trial	N = 19 Children (4 mo–3 y)	Yes, SASSAS No difference between groups; all improved Mild population: only HC 1% required
Dabade et al,[35] 2012	Retrospective observational inpatient comparison	N = 218 Children (2 mo–17 y)	No, IGA: no objective score >90% improvement in WWT
Devillers et al,[36] 2002	Retrospective observational inpatient side-to-side comparison	N = 26 14 children (6 mo–10 y) and 12 adults	Yes, SCORAD Improved modified objective SCORAD index in WWT
Foelster-Holst et al,[37] 2006	Prospective randomized controlled trial, left or right study	N = 24 Adults (18–63 y) and children (6–16 y)	Yes, SCORAD Improved SCORAD index both treatment arms significantly better in WWT
Goodyear et al,[31] 1991	Prospective observational	N = 30 Children (9 m–16 y)	No, IGA >90% clear in WWT
Hindley et al,[38] 2006	Prospective randomized controlled trial	N = 50 Children (4–27 mo)	Yes, SCORAD Improved SCORAD index in all treatment arms; moderate to severe wraps varied 12–24 h vs none; 4-wk trial
Hon et al,[39] 2007	Prospective observational case studies	N = 6 Children (3–15 y)	Yes, SCORAD Improved SCORAD index in WWT
Leloup et al,[32] 2015	Prospective open-label	N = 17 Children (<18 y)	Yes, SCORAD and subject questionnaire Improved SCORAD "satisfied & tolerated"

Study	Study design	Sample	Outcome
Janmohamed et al,[40] 2014	Prospective, randomized controlled trial, double-blind, placebo-controlled trial	N = 39, Children (6 mo–10 y)	Yes, SCORAD; Improved SCORAD WWT with diluted corticosteroids more than WWT with emollients
Mallon et al,[41] 1994	Prospective observational	N = 21, Children (4 mo–10 y)	No, IGA and parental questionnaire "All responded well"
Nicol et al,[30] 2014	Retrospective observational-nurse supervised	N = 72, Children (6 mo–12.8 y)	Yes, SCORAD; Improved SCORAD index in WWT; lasting benefit 1 mo after discontinuing WWT intervention
Oranje & de Waard-van der Spek,[42] 1999	Prospective observational	N = 7, 3 children (6 mo–4 y) and 4 adults	Yes, SCORAD; Improved modified objective SCORAD index with WWT
Pei et al,[43] 2001	Prospective randomized controlled trial	N = 40, Children (1–15 y)	No, CSS and parental questionnaire; Improved CSS and parental questionnaire in both groups using different topical steroid and WWT
Schnopp et al,[44] 2002	Randomized controlled trial; inpatient comparison side-to-side	N = 20, Children (2–17 y)	Yes, SCORAD; Improved Regional SCORAD index and TEWL in steroid-containing WWT vs vehicle WWT
Tang & Chan,[45] 1999	Prospective observational	N = 12, Children (3–12 y)	No, CSS and self-assessment; WWT effective
Tang,[46] 2000	Prospective observational	N = 10, Children (4–15 y)	No, IGA and parental assessment WWT "good"
Wolkerstorfer et al,[47] 2000	Prospective observational; comparison of 3 arms	N = 31, Children (5 mo–13 y)	Yes, SCORAD; Improved modified objective SCORAD index with WWT

Abbreviations: CSS, clinical severity scoring; IGA, investigator's global assessment; SASSAD, six area, six sign atopic dermatitis.

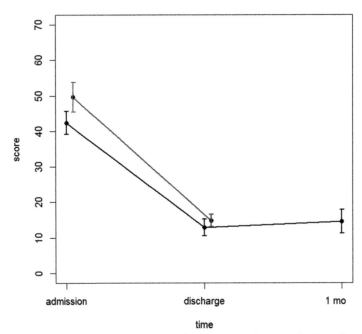

Fig. 4. Sustained improvement in severity of AD (SCORAD) 1 month after discontinuing WWT as measured by ADQ. Mean ADQ (*lower line*) versus SCORAD (*top line*), with 95% confidence limits. (*From* Nicol NH, Boguniewicz M, Strand M, et al. Wet wrap therapy in children with moderate to severe atopic dermatitis in a multidisciplinary treatment program. J Allergy Clin Immunol Pract 2014;2(4):405; with permission.)

Importantly, WWT was used as an acute treatment intervention, not part of a maintenance regimen.

SUMMARY

National and international AD guidelines address AD care in a stepwise fashion. The literature, as well as the authors' experience, suggests that WWT plays an important role as an acute therapeutic intervention for management of moderate to severe AD used with undiluted topical corticosteroids of appropriate potency. Simplifying WWT by using clothing in place of bandages makes this treatment simpler, less time intensive, and less expensive. Education of patients and caregivers is critical to the success of WWT. WWT methodology needs to become more standardized. Future WWT studies need to carefully describe all components of WWT procedures. Incorporation of the SCORAD index or other validated outcomes tools would help with interpretation of future studies using WWT. WWT should be considered as a treatment option ahead of systemic immunosuppressive therapies for patients failing conventional topical therapy.

ACKNOWLEDGMENTS

The authors thank the multidisciplinary team in the Day Program at National Jewish Health for their exceptional dedication to our patients and families. We also thank our patients and caregivers for their enthusiastic support for our program. A special thanks to our biomedical photographer Beth Woods for contributing the patient photos in this article.

REFERENCES

1. Shaw TE, Currie GP, Koudelka CW, et al. Eczema prevalence in the United States: data from the 2003 national survey of children's health. J Invest Dermatol 2011; 131(1):67–73.
2. Silverberg JI, Hanifin JM. Adult eczema prevalence and associations with asthma and other health and demographic factors: a US population-based study. J Allergy Clin Immunol 2013;132(5):1132–8.
3. Odhiambo JA, Williams HC, Clayton TO, et al. Global variations in prevalence of eczema symptoms in children from ISAAC phase three. J Allergy Clin Immunol 2009;124(6):1251–8.e23.
4. Margolis JS, Abuabara K, Bilker W, et al. Persistence of mild to moderate atopic dermatitis. JAMA Dermatol 2014;150(6):593–600.
5. Kapoor R, Menon C, Hoffstad O, et al. The prevalence of atopic triad in children with physician-confirmed atopic dermatitis. J Am Acad Dermatol 2008;58(1): 68–73.
6. Boguniewicz M, Leung DY. Atopic dermatitis: a disease of altered skin barrier and immune dysregulation. Immunol Rev 2011;242(1):233–46.
7. Cork MJ, Robinson DA, Vasilopoulos Y, et al. New perspectives on epidermal barrier dysfunction in atopic dermatitis: gene-environment interactions. J Allergy Clin Immunol 2006;118(1):3–21.
8. Boguniewicz M, Leung DYM. Recent insights into AD and implications for management of infectious complications. J Allergy Clin Immunol 2010;125(1):4–13.
9. Schneider L, Tilles S, Lio P, et al. Atopic dermatitis: a practice parameter update 2012. J Allergy Clin Immunol 2013;131(2):295–9.
10. Chamlin SL. The psychosocial burden of childhood atopic dermatitis. Dermatol Ther 2006;19(2):104–7.
11. Bhanegaonkar A, Horodniceanu EG, Ji X, et al. Economic burden of atopic dermatitis in high-risk infants receiving cow's milk or partially hydolyzed 100% whey-based formula. J Pediatr 2015;166:1145–51.e3.
12. Boguniewicz M, Nicol N, Kelsay K, et al. A multidisciplinary approach to evaluation and treatment of atopic dermatitis. Semin Cutan Med Surg 2008;27(2): 115–27.
13. Nicol NH. Atopic dermatitis: the (wet) wrap-up. Am J Nurs 1987;87(12):1560–3.
14. Nicol NH, Ersser SJ. The role of the nurse educator in managing atopic dermatitis. Immunol Allergy Clin North Am 2010;30(3):369–83.
15. Nicol NH, Boguniewicz M. Successful strategies in atopic dermatitis management. Dermatol Nurs 2008;Suppl:3–18.
16. Boguniewicz M, Nicol N. Conventional therapy for atopic dermatitis. Immunol Allergy Clin N Am 2002;22:107–24.
17. Nicol NH, Boguniewicz M. Understanding and treating atopic dermatitis. Nurse Pract Forum 1999;10(2):48–55.
18. Bender BG, Ballard R, Canono B, et al. Disease severity, scratching, and sleep quality in patients with atopic dermatitis. J Am Acad Dermatol 2008;58(3):415–20.
19. Eichenfield LF, Tom WL, Berger TG, et al. Guidelines of care for the management of atopic dermatitis: section 2. Management and treatment of atopic dermatitis with topical therapies. J Am Acad Dermatol 2014;71(1):116–32.

20. Akdis CA, Akdis M, Bieber T, et al. Diagnosis and treatment of atopic dermatitis in children and adults: European Academy of Allergology and Clinical Immunology/American Academy of Allergy, Asthma and Immunology/PRACTALL Consensus Report. J Allergy Clin Immunol 2006;118(1):152–69.
21. Nicol NH. Use of moisturizers in dermatologic disease: the role of healthcare providers in optimizing treatment outcomes. Cutis 2005;76(6 Suppl):26–31.
22. Sidbury R, Davis DM, Cohen DE, et al. Guidelines of care for the management of atopic dermatitis: section 3. Management and treatment with phototherapy and systemic agents. J Am Acad Dermatol 2014;71(2):327–49.
23. Ersser SJ. Annotated bibliography of the dermatological nursing literature. In: Ersser SJ, editor. The book title is Annotated Bibliography of the Dermatologic Nursing Literature. Oxford (England): Oxford Centre for Health Care Research and Development; 1998. p. 49.
24. Andersen RM, Thyssen JP, Maibach HI. The role of wet wrap therapy in skin disorders a literature review. Acta Derm Venereol 2015;95(8):933–9.
25. Braham SJ, Pugasjetti R, Koo J, et al. Occlusive therapy in atopic dermatitis: overview. J Dermatolog Treat 2010;21:62–72.
26. Devillers AC, Oranje AP. Efficacy and safety of 'wet-wrap' dressings as an intervention treatment in children with severe and/or refractory atopic dermatitis: a critical review of the literature. Br J Dermatol 2006;154(4):579–85.
27. Lee JH, Lee SJ, Kim D, et al. The effect of wet-wrap dressing on epidermal barrier in patients with atopic dermatitis. J Eur Acad Dermatol Venereol 2007;21(10):1360–8.
28. Aly R, Shirley C, Cunico B, et al. Effect of prolonged occlusion on the microbial flora, pH, carbon dioxide and transepidermal water loss on human skin. J Invest Dermatol 1978;71(6):378–81.
29. Oranje AP, Devillers AC, Kunz B, et al. Treatment of patients with atopic dermatitis using wet-wrap dressings with diluted steroids and/or emollients. An expert panel's opinion and review of the literature. J Eur Acad Dermatol Venereol 2006;20(10):1277–86.
30. Nicol NH, Boguniewicz M, Strand M, et al. Wet wrap therapy in children with moderate to severe atopic dermatitis in a multidisciplinary treatment program. J Allergy Clin Immunol Pract 2014;2(4):400–6.
31. Goodyear HM, Spowart K, Harper JI. 'Wet-wrap' dressings for the treatment of atopic eczema in children. Br J Dermatol 1991;125(6):604.
32. Leloup P, Stalder JF, Barbarot S. Outpatient home-based wet wrap dressings with topical steroids with children with severe recalcitrant atopic dermatitis: a feasibility pilot study. Pediatr Dermatol 2015;32(4):e177–8.
33. Abeck D, Brockow K, Mempel M, et al. Treatment of acute exacerbated atopic eczema with emollient-antiseptic preparations using the "wet wrap" ("wet pajama") technique. Hautarzt 1999;50(6):418–21.
34. Beattie PE, Lewis-Jones MS. A pilot study on the use of wet wraps in infants with moderate atopic eczema. Clin Exp Dermatol 2004;29(4):348–53.
35. Dabade TS, Davis DM, Wetter DA, et al. Wet dressing therapy in conjunction with topical corticosteroids is effective for rapid control of severe pediatric atopic dermatitis: experience with 218 patients over 30 years at Mayo Clinic. J Am Acad Dermatol 2012;67(1):100–6.
36. Devillers AC, de Waard-van der Spek FB, Mulder PG, et al. Treatment of refractory atopic dermatitis using 'wet-wrap' dressings and diluted corticosteroids: results of standardized treatment in both children and adults. Dermatology 2002;204(1):50–5.

37. Foelster-Holst R, Nagel F, Zoellner P, et al. Efficacy of crisis intervention treatment with topical corticosteroid prednicarbat with and without partial wet-wrap dressing in atopic dermatitis. Dermatology 2006;212(1):66–9.
38. Hindley D, Galloway G, Murray J, et al. A randomised study of "wet wraps" versus conventional treatment for atopic eczema. Arch Dis Child 2006;91(2):164–8.
39. Hon KL, Wong KY, Cheung LK, et al. Efficacy and problems associated with using a wet-wrap garment for children with severe atopic dermatitis. J Dermatolog Treat 2007;18(5):301–5.
40. Janmohamed SR, Oranje AP, Devillers AC, et al. The proactive wet-wrap method with diluted corticosteroids versus emollients in children with atopic dermatitis: a prospective, randomized, double-blind, placebo-controlled trial. J Am Acad Dermatol 2014;70(6):1076–82.
41. Mallon E, Powell S, Bridgman A. "Wet-wrap" dressings for the treatment of atopic eczema in the community. J Dermatolog Treat 1994;5:97–8.
42. Oranje AP, de Waard-van der Spek FB. Treatment of erythrodermic atopic dermatitis with "wet-wrap" fluticasone propionate 0.05% cream/emollient 1: 1 dressings. J Dermatolog Treat 1999;10(1):73–4.
43. Pei AY, Chan HH, Ho KM. The effectiveness of wet wrap dressings using 0.1% mometasone furoate and 0.005% fluticasone proprionate ointments in the treatment of moderate to severe atopic dermatitis in children. Pediatr Dermatol 2001;18(4):343–8.
44. Schnopp C, Holtmann C, Stock S, et al. Topical steroids under wet-wrap dressings in atopic dermatitis—a vehicle-controlled trial. Dermatology 2002;204(1): 56–9.
45. Tang W, Chan H. Outpatient, short-term, once-daily, diluted, 0.1 mometasone furoate wet-wraps for childhood atopic eczema. J Dermatolog Treat 1999;10: 157–63.
46. Tang WY. Diluted steroid facial wet wraps for childhood atopic eczema. Dermatology 2000;200(4):338–9.
47. Wolkerstorfer A, Visser RL, de Waard van der Spek FB, et al. Efficacy and safety of wet-wrap dressings in children with severe atopic dermatitis: influence of corticosteroid dilution. Br J Dermatol 2000;143(5):999–1004.
48. Carel K, Bratton DL, Miyazawa N, et al. The Atopic Dermatitis Quickscore (ADQ): validation of a new parent-administered atopic dermatitis scoring tool. Ann Allergy Asthma Immunol 2008;101(5):500–7.

Allergic Contact Dermatitis

Lisa Kostner, MD[a], Florian Anzengruber, MD[a],
Caroline Guillod, MD[a], Mike Recher, MD[b], Peter Schmid-Grendelmeier, MD[a],
Alexander A. Navarini, MD, PhD[a],*

KEYWORDS

- Contact • Dermatitis • Allergen • T cell • Patch • Work related

KEY POINTS

- Allergic contact dermatitis (ACD) is one of the most common work-related conditions.
- Clinical features of chronic ACD and irritant contact dermatitis may overlap.
- Identification of the offending allergen in ACD is often circumstantial.
- New techniques are required to overcome these challenges.

INTRODUCTION

Allergic contact dermatitis (ACD) seems a straightforward and simple disease. The problem is easily defined: it is a cutaneous immune reaction against 1 or more nontoxic allergens that come in contact with the skin. All the patient should need to do is to get rid of the allergen. However, detection, allergen avoidance, and therapy are often very difficult. Therefore, ACD can affect patients for years and is a grave socioeconomic problem.

ACD and irritant contact dermatitis (ICD) can lead to mostly similar clinical phenotypes, even though the latter is much more common and not caused by an immune reaction to well-defined allergens. Together they make up more than 90% of occupational skin disorders. Affected patients have great impairment in their quality of life and experience long periods of sick leave, which has an important socioeconomic impact.

The 1-year prevalence for allergic contact eczema is about 15%.[1,2] Therefore, it concerns groups of all ages with high prevalence and incidence, even though elderly people are often affected because of impaired epidermal barriers or alterations of immune reactivity.[3] The 2 main groups of contact eczema coexist in many cases and differentiating between them often proves to be difficult. Both diseases can have similar clinical and histologic aspects.

[a] Department of Dermatology, University Hospital Zurich, Gloriastrasse 31, 8091, Zurich, Switzerland; [b] Immunodeficiency Clinic, Medical Outpatient Unit and Immunodeficiency Lab, Department Biomedicine, University Hospital, Petersgraben 4, 4031, Basel, Switzerland
* Corresponding author.
E-mail address: alexander.navarini@usz.ch

Immunol Allergy Clin N Am 37 (2017) 141–152
http://dx.doi.org/10.1016/j.iac.2016.08.014
0889-8561/17/© 2016 Elsevier Inc. All rights reserved.
immunology.theclinics.com

EPIDEMIOLOGY

Between 4% and 7% of all dermatology consultations are for contact dermatitis. In Sweden, about 10% to 12% of adults had hand eczema during a period of 1 year. However, the tendency for ACD is decreasing slightly, and is inversely mirrored by the increase of atopic dermatitis. The point prevalence of contact sensitivity is 15.2% in teenagers. In adults, this is much higher and can reach 18.6%. This higher rate may be mostly caused by the cumulative opportunities of sensitization rather than an effect of age, because the latter does not have a direct influence on capability for sensitization. The prevalence of pure ACD is difficult to measure because ACD and ICD usually coexist. The incidence of occupational dermatitis per 1000 workers per year is about 0.5 to 1.9 in most European countries.

PATHOMECHANISM

ACD develops only after an initial sensitization[4] phase with usually innocuous substances; usually small molecules that cannot be recognized on their own by the adaptive immune system. However, when they are bound to cutaneous proteins they can associate with major histocompatibility complex (MHC) class II antigens (MHC II). Some chemicals can also directly bind to MHC II that are present on Langerhans cells and other epidermal antigen-presenting cells, mostly of dendritic origin. After application, it takes about 6 hours until the allergen is presented on these cells. Additional signals such as inflammatory cytokines (eg, tumor necrosis factor alpha, interleukin [IL] 1-β) can support sensitization and could arise from irritation of the skin, perhaps explaining the close connection of allergy and irritation in this disease. Also, MHC molecules are upregulated. The activation (priming) of specific T cells takes place in the lymph nodes. The antigen-presenting cells migrate there and depending on the nature of the antigen present it on MHC II (ie, a polar hapten) or MHC I (ie, the small lipid soluble molecule urushiol). T cells then proliferate in the lymph nodes, primed T-cell clones start to disseminate throughout the skin, and cutaneous lymphocyte antigen–positive T cells thereafter stay in the skin for long periods of time.[5] Activated T cells produce cytokines such as interferon gamma, IL-2, and IL-17. They are attracted to the locus of inflammation by keratinocyte-derived CCL27, which binds to their CCR10. T cells have an apoptotic effect on keratinocytes because of their FasL and perforin expression. These combined effects ultimately lead to the clinical phenotype of ACD. Taken together, the delayed hypersensitivity reaction is caused by the previously activated T cells, which only at second contact cause rapid inflammation.[6,7] As an exception, a single, prolonged contact with an allergen may lead to ACD, but this should require several days to develop. The sensitization phase is specific for ACD and is not a feature of ICD, even though similar clinical features develop in both conditions. In ICD, the inflammation is caused by the irritant, which (somewhat in contrast with ACD) is dose dependent.

CLINICAL FEATURES

ACD presents with erythema, edema, vesicles, oozing, and notably intense pruritus. In the mildest form, only erythema is visible at the site of contact; sometimes, the type of substance can be already suspected (ie, when liquid tracks are visible). Stronger reactions include spongiotic vesicles that itch and burst quickly, weeping intensively and crusting thereafter (**Fig. 1**A, B). In ACD caused by a single exposure, all lesions are at the same stage in this process.[8] When it becomes chronic, the term eczema is used and features such as hyperkeratosis, desquamation, lichenification, and

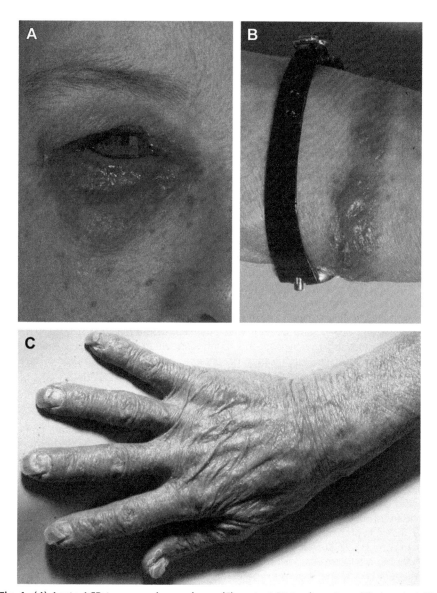

Fig. 1. (*A*) Acute ACD to neomycin eye drops; (*B*) acute ACD to chromium; (*C*) chronic ACD.

fissuring become more prominent[9] (**Fig. 1**C). The lesion is then less sharply circumscribed, infiltration and thickness of skin increase, lichenification marks develop, and regional differences in the stage of the inflammation can be seen. The localization plays an important role in the morphology of ACD, even though it can occur on every part of the body. Also, the body site gives important clues to the cause of ACD and is the starting point for detailed history taking, which is crucial to guide patch testing for identification of the responsible allergen. In delicate areas with a thin stratum corneum, such as the eyelids, penis, and scrotum, erythema and edema usually outweigh papules and vesicles. The same clinical features develop in allergic contact stomatitis and vulvitis.[9] An allergic contact reaction is typically not sharply limited. It is predominant in the area of contact, but can widely spread to other areas. In ectopic ACD, the allergen reaches the patients' skin by exceptional routes[7]:

- Autotransfer: for example, with nail lacquer located on the eyelids or on the neck (transfer by fingers)
- Heterotransfer: transfer of the allergen to another person, mainly the partner, also known as connubial ACD
- Airborne ACD: transport of the contact allergen by air (dust particles, vapors, or gasses; eg, from wall paint or pollen), typically clinical lesions on uncovered areas
- Photoallergic ACD: from ultraviolet (UV) light, clinical lesions on light-exposed zones; typically spares areas covered with clothes or shaded by hair, such as ears or scalp

Sometimes, generalized contact dermatitis occurs. The pathomechanism remains unclear. Exposure to high doses of allergens, dissemination via blood vessels, or a generalized activation of immunologic effector cells have all been suggested as potential explanations.[10] Atypical forms of ACD are dyshidrotic and pompholyx-type contact dermatitis, erythema multiforme–like reactions, pigmented purpura, pustular reactions, granulomas, and sclerodermalike lesions.[8]

In contrast, acute irritative-toxic dermatitis can present, apart from edema, erythema, vesicles, bullae, and oozing, with pustules, ulceration, and necrosis. It can also be characterized by dryness and roughness, whereas the chronic stadium is similar to chronic ACD. Pruritus may be present, but the main symptoms may be burning and pain. It is usually sharply defined and does not disseminate.[9]

DIFFERENTIAL DIAGNOSES

Numerous differentials must be considered, the primary one being various types of dermatitis of different causes, including irritative-toxic dermatitis, atopic dermatitis, dyshidrotic dermatitis, nummular dermatitis, stasis dermatitis, and lichen simplex chronicus.[11] Imitators of ACD that differ in pathophysiology and response to treatment include psoriasis, seborrheic dermatitis, pityriasis rosea, palmoplantar pustulosis, lichenoid dermatitis, lymphoma, and tinea manuum.[12] Eczema can also occur as a secondary phenomenon, such as in scabies, in which it occurs as a reaction to the mites' feces; in phthiriasis; mycoses, including candidiasis; and in impetiginous infections. In contrast, ACD can, rarely, also be concealed by noneczematous lesions such as erythema multiform–like lesions,[13,14] urticarial papular plaques, lichen planus–like and lichenoid eruptions,[15] purpuric petechial reactions,[16] dermal reactions,[17] lymphomatoid contact dermatitis,[18] granulomatous and pustular reactions,[19] and pemphigoidlike lesions.[20]

DIAGNOSIS

Because it is difficult to differentiate clinically between the various eczema entities, the collection of a precise medical history and a correct assignment of the morphologic patterns are the fundamental steps leading to a proper diagnosis and guiding subsequent patch tests.

A useful history should include:
- Time of onset and possible contact with allergens or irritants (temporal relationship)

- Contact area corresponding with reaction area
- Initial clinical patterns and evolution of morphology
- Working environment: exposure to potential allergens (even unexpected allergens, such as phone cards[21]); dose; frequency; duration; protective measures, such as gloves, masks, and barrier creams; and concomitant factors, such as humidity, temperature, occlusion, friction
- Similar situation in coworkers
- Leisure activities
- Domestic products, protective measures used while cleaning
- Skin care products, fragrances, nail and hair products
- Jewelry and clothing, communication devices
- Suspicion regarding autotransfer, heterotransfer (eg, connubial dermatitis), aerogen dermatitis, photoallergic dermatitis
- History of previous dermatitis (past contact dermatitis, patch testing, atopic diathesis, family history)

The clinical investigation should always register the body site and try to differentiate between probably primary site and spreading. It should be noted whether symmetry is present, erythema, fragile vesicles or dyshidrosiform sago-type vesicles, papules, scales, hyperkeratosis, lichenification, or infiltration. Lesions compatible with a differential of ACD should be sought, including for lichen planus and scabies. The nails must be examined for signs of dystrophy, onychomycosis, or psoriasis (oil spots).

ACD and ICD are often coexistent. It is also known that an ACD often develops from an ICD. Constant irritation may lead to increased penetration of potential allergens. The detailed evaluation of a patient's medical history and clinical features guides the selection of allergens for the patch test, which is the gold standard for diagnosis. Even though type I hypersensitivity reactions such as the protein contact allergy rarely occur,[22] the overwhelming part of ACD is caused by T cell–mediated delayed type IV reactions.

PATCH TEST

Patch testing is now the gold standard in diagnosing allergic contact eczema. It is the in vivo proof of the disease-causing effect of renewed contact with the allergen and evokes on a small scale the elicitation phase of a delayed hypersensitivity (type IV) reaction. It involves the application of a series of allergens in specific chambers directly on the skin (mostly the upper back).

Usually the specific allergens are carried on petrolatum-based vehicles in hypoallergenic chambers, which are attached on the patient's upper back. The standard series includes the most common allergens according to the German Contact Dermatitis Research Group (**Table 1**). A commercially available ready-made chamber system is called the TRUE Test, which guarantees an exact standardized dosage and a high bioavailability for the allergens. Bioavailability depends on many factors, such as intrinsic penetration capacity, concentration, vehicle, occlusivity of the patch test system and tape, and on the exposure time. The standardized TRUE system therefore is a good option to avoid biased results,[23,24] even though it is limited to a standard series of 35 common allergens and shows only partial overlap with the recommended standard series.[3]

In addition, the patients' history and clinical features should prompt selection of additional panels for testing, as well as the patient's own products in case of suspicion. Furthermore, an obligate irritant, such as sodium lauryl sulfate 0.25% or nonionic acid, can be applied as a positive control to check the skin's irritability at the time of

Table 1
Standard patch test series recommended by the German Contact Dermatitis Research Group

Substance	Vehicle	Concentration
Potassium dichromate	PET	0.5%
Thiuram mix	PET	1%
Cobalt (II) chloride, 6(H_2O)	PET	1%
Balsam of Peru	PET	25%
Colophony	PET	20%
N-Isopropyl-N'-phenyl paraphenylenediamine	PET	0.1%
Wool alcohols	PET	30%
Mercapto mix without MBT (only CBS, MBTS, MOR)	PET	1%
Epoxy resin	PET	1%
Nickel (II) sulfate, 6(H_2O)	PET	5%
Para tertiary butyl phenol formaldehyde resin	PET	1%
Formaldehyde	AQU	1%
Fragrance mix	PET	8%
Turpentine	PET	10%
(Chloro)-methylisothiazolinone (MCI/MI)	AQU	100 ppm
Paraben mix	PET	16%
Cetyl stearyl alcohol	PET	20%
Zinc bis(diethyldithiocarbamate)	PET	1%
Dibromodicyanobutane (methyldibromo glutaronitrile)	PET	0.2%
Propolis	PET	10%
Bufexamac	PET	5%
Compositae mix II	PET	5%
Mercaptobenzothiazole	PET	2%
Hydroxymethylpentylcyclohexenecarboxaldehyde (Lyral)	PET	5%
Bronopol (2-bromo-2-nitropropane-1,3-diol)	PET	0.5%
Fragrance mix II	PET	14%
Sodium lauryl sulfate	AQU	0.25%
Ylang-ylang (I + II) oil	PET	10%
Sandalwood oil	PET	10%
Jasmine absolute	PET	5%

Abbreviations: CBS, N-Cyclohexyl-2-benzothiazole-sulenamide; MBT, Mercaptobenzothiazole; MBTS, Mercapto Benzo Thiazole Sulphate; MOR, Morpholinylmercaptobenzothiazole; PET, Petrolatum.
   Data from German Dermatological Society, Erlangen, Germany. Available at: http://dkg.ivdk.org/dkgblo.html. Accessed October 2016.

exposure. A positive reaction to the sodium lauryl sulfate does not indicate an allergic reaction because it is purely irritant.[25] Patients under immunosuppression (including systemic steroids or active phototherapy at the side of testing) should not be tested because of false-negative results. This requirement is even more important because the patch test does not include a positive control.

   The first reading of the test is performed at 48 hours, when the patches are removed again. In some clinics, patches have already been removed at 24 hours. There is no strict agreement whether to keep it on for 24 hours or 48 hours. The reading should be done about half an hour after removing the test (after 48 hours, see earlier discussion), then after 72 hours, and at another time after 96 hours, especially if there are questionably positive results at 72 hours. A repeated reading after 1 week is highly suggested in order to avoid missing a delayed reaction (eg, neomycin, corticosteroids).[9] For the analysis, there are several scoring systems, but a commonly used evaluation method is the system described by Wilkinson and colleagues[26] (**Table 2**). Reading and scoring have to be repeated at each visit to check the progression or regression of the reaction (day 2, day 3, day 4, or day 7). A modification version has been proposed by Menné and White[27] (**Table 3**), but, to date, a worldwide consensus is lacking. Follicular reactions are common, such as to metals, and can be noted with an "f" beside the reaction intensity.

An increasing reaction (crescendo) in patch testing is compatible with an ACD; an initially positive and subsequently waning reaction (decrescendo) suggests an irritative cause.

Positive reactions to chemically similar allergens may indicate cross reactions. Positive reactions to more than 5 nonrelated substances can indicate polysensibilization,[28] but a so-called angry back/excited skin syndrome must be considered as well.[29,30] Angry back/excited skin syndrome can be ruled out by repeat testing of selected allergens about 2 months later.

LIMITATIONS OF PATCH TESTING

Pooling of data and objective comparisons are limited by the current lack of standardization, which includes the source and amount of allergens, variation in materials (chambers, vehicles), variation in the type of occlusion, the duration of application, reading times, and the score grading of patch test reactions.

The amount of allergen is important, because the reactions can provoke either false-positive (eg, by using an increased quantity of the allergen, causing an irritation instead of an allergic reaction) or false-negative reactions (eg, by using too little of the allergen). Ready-made tests or testing preparations seek to overcome this problem. Petrolatum is the most commonly used carrier for allergens, with the exception of the TRUE system, which takes advantage of a dried-in-gel vehicle such as polyvidone or a cellulose derivate. Not all allergens are stable over time; several have a unsatisfactory chemical stability because of oxidation.[9] The highest objectivity in reading and scoring can be achieved by detailed description of the reaction seen, as well as using a standardized score.

Table 2 Scoring of patch test reactions according to Wilkinson and colleagues[26] on behalf of the International Contact Dermatitis Research Group	
Score	**Interpretation**
−	Negative reaction
?+	Doubtful reaction; faint erythema only, not considered proven allergic reaction
+	Weak (nonvesicular) reaction; erythema, slight infiltration
++	Strong (edematous or vesicular) reaction; erythema, infiltration, vesicles
+++	Extreme (bullous or ulcerative)
IR	Irritant reactions of different types
NT	Not tested

From Wilkinson DS, Fregert S, Magnusson B, et al. Terminology of contact dermatitis. Acta Derm Venereol 1970;50(4):287–92; with permission.

Table 3
Scoring of patch test reactions, on behalf of European Contact Dermatitis Society and European Environmental and Contact Dermatitis Research Group

Score	Interpretation
+	Homogeneous redness in the test area with scattered papules
++	Homogeneous redness and homogeneous infiltration in the test area
+++	Homogeneous redness and infiltration with vesicles
++++	Homogeneous redness and infiltration with coalescing vesicles

From Menné T, White I. Standardization in contact dermatitis. Contact Dermatitis 2008;58(6):321; with permission.

Other disadvantages in patch testing are the possibilities to induce or reactivate hypersensitivity in sensibilized patients. Also, it can only be performed if there is no more active inflammation, otherwise the result could be a false-positive. No florid eczema or intense exposition to UV light should precede the test. There are no data available regarding patch testing in pregnancy. For this reason, the International Contact Dermatitis Research Group advises against testing pregnant women.[7] For medicaments and patch testing there are only unclear or controversial data available. For corticosteroids there is no consensus yet, but, according to Lachapelle and Maibach,[7] patch testing in patients undergoing corticosteroid therapy requires caution in the evaluation phase and we advise against it (see earlier). For antihistamines there is no general agreement, so in most centers treatment with antihistamines is paused during testing.[31] In addition, immunomodulators may alter the results[32] so, whenever possible, they should be avoided during testing.

SURVEY OF PATCH TEST REACTIONS VIA DIGITAL IMAGING

A recent pilot study by Boone and colleagues[33] was designed to distinguish doubtful (+?) allergic contact reactions from irritant reactions. High-definition optical coherence tomography (HD-OCT) offers noninvasive, in vivo, real-time, three-dimensional measurement of the epidermal thickness, and it showed that an increased thickness of the epidermis correlates with irritant reactions, which may be counterintuitive for some experts. Furthermore, specific HD-OCT features corresponded with the severity of visual scoring. This peculiarity might lead to more objectivity in the scoring of inflammatory reactions. Standard three-dimensional photography may soon be available at sufficient resolution to reliably allow grading of reactions.

MODIFICATIONS OF PATCH TESTING

1. Strip patch testing: can increase the sensitivity of patch testing by decreasing the thickness of the stratum corneum, which results in a higher penetration of the allergens
2. Repeated open application test: repeated open application of an allergen over a few days; for example, when patch testing is negative but ACD from a specific allergen is highly probable
3. Atopy patch testing: for the diagnosis of aerogenic or alimentary allergens in patients with atopic history; not yet sufficiently validated
4. Scratch testing[34]
5. Prick testing: in suspicion of type I allergy, such as protein contact allergy[3]

IN VITRO TESTS

In vitro lymphocyte stimulation tests expose blood-derived lymphocytes to controlled, purified amounts of allergens. A proliferation (traditionally measured with H_3 thymidine incorporation) correlating with increasing titers of allergen is interpreted as allergen-specific reaction. Especially for metal salts, these assays are very well validated. In vitro assays allow more control but have several disadvantages. First, allergens must be free of nonspecific stimulatory compounds, such as lipopolysaccharide. Second, a proliferation to an allergen does not allow the conclusion that a manifest allergy is present. Third, newer data[35] have shown that most allergen-specific T cells are in the skin. Thus, the sensitivity of tests with peripheral blood mononuclear cells may not be high. Fourth, the in vitro tests are very labor intensive and have limited sensitivity and specificity. They are not standardized enough to be available as kits; instead, the tests must be performed by experienced, specialized laboratories and results must be carefully evaluated. Thus, they are not used for routine diagnostics for ACD.[3,36]

TREATMENT

One of the most important measures in the prevention of ACD is avoidance of contact with the respective allergens. Often this is not feasible because of work or environmental circumstances. In these cases, patients need to be carefully instructed about protective arrangements, such as the wearing of appropriate clothes (eg, gloves, masks) and barrier creams.

Most frequently, acute and chronic ACD are treated with topical corticosteroids (class II–III, most usually mometasone furoate or betamethasone). Even though palms and soles are not considered high-risk regions for steroid-induced atrophy, some atrophy is often observed after long-term treatment and may contribute to the areas' risk of being a minoris locus resistentiae to eczema. In these situations, and especially in areas with thin epidermis, such as intertriginous areas, topical calcineurin inhibitors (eg, tacrolimus, pimecrolimus) are good choices for maintenance therapy after a short spell of steroids to reduce inflammation. They do not cause skin atrophy and have been shown to be useful to dampen chronic inflammation in atopic dermatitis.[37] In some cases, antihistamines can also reduce pruritus.

Individuals with chronic ACD may benefit from narrow-band UV-B phototherapy or psoralen plus UV-A (PUVA) treatments. Systemic retinoids, especially the new retinoid alitretinoin but also acitretin, are very successful in treating eczema.[38]

Because of their teratogenicity, contraception is key. In special cases, a short course of systemic corticosteroid therapy can be useful, particularly in cases of systemic contact allergies as a result of hematogenic dissemination. Rarely, immunosuppressive agents such as cyclosporine, azathioprine, or mycophenolate are also used in chronic ACD.[3] It remains unknown whether biologics such as the IL-4/IL-13 antagonist dupilumab or the IL-6 antagonist tocilizumab[39] are beneficial in ACD.

CURRENT CONTROVERSIES

There are few fields more controversial than ACD and its diagnostic techniques. Since the conception of the patch test by Josef Jadassohn (1863–1936) and further development by Bruno Bloch (1878–1933), every aspect of diagnosis and test has been challenged.

Who should be patch tested? Every eczematous dermatosis? A general rule is that patch testing should produce positive test results between 30% and 65% of the time.[40] This guide may help clinicians to adjust their thresholds of ordering patch tests, but is little help in deciding whether a given patient should be patch tested or not. The most promising candidates for patch testing are eczematous disorders in which ACD is suspected or failing to respond to treatment, chronic hand and foot dermatitis, or stasis eczema, and also scattered generalized distribution of dermatitis.

What standard series should be used? It is different in every country. This question is controversial and not all selections seem to be strictly evidence based and in accord with locally prevalent allergies. Also, minor factors, such as the size of testing chambers, can affect the outcome of patch testing.

Interpretation of the relevance of positive patch test reactions is a challenge for dermatologists.[41] The circumstantial nature of the patch test does not allow a direct conclusion on the allergen causing the ACD, therefore each reaction must be considered in the context of the patient's history and clinical features.

Understanding of the pathophysiology of ACD may soon change. In the past, ACD was thought to depend on the systemic presence of primed T cells that were expected to be everywhere in the skin. Therefore, a negative reaction in a patch test was usually interpreted as an absence of sensitized T cells against the respective allergen in the tested patient. However, because newer data showed predominant numbers of T cells residing in the skin and staying locally for prolonged periods of time, it could be that some contact allergies are local phenomena.

The reasons for irritant and allergic reactions showing similar histologic (including T-cell infiltrates) and clinical patterns remain unclear. It could be that latent, perhaps nonspecific, T cells are expanded on irritation of the skin, but this remains largely unproved.

Taken together, the study of ACD continues to thrive and evolve. These conditions affect a high percentage of the population and are ideal targets for further investigation for prevention and treatment. In the future, new forms of contact allergy diagnostics and, it is hoped, standardized procedures for testing and interpretation of the relevance of positive findings may be developed.

REFERENCES

1. Johannisson A, Ponten A, Svensson A. Prevalence, incidence and predictive factors for hand eczema in young adults - a follow-up study. BMC Dermatol 2013;13: 14.
2. Hermann-Kunz E. Incidence of allergic diseases in East and West Germany. Gesundheitswesen 1999;61(Spec No):S100–5 [in German].
3. Brasch J, Becker D, Aberer W, et al. Guideline contact dermatitis: S1-Guidelines of the German Contact Allergy Group (DKG) of the German Dermatology Society (DDG), the Information Network of Dermatological Clinics (IVDK), the German Society for Allergology and Clinical Immunology (DGAKI), the Working Group for Occupational and Environmental Dermatology (ABD) of the DDG, the Medical Association of German Allergologists (AeDA), the Professional Association of German Dermatologists (BVDD) and the DDG. Allergo J Int 2014;23(4):126–38.
4. Bonneville M, Chavagnac C, Vocanson M, et al. Skin contact irritation conditions the development and severity of allergic contact dermatitis. J Invest Dermatol 2007;127(6):1430–5.
5. Clark RA, Chong B, Mirchandani N, et al. The vast majority of CLA+ T cells are resident in normal skin. J Immunol 2006;176(7):4431–9.
6. Martin SF. Allergic contact dermatitis: xenoinflammation of the skin. Curr Opin Immunol 2012;24(6):720–9.

7. Lachapelle JM, Maibach HI. Patch testing and prick testing, vol. 3. Germany: Springer; 2012.

8. Brasch J, Becker D, Aberer W, et al. Contact dermatitis. J Dtsch Dermatol Ges 2007;5(10):943–51.

9. Ale IS, Maibacht HA. Diagnostic approach in allergic and irritant contact dermatitis. Expert Rev Clin Immunol 2010;6(2):291–310.

10. Veien NK. Systemic contact dermatitis. Int J Dermatol 2011;50(12):1445–56.

11. Becker D. Allergic contact dermatitis. J Dtsch Dermatol Ges 2013;11(7):607–19 [quiz: 620-1].

12. Quah CH, Koh D, How CH, et al. Approach to hand dermatitis in primary care. Singapore Med J 2012;53(11):701–4 [quiz: p 705].

13. Kerre S, Busschots A, Dooms-Goossens A. Erythema-multiforme-like contact dermatitis due to phenylbutazone. Contact Dermatitis 1995;33(3):213–4.

14. Stingeni L, Caraffini S, Assalve D, et al. Erythema-multiforme-like contact dermatitis from budesonide. Contact Dermatitis 1996;34(2):154–5.

15. Yiannias JA, el-Azhary RA, Hand JH, et al. Relevant contact sensitivities in patients with the diagnosis of oral lichen planus. J Am Acad Dermatol 2000;42(2 Pt 1):177–82.

16. Roed-Petersen J, Clemmensen OJ, Menné T, et al. Purpuric contact dermatitis from black rubber chemicals. Contact Dermatitis 1988;18(3):166–8.

17. Katoh N, Hirano S, Kishimoto S, et al. Dermal contact dermatitis caused by allergy to palladium. Contact Dermatitis 1999;40(4):226–7.

18. Orbaneja JG, Diez LI, Lozano JL, et al. Lymphomatoid contact dermatitis: a syndrome produced by epicutaneous hypersensitivity with clinical features and a histopathologic picture similar to that of mycosis fungoides. Contact Dermatitis 1976;2(3):139–43.

19. Sanchez-Motilla JM, Pont V, Nagore E, et al. Pustular allergic contact dermatitis from minoxidil. Contact Dermatitis 1998;38(5):283–4.

20. Stransky L. The so-called contact dermatoses. Contact Dermatitis 1998;38(4):216–7.

21. Schmid-Grendelmeier P, Elsner P. Contact dermatitis due to occupational dibutylthiourea exposure: a case of phonecard dermatitis. Contact Dermatitis 1995;32(5):308–9.

22. Levin C, Warshaw E. Protein contact dermatitis: allergens, pathogenesis, and management. Dermatitis 2008;19(5):241–51.

23. Fischer T, Maibach H. Patch test allergens in petrolatum: a reappraisal. Contact Dermatitis 1984;11(4):224–8.

24. Fischer TI, Maibach HI. The thin layer rapid use epicutaneous test (TRUE-test), a new patch test method with high accuracy. Br J Dermatol 1985;112(1):63–8.

25. Loffler H, Becker D, Brasch J, et al. Simultaneous sodium lauryl sulphate testing improves the diagnostic validity of allergic patch tests. Results from a prospective multicentre study of the German Contact Dermatitis Research Group (Deutsche Kontaktallergie-Gruppe, DKG). Br J Dermatol 2005;152(4):709–19.

26. Wilkinson DS, Fregert S, Magnusson B, et al. Terminology of contact dermatitis. Acta Derm Venereol 1970;50(4):287–92.

27. Menné T, White I. Standardization in contact dermatitis. Contact Dermatitis 2008;58(6):321.

28. Carlsen BC, Andersen KE, Menné T, et al. Patients with multiple contact allergies: a review. Contact Dermatitis 2008;58(1):1–8.

29. Brasch J, Geier J, Schnuch A, et al. A high-positive patch test load correlates with further positive patch test reactions irrespective of their location. Allergy 2006; 61(12):1411–5.

30. Schnuch A, Brasch J, Lessmann H, et al. A further characteristic of susceptibility to contact allergy: sensitization to a weak contact allergen is associated with polysensitization. Results of the IVDK. Contact Dermatitis 2007;56(6):331–7.

31. Elston D, Licata A, Rudner E, et al. Pitfalls in patch testing. Am J Contact Dermat 2000;11(3):184–8.

32. Wee JS, White JM, McFadden JP, et al. Patch testing in patients treated with systemic immunosuppression and cytokine inhibitors. Contact Dermatitis 2010; 62(3):165–9.

33. Boone MA, Jemec GB, Del Marmol V. Differentiating allergic and irritant contact dermatitis by high-definition optical coherence tomography: a pilot study. Arch Dermatol Res 2015;307(1):11–22.

34. Indrajana T, Spieksma FT, Voorhorst R. Comparative study of the intracutaneous, scratch and prick tests in allergy. Ann Allergy 1971;29(12):639–50.

35. Gaide O, Emerson RO, Jiang X, et al. Common clonal origin of central and resident memory T cells following skin immunization. Nat Med 2015;21(6):647–53.

36. Renz H, Becker WM, Bufe A, et al. In vitro allergy diagnosis. Guideline of the German Society of Asthma and Immunology in conjunction with the German Society of Dermatology. J Dtsch Dermatol Ges 2006;4(1):72–85 [in German].

37. Wong E, Kurian A. Off-label uses of topical calcineurin inhibitors. Skin Therapy Lett 2016;21(1):8–10.

38. Ruzicka T, Lynde CW, Jemec GB, et al. Efficacy and safety of oral alitretinoin (9-cis retinoic acid) in patients with severe chronic hand eczema refractory to topical corticosteroids: results of a randomized, double-blind, placebo-controlled, multicentre trial. Br J Dermatol 2008;158(4):808–17.

39. Navarini AA, French LE, Hofbauer GF. Interrupting IL-6-receptor signaling improves atopic dermatitis but associates with bacterial superinfection. J Allergy Clin Immunol 2011;128(5):1128–30.

40. Cronin E. Clinical prediction of patch test results. Trans St Johns Hosp Dermatol Soc 1972;58(2):153–62.

41. Kligman AM. A personal critique of diagnostic patch testing. Clin Dermatol 1996; 14(1):35–40.

Mastocytosis and Anaphylaxis

Anna Schuch, MD, Knut Brockow, MD*

KEYWORDS

- Mastocytosis • Mast cell activation syndrome • Anaphylaxis • Risk factors
- Triggers • Hymenoptera venom anaphylaxis • Drug-induced anaphylaxis

KEY POINTS

- There are two major forms of indolent systemic mastocytosis associated with anaphylaxis: the classical form with mastocytosis in the skin, and a form without skin lesions becoming apparent only through the occurrence of anaphylactic reactions.
- Anaphylactic reactions in mastocytosis mostly are associated with Hymenoptera stings, but also may be occasionally labeled idiopathic anaphylaxis or triggered by food or drugs.
- In children anaphylaxis is uncommon, mostly idiopathic, and manifests normally during active blistering episodes in those with extensive skin involvement and high serum, whereas adults with systemic mastocytosis carry a 20%–50% risk for anaphylaxis, but with less defined risk factors.
- Because mastocytosis is a well-recognized basis for anaphylaxis, emergency preparedness, including availability and use of emergency medications and, if indicated, life-long venom immunotherapy, is necessary.

INTRODUCTION

Mastocytosis (MC) is a proliferative disorder of hematopoetic mast cell progenitors,[1] which leads to an expansion and accumulation of excessive numbers of mast cells in one or more organs, such as skin, bone marrow, gastrointestinal tract, liver, and spleen.[1,2] The basis of the disease is an activating mutation in the mast cell growth receptor KIT, a protein tyrosine kinase receptor, most commonly a point mutation with exchange of aspartic acid to valine in codon 816 (D816V).[3] More than 80% of all patients with systemic mastocytosis (SM) carry the D816V mutation.[4]

Whereas in most children only the skin seems to be involved (cutaneous MC [CM]), in adults, other organs are also affected (SM). To diagnose SM, according to the World

Disclosure Statement: The authors have nothing to disclose.
Department of Dermatology and Allergy Biederstein, Technische Universität München, Munich, Germany
* Corresponding author. Department of Dermatology and Allergy Biederstein, Technische Universität München, Biedersteiner Straße 29, Munich 80802, Germany.
E-mail address: knut.brockow@tum.de

Immunol Allergy Clin N Am 37 (2017) 153–164
http://dx.doi.org/10.1016/j.iac.2016.08.017   immunology.theclinics.com

Health Organization, several criteria have to be fulfilled. In detail, there are one major and four minor criteria for SM (**Box 1**), of which one major and one minor or three minor criteria are required for diagnosing SM.[2,5]

The overall prevalence of SM in all adults with MC has been reported to be more than 95%.[6,7] In adult SM, there is a subfraction of patients without presence of skin lesions. Comparing these patients with and without MC in the skin (MIS) there is a male predominance and history of insect-sting anaphylaxis in those without MIS.[8] A study, for which patients with classical skin lesions and patients with insect-sting or idiopathic anaphylaxis were recruited, showed almost equal numbers of patients with indolent SM (ISM) with and without skin lesions.[9]

SM is subdivided into different clinical forms according to aggressiveness and prognosis. The most common form (90%–95% of all patients) is ISM. Rare advanced forms are SM with an associated hematologic non–mast cell disorder, aggressive SM and mast cell leukemia.[10] The cumulative probability of disease progression in patients with ISM is low (calculated to be 1.7% in 10 years) and patients with ISM carry a normal life expectancy.[7]

Anaphylaxis is a systemic or generalized life-threatening and potentially fatal systemic hypersensitivity reaction.[11] Clinically, criteria for anaphylaxis have been defined.[12] Typically, it occurs after contact to a known allergen (eg, peanut ingestion) and involves at least two out of the four organ systems: skin (eg, flush, urticaria, angioedema), gastrointestinal tract (eg, abdominal pain, nausea, diarrhea), pulmonary system (eg, wheezing, dyspnea), and cardiovascular system (eg, hypotension, shock).[12]

In addition to patients with SM, there are patients with anaphylaxis that carry clonal mast cells expressing the D816V KIT mutation, but that do not meet enough criteria to diagnose MC. This condition has been named monoclonal mast cell activation syndrome (MMCAS).[13,14]

EPIDEMIOLOGY
Prevalence of Mastocytosis

In 1997 it was calculated that 1 in 1000 to 8000 new patients in dermatology outpatient departments may have some form of MC.[15] More recent studies found a prevalence of ISM of 9.6 to 13 in 100,000 people and an incidence for all subtypes of SM of 0.89 per 100,000 per year.[16,17]

Box 1
Criteria for the diagnosis of systemic mastocytosis

Major criterion

- Multifocal dense aggregates of ≥15 mast cells in bone marrow and/or other extracutaneous tissues

Minor criteria

- Morphologically atypical mast cells in smears of biopsy sections of bone marrow or other extracutaneous organs
- Aberrant expression of CD25 and/or CD2 by mast cells in the bone marrow
- D816V KIT mutation in bone marrow, blood, or other extracutaneous organs
- Serum tryptase levels >20 μg/L

Prevalence of Atopy and Allergy in Mastocytosis

Smaller studies have reported that the prevalence of atopy in patients with MC is similar to that of the general population.[18,19] In addition, a comparison of prevalence rates of IgE-mediated allergy among patients with MC and in the general population has shown no significant difference.[2]

Prevalence of Anaphylaxis in General Population

The general prevalence of anaphylaxis can only been estimated using data from different studies. One study based on a survey of 1000 US citizens selected at random suggests that the lifetime risk of systemic anaphylaxis may be at least 1.6%.[20] A more conservative systematic review has estimated a cumulative lifetime prevalence of 0.3% and the incidence to be about 5 per 100,000 person years.[21]

Prevalence of Anaphylaxis in Patients with Mastocytosis

In children with MC, the percentage of anaphylaxis has been reported to be between 6%[19] and 9%.[22] In adults, the cumulative prevalence of anaphylaxis is much higher, estimated to be 22%,[19] 43%,[23] and 49%[22] in different study populations, which may be roughly 100-times as much as in the general population. The overall risk for anaphylactic reactions is increased for patients with SM compared with patients with MC limited to the skin.[22] Anaphylaxis also seems to occur more often in patients with ISM without cutaneous involvement.[2,22,23] This, however, is no surprise, because the symptom leading to the diagnosis of SM in most patients without skin involvement is anaphylaxis, whereas skin lesions are the leading manifestation in those with MIS and the prevalence of anaphylaxis in this group is lower than 50%.

According to the previously mentioned prevalence rates, the cumulative lifetime prevalence of MC together with anaphylaxis in adults may be estimated to be between 0.002% and 0.006%.

RISK FACTORS FOR ANAPHYLAXIS IN PATIENTS WITH MASTOCYTOSIS

In one study in children with MC, the most common systemic symptoms were diarrhea and abdominal pain, whereas anaphylaxis was only present in 1.5%.[24] In addition to the number of skin lesions, the number of skin symptoms, such as itching, blistering, and flushing, were significant predictors of the number of systemic symptoms, showing a linear correlation.[24] The extent and density of skin lesions and higher serum tryptase values have also been identified as risk factors for anaphylaxis in children (**Table 1**).[22] Moreover, it was shown that diffused CM, the most severe form of CM, is a risk factor for more severe anaphylaxis.[25]

Another study with 111 children suffering from MIS, which was designed to find predictors for severe mast cell activation episodes mostly resembling anaphylaxis, showed that all 12 children with severe symptoms who required hospitalization had extensive cutaneous disease, more than 90% of the body surface area involved, and significantly higher levels of serum tryptase compared with the other children without such severe reactions.[26] In addition, blistering episodes seemed to be a risk factor for hospitalization.[27] Thus, severe systemic symptoms often fulfilling the criteria for anaphylaxis in children with MIS are likely to develop in those patients with a severe skin involvement with MC lesions, high serum tryptase levels, blistering episodes, and diffused CM, whereas the risk in the remainder seems low.

Anaphylaxis in adults was more common in those with SM than in patients with CM.[22] In patients with SM and MIS, the extent and density of skin involvement was not associated with a higher risk of anaphylaxis.[22,23,28] Baseline serum tryptase has

Table 1
Possible risk factors for anaphylaxis in patients with mastocytosis

Patient Group	Risk Factor	Outcome	Study
Children	Extent and density of skin lesions	Anaphylaxis in those with extent >45% and density >15%	Brockow et al,[22] 2008
	Serum tryptase	Significantly elevated in patients with anaphylaxis	Brockow et al,[22] 2008
		Correlation with severity	Alvarez-Twose et al,[26] 2012
	Skin involvement >90%	Risk factor for hospitalization[a]	Alvarez-Twose et al,[26] 2012
	Blistering	Risk factor for hospitalization[a]	Brockow et al,[27] 2012
	Diffuse cutaneous mastocytosis	Risk factor for hospitalization[a]	Alvarez-Twose et al,[26] 2012
Adults	Extent and density of skin lesions	Not significant	Brockow et al,[22] 2008 Gülen et al,[23] 2014
	Serum tryptase	Elevated in patients with anaphylaxis (high overlap)	Brockow et al,[22] 2008
	Form of systemic mastocytosis	Mostly in indolent systemic mastocytosis	Gülen et al,[23] 2014
	D816V allele burden	No difference	Broesby-Olsen et al,[31] 2013

[a] Hospitalization because of severe mast cell activation episodes.

been reported to be higher in those with as compared with those without anaphylaxis, however, with a large overlap.[22] Male sex, tryptase levels greater than 25 ng/mL, anaphylaxis with cardiovascular symptoms (eg, dizziness, syncope) in the absence of urticaria or angioedema, and anaphylaxis to Hymenoptera venom have been described as indicators for MC in unselected patients with anaphylaxis.[29] The correlation between the risk of anaphylaxis and serum tryptase values does not seem to be linear. The prevalence of Hymenoptera venom allergy in adults was rising with basal serum tryptase levels up to a peak of around 28 ng/mL and decreasing with higher levels.[30]

The highest risk for anaphylactic reactions comes with the diagnosis of ISM.[23,28] Surprisingly, there is no evidence that anaphylaxis is more common in patients with more advanced SM (eg, mast cell leukemia, aggressive SM). On the contrary, in our experience it seems to be less common. Furthermore, the allele burden of KIT D816V mutation measured by quantitative real-time polymerase chain reaction was not different between adults with or without anaphylaxis.[31]

PATHOPHYSIOLOGY

The tyrosine kinase receptor KIT and its ligand stem cell factor controls differentiation and proliferation of mast cells.[32] In MC, mast cells carrying an activating D816V mutation are a basis for the disease. The mutation causes a ligand-independent activation of the receptor, leading to expansion of the mast cell population.[3] It has been speculated that these cells also may be hyperactive to external triggers, such as allergens, which may result in a lower threshold for anaphylaxis. This, however, has not yet been proven. In addition, because MC is associated with an increased number of body mast cells, that is, a higher number of potential effector cells for immediate-type allergies, this could result in potentially higher mediator release and more severe symptoms of anaphylaxis (**Fig. 1**).

CLINICAL FEATURES

Anaphylaxis in patients with MC principally presents with the same symptoms and manifestations as in patients without MC. However, cardiovascular symptoms, such as dizziness, tachycardia, hypotension, and/or syncope, tend to be more common and skin reactions, such as urticaria and angioedema, respiratory symptoms, and gastrointestinal reactions less frequent.[22,23] In comparison with patients with idiopathic anaphylaxis without MC, in patients with ISM, hypotension in the absence of urticaria occurred significantly more often.[33] The severity of anaphylaxis in adults with ISM seems to be increased. In one study, 48% of reactions were classified as severe and 38% resulted in unconsciousness[22]; another study reported unconsciousness in 72% of patients.[23]

TRIGGERS OF ANAPHYLAXIS IN MASTOCYTOSIS

Most frequently reported triggers for anaphylaxis in adults with MC are Hymenoptera stings, whereas food and medication are reported less frequently.[22] In unselected patients with food or drug anaphylaxis, elevated basal serum tryptase levels and MC are uncommon.[34] Physical stimuli, such as exposition to heat or cold, fast changes of temperature, rubbing of skin lesions (Darier sign), or stress and anxiety can lead to mast cell activation.[2] Anaphylaxis after jumping into cold water has been reported anecdotally. If no potential trigger is found, idiopathic anaphylaxis is diagnosed.[35]

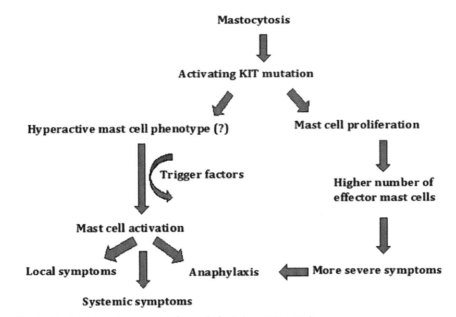

Fig. 1. Model for pathogenesis of anaphylaxis in mastocytosis.

Hymenoptera Venom Anaphylaxis in Mastocytosis

Elevated baseline tryptase levels or urticaria pigmentosa have been found in about 5% to 15% of those patients with Hymenoptera venom anaphylaxis (HVA),[36,37] both indicating a possible underlying mast cell disease, such as SM. Most patients with SM without MIS are diagnosed in the follow-up of Hymenoptera venom allergy and elevated tryptase levels. MC has been identified to be a risk factor for severe anaphylaxis to Hymenoptera venom[37] and in patients with honey bee or vespid venom allergy, elevated baseline serum tryptase values were associated with the risk of severe anaphylaxis.[38]

Having an increased risk of severe reactions, the correct diagnosis and therapy for HVA is important for patients with SM. Unfortunately, in MC total sIgE levels are often lower, which leads more often to negative sIgE and negative skin tests compared with patients with HVA without MC.[39] Thus, it might be necessary to use recombinant allergens (Ves v1/5 and Api m1-4/10) and a diagnostic cutoff of 0.1 KU/L in patients with low total sIgE to diagnose HVA correctly.[40] An additional diagnostic tool to use in these patients is the basophil activation test, which is sometimes able to confirm sensitization or to identify the culprit insect.[41]

Idiopathic Anaphylaxis in Mastocytosis

Idiopathic anaphylaxis is common in patients with MC.[23] No trigger factors are found in about 67% of all anaphylactic reactions in children and in 13% of the adult cases.[22] Before idiopathic anaphylaxis is diagnosed, all potential triggers have to be ruled out.

Food Anaphylaxis in Mastocytosis

Whereas many adult patients with MC suspect foods as triggers of anaphylaxis, in only few of them can these triggers be confirmed.[19,22,23] Nevertheless, recently published cases indicate that food allergy has to be considered in patients with MC. One patient with ISM presented with greater than 10 anaphylactic episodes after eating meat. In this patient, the provocation test with pork resulted in delayed occurring severe anaphylaxis despite low levels of specific IgE to meats and galactose-α-1,3-galactose.[42] Two other cases of IgE-mediated fish- and crustacean-induced anaphylaxis were reported, where further assessment showed an underlying ISM.[43]

Anaphylaxis Caused by Drugs

Only a minority of cases with drug-induced anaphylaxis are associated with MC. Many of them were related to general anesthesia, others to nonsteroidal anti-inflammatory drugs (NSAIDs), opioids, contrast media, β-lactams, or other drugs typically leading to anaphylaxis.[44] Anaphylaxis during general anesthesia is an area of concern.[45,46] In patients with MC who underwent different kinds of anesthetic techniques (general, local, and epidural anesthesia or sedation) 2% of the adult cases and 4% of the pediatric cases have been reported to develop perioperative symptoms related to mast cell activation, resulting in anaphylaxis in 0.4% of the adults and in 1 out of 40 children.[47] Symptoms presenting in adults were hypotension, cardiorespiratory arrest, coagulopathy, generalized urticaria, and loss of consciousness, whereas bronchospasm and generalized erythema was present in the pediatric case. Severe anaphylaxis has anecdotally been reported in patients with SM after intake of acetylsalicylic acid.[48]

However, MC was an uncommon diagnosis when patients with hypersensitivity reactions to NSAIDs were analyzed. In patients with NSAID hypersensitivity, no association to elevated basal serum tryptase levels was found, which is in contrast to patients with HVA.[49]

Anaphylaxis in the Context of Mast Cell Activation Syndrome

For some patients and clinicians the term "mast cell activation syndrome" (MCAS) may be confusing. It has been introduced to propose a global unifying classification of all mast cell disorders.[50] The classification includes three distinct types of MCAS. (1) MC and MMCAS constitute primary MCAS. Patients with MMCAS have the same triggers for anaphylaxis as patients with MC (described previously).[13,14,36] (2) Type I allergies are the main cause for secondary MCAS. (3) Idiopathic MCAS is the diagnosis, when no primary MCAS or trigger for secondary MCAS is found despite confirmed episodes with mast cell activation. Typical examples are idiopathic anaphylaxis or chronic sporadic urticaria. Thus, if a patient had MC, HVA anaphylaxis, and idiopathic anaphylaxis together, he or she would fulfill criteria for primary, secondary, and idiopathic MCAS. However, there is no additional benefit in calling anaphylaxis secondary (allergic) or idiopathic MCAS, because it is a well-recognized and well-described entity itself. Patients believing to suffer from idiopathic MCAS with polysymptomatic symptoms compatible with mast cell activation (eg, chronic diarrhea, headache, pruritus) do not seem to have an obviously increased risk for anaphylaxis.

ACUTE MANAGEMENT

Because patients with MC have a high risk for anaphylactic reactions and often present more severe symptoms than patients without MC, immediate therapy is necessary and delay may result in fatal reactions.[51] The first-line medication is epinephrine, administered at a dose of 0.3 mg to 0.5 mg in adults and 0.01 mg/kg in children. This should be primarily administered intramuscularly and can be repeated every 5 to 15 minutes, if necessary.[11,52] In cases of severe hypotension or cardiac arrest an intravenous bolus infusion under monitoring cardiac response is suggested (eg, 1–10 μg/min). Supporting measures are high-flow oxygen, positioning the patient in the flat Trendelenburg position, and volume replacement.

Bronchospasm responds best to inhaled β-agonists (eg, salbutamol) or epinephrine. Other therapeutics are H_1 and H_2 antihistamines. Steroids are often given; however, their action seems to be on the prevention of protracted or biphasic reactions than in the acute management of anaphylactic reactions because of their slow onset of action.[11]

CHRONIC MANAGEMENT
Emergency Preparedness

Adults with MC and children with extensive skin involvement or high levels of serum tryptase have a high risk of anaphylaxis. For these patients it is recommended to carry an epinephrine autoinjector at all times.[53] In German-speaking countries, emergency kits also contain a rapid-acting H_1 antihistamine (eg, dimethindene or cetirizine) and a corticosteroid (eg, betamethasone), both for oral use.[54] When handing out an emergency kit, it is important to provide an appropriate instruction how to use the emergency medication, or even better an anaphylaxis education.[55] It should be ensured that the patient and his or her close environment recognize anaphylaxis, can use the epinephrine autoinjector correctly, and are instructed to call for professional help immediately.[56] In Germany an MC pass is handed out to the patient with information on acute treatment, prescribed emergency medication, and drugs to avoid or to be given under medical supervision.

Venom Immunotherapy in Mastocytosis

Venom immunotherapy (VIT) is recommended for all patients with Hymenoptera allergy (general urticaria, angioedema, or anaphylaxis) and MC. In patients with MC side effects are more frequent than in general patients with HVA, especially in those with yellow jacket venom allergy.[57] Systemic reactions to VIT seem to happen in 18%[58] to 24%[59] of treated patients with SM, whereas VIT was generally tolerated without any side effects in patients with CM.[60] Moreover, in MC the efficacy of VIT is slightly reduced, indicated by higher rates of systemic reactions to sting challenges during the first year of VIT.[58] Most of those patients are protected by an increase of the maintenance dose to 150 μg or 200 μg.[61] In patients with SM who discontinued VIT after uneventful treatment, cases of fatal anaphylactic reactions have been described after being restung by the culprit insect. This has been described for yellow jacket and honey bee venom allergy.[62,63]

In summary, VIT is highly recommended for patients with Hymenoptera allergy and SM. It should be optimally performed either with a sting challenge to control efficacy or with an increased maintenance dose of 200 μg and should best be carried out lifelong.

Anesthesia in Patients with Mastocytosis

MC is not a contraindication for anesthesia. Most patients with anaphylaxis after anesthesia had previously unrecognized SM. If this diagnosis is known, precautions may be taken and emergency preparedness may be achieved. It has been recommended to administer a prophylactic premedication before anesthesia. Most premedications include an H_1 (and possibly an H_2 antihistamine) and/or corticosteroids. However, the efficacy of such a premedication in this setting has not been proven. In one study in children with severe CM where no specific premedication had been given, but where the anesthesiologists chose the appropriate conditions, no serious adverse event occurred out of 29 diagnostic and surgical procedures.[64] Thus, deviations from routine anesthesia techniques are not necessarily warranted. However, a meticulous preparation and understanding of anesthetic implications are advised. For example, it may be considered to reduce stress and anxiety by the use of benzodiazepines and to avoid temperature changes and mechanical stimulation for the patient.[2,47]

Further Treatment Options for Severe Cases of Recurrent Anaphylaxis

Recent publications show that omalizumab has proven to prevent symptoms, such as urticaria, gastrointestinal affliction, and hypotension, and can help to reduce adverse events during VIT.[65] This therapy has also shown to be effective in patients with idiopathic anaphylaxis and MC. The first approach, however, may be to administer high doses of antimediator therapy (H_1 and H_2 antihistamines, cromoglycate, montelukast), which is often sufficient (authors' personal experience).

In patients with recurrent severe life-threatening anaphylactic episodes caused by mast cell activation and a huge mast cell burden, cytoreductive therapy has been considered. It was shown that the frequency of such episodes was decreased after cladribine (2CdA) therapy.[66] Another therapy is tyrosine kinase inhibitors targeting the mast cell growth receptor KIT. A recently published study showed efficacy of the multikinase inhibitor midostaurin in patients with advanced SM, being able to reduce organ damage and disease progression.[67] However, data are not yet sufficient to recommend such an approach for anaphylaxis treatment. Another future therapy option may be the development of blocking antibodies directed against cell surface antigens expressed on mast cells, such as CD25, CD30, CD33, or CD52.[68]

REFERENCES

1. Theoharides TC, Valent P, Akin C. Mast cells, mastocytosis, and related disorders. N Engl J Med 2015;373(2):163–72.
2. Escribano L, Orfao A. Anaphylaxis in mastocytosis. In: Castells MC, editor. Anaphylaxis and hypersensitivity reactions. New York: Springer Science+Business Media, LLC; 2011. p. 257–70.
3. Nagata H, Worobec AS, Oh CK, et al. Identification of a point mutation in the catalytic domain of the protooncogene c-kit in peripheral blood mononuclear cells of patients who have mastocytosis with an associated hematologic disorder. Proc Natl Acad Sci U S A 1995;92(23):10560–4.
4. Hägglund H, Sander B, Ahmadi A, et al. Analysis of V600E BRAF and D816V KIT mutations in systemic mastocytosis. Med Oncol 2014;31(8):123.
5. Valent P, Horny HP, Escribano L, et al. Diagnostic criteria and classification of mastocytosis: a consensus proposal. Leuk Res 2001;25:603–25.
6. Brockow K, Ring J. Update on diagnosis and treatment of mastocytosis. Curr Allergy Asthma Rep 2011;11:292–9.
7. Escribano L, Alvarez-Twose I, Sanchez-Munoz L, et al. Prognosis in adult indolent systemic mastocytosis: a long-term study of the Spanish Network on Mastocytosis in a series of 145 patients. J Allergy Clin Immunol 2009;124:514–21.
8. Alvarez-Twose I, Zanotti R, Gonzalez-de-Olano D, et al. Nonaggressive systemic mastocytosis (SM) without skin lesions associated with insect-induced anaphylaxis shows unique features versus other indolent SM. J Allergy Clin Immunol 2014;133(2):520–8.
9. Zanotti R, Bonadonna P, Bonifacio M, et al. Isolated bone marrow mastocytosis: an underestimated subvariant of indolent systemic mastocytosis. Haematologica 2011;96(3):482–4.
10. Valent P, Arock M, Akin C, et al. The classification of systemic mastocytosis should include mast cell leukemia (MCL) and systemic mastocytosis with a clonal hematologic non-mast cell lineage disease (SM-AHNMD). Blood 2010;116:850–1.
11. Simons FE, Ardusso LR, Bilò MB, et al. World Allergy Organization anaphylaxis guidelines: summary. J Allergy Clin Immunol 2011;127(3):587–93.
12. Sampson HA, Munoz-Furlong A, Campbell RL, et al. Second symposium on the definition and management of anaphylaxis: summary report – Second National Institute of Allergy and Infectious Disease/Food Allergy and Anaphylaxis Network symposium. J Allergy Clin Immunol 2006;117(2):391–7.
13. Sonneck K, Florian S, Mullauer L, et al. Diagnostic and subdiagnostic accumulation of mast cells in the bone marrow of patients with anaphylaxis: monoclonal mast cell activation syndrome. Int Arch Allergy Immunol 2007;142:158–64.
14. Akin C, Scott LM, Kocabas CN, et al. Demonstration of an aberrant mast-cell population with clonal markers in a subset of patients with "idiopathic" anaphylaxis. Blood 2007;110:2332–3.
15. Golkar L, Bernhard JD. Mastocytosis. Lancet 1997;349:1379–85.
16. van Doormaal JJ, Arends S, Brunekreeft KL, et al. Prevalence of indolent systemic mastocytosis in a Dutch region. J Allergy Clin Immunol 2013;131:1429–31.
17. Cohen SS, Skovbo S, Vestergaard H, et al. Epidemiology of systemic mastocytosis in Denmark. Br J Haematol 2014;166(4):521–8.
18. Brockow K, Akin C, Huber M, et al. Assessment of the extent of cutaneous involvement in children and adults with mastocytosis: relationship to

symptomatology, tryptase levels and bone marrow pathology. J Am Acad Dermatol 2003;48:508–16.

19. González-de-Olano D, de la Hoz B, Nunez-Lopez R, et al. Prevalence of allergy and anaphylactic symptoms in 210 adults and pediatric patients with mastocytosis in Spain: a study of the Spanish network on mastocytosis (REMA). Clin Exp Allergy 2007;37:1547–55.

20. Wood RA, Camargo CA Jr, Lieberman P, et al. Anaphylaxis in America: the prevalence and characteristics of anaphylaxis in the United States. J Allergy Clin Immunol 2014;133(2):461–7.

21. Panesar SS, Javad S, de Silva D, et al. The epidemiology of anaphylaxis in Europe: a systematic review. Allergy 2013;68(11):1353–61.

22. Brockow K, Jofer C, Behrendt H, et al. Anaphylaxis in patients with mastocytosis: a study on history, clinical features and risk factors in 120 patients. Allergy 2008; 63:226–32.

23. Gülen T, Hägglund H, Dahlén B, et al. High prevalence of anaphylaxis in patients with systemic mastocytosis: a single-centre experience. Clin Exp Allergy 2014; 44(1):121–9.

24. Barnes M, Van L, DeLong L, et al. Severity of cutaneous findings predict the presence of systemic symptoms in pediatric maculopapular cutaneous mastocytosis. Pediatr Dermatol 2014;31(3):271–5.

25. Matito A, Carter M. Cutaneous and systemic mastocytosis in children: a risk factor for anaphylaxis? Curr Allergy Asthma Rep 2015;15(5):22.

26. Alvarez-Twose I, Vano-Galvan S, Sanchez-Munoz L, et al. Increased serum baseline tryptase levels and extensive skin involvement are predictors for the severity of mast cell activation episodes in children with mastocytosis. Allergy 2012;67: 813–21.

27. Brockow K, Ring J, Alvarez-Twose I, et al. Extensive blistering is a predictor for severe complications in children with mastocytosis. Allergy 2012;67(10):1323–4.

28. Górska A, Niedoszytko M, Lange M, et al. Risk factors for anaphylaxis in patients with mastocytosis. Pol Arch Med Wewn 2015;125(1–2):46–53.

29. Alvarez-Twose I, González de Olano D, Sánchez-Munos L, et al. Clinical, biological and molecular characteristics of clonal mast cell disorders presenting with systemic mast cell activation symptoms. J Allergy Clin Immunol 2010;125(6): 1269–78.

30. van Anrooij B, van der Veer E, de Monchy JG, et al. Higher mast cell load decreases risk of Hymenoptera venom-induced anaphylaxis in patients with mastocytosis. J Allergy Clin Immunol 2013;132:125–30.

31. Broesby-Olsen S, Kristensen T, Vestergaard H, et al. KIT D816V mutation burden does not correlate to clinical manifestations of indolent systemic mastocytosis. J Allergy Clin Immunol 2013;132(3):723–8.

32. Grabbe J, Welker P, Dippel E, et al. Stem cell factor, a novel cutaneous growth factor for mast cells and melanocytes. Arch Dermatol Res 1994;287(1):78–84.

33. Koterba A, Akin C. Differences in the clinical presentation of anaphylaxis in patients with indolent systemic mastocytosis versus idiopathic anaphylaxis [abstract]. J Allergy Clin Immunol 2008;121:S68.

34. Bonadonna P, Zanotti R, Pagani M, et al. How much specific is the association between Hymenoptera venom allergy and mastocytosis? Allergy 2009;64(9): 1379–82.

35. Worobec AS. Treatment of systemic mast cell disorders. Hematol Oncol Clin North Am 2000;14:659–87.

36. Bonadonna P, Perbellini O, Passalacqua G, et al. Clonal mast cell disorders in patients with systemic reactions to Hymenoptera stings and increased serum tryptase levels. J Allergy Clin Immunol 2009;123:680–6.
37. Ludolph-Hauser D, Rueff F, Fries C, et al. Constitutively raised serum concentrations of mast-cell tryptase and severe anaphylactic reactions to Hymenoptera stings. Lancet 2001;357:361–2.
38. Rueff F, Przybilla B, Biló MB, et al. Predictors of severe systemic anaphylactic reactions in patients with Hymenoptera venom allergy: importance of baseline serum tryptase. A study of the European Academy of Allergology and clinical immunology interest group on insect venom hypersensitivity. J Allergy Clin Immunol 2009;124:1047–54.
39. Potier A, Lavigne C, Chappard D, et al. Cutaneous manifestations in Hymenoptera and Diptera anaphylaxis: relationship with basal serum tryptase. Clin Exp Allergy 2009;39:717–25.
40. Michel J, Brockow K, Darsow U, et al. Added sensitivity of component-resolved diagnosis in Hymenoptera venom-allergic patients with elevated serum tryptase and/or mastocytosis. Allergy 2016;71(5):651–60.
41. González-de-Olano D, Alvarez-Twose I, Morgado JM, et al. Evaluation of basophil activation in mastocytosis with Hymenoptera venom anaphylaxis. Cytometry B Clin Cytom 2011;80(3):167–75.
42. Roenneberg S, Boehner A, Brockow K, et al. Alpha-Gal: a new clue for anaphylaxis in mastocytosis. J Allergy Clin Immunol Pract 2016;4(3):531–2.
43. Prieto-García A, Álvarez-Perea A, Matito A, et al. Systemic mastocytosis presenting as IgE-mediated food-induced anaphylaxis: a report of two cases. J Allergy Clin Immunol Pract 2015;3(3):456–8.
44. Brockow K, Bonadonna P. Drug allergy in mast cell disease. Curr Opin Allergy Clin Immunol 2012;12:354–60.
45. Vaughan STA, Jones GN. Systemic mastocytosis presenting as profound cardiovascular collapse during anaesthesia. Anaesthesia 1993;53:804–7.
46. Tirel O, Chaumont A, Ecoffey C. Circulatory arrest in the course of anaesthesia for a child with mastocytosis. Ann Fr Anesth Reanim 2001;20:874–5 [in French].
47. Matito A, Morgado JM, Sánchez-López P, et al. Management of anesthesia in adult and pediatric mastocytosis: a study of the Spanish network on mastocytosis (REMA) based on 726 anesthetic procedures. Int Arch Allergy Immunol 2015;167(1):47–56.
48. Yocum MW, Butterfield JH, Gharib H. Increased plasma calcitonin levels in systemic mast cell disease. Mayo Clin Proc 1994;69(10):987–90.
49. Seitz CS, Brockow K, Hain J, et al. Non-steroidal anti-inflammatory drug hypersensitivity: association with elevated basal serum tryptase? Allergy Asthma Clin Immunol 2014;10(1):19.
50. Valent P, Akin C, Arock M, et al. Definition, criteria and global classification of mast cell disorders with special reference to mast cell activation syndromes: a consensus proposal. Int Arch Allergy Immunol 2012;157:215–25.
51. Haeberli G, Bronnimann M, Hunziker T, et al. Elevated basal serum tryptase and Hymenoptera venom allergy: relation to severity of sting reactions and to safety and efficacy of venom immunotherapy. Clin Exp Allergy 2003;33:1216–20.
52. Irani AM, Akl EG. Management and prevention of anaphylaxis. F1000Res 2015;22:4.
53. Simons FE. Anaphylaxis: recent advances in assessment and treatment. J Allergy Clin Immunol 2009;124(4):625–36.
54. Przybilla B, Rueff F, Fuchs T, et al. Insektengiftallergie. Allergo J 2004;13:186–90.

55. Brockow K, Schallmayer S, Beyer K, et al. Effects of a structured educational intervention on knowledge and emergency management in patients at risk for anaphylaxis. Allergy 2015;70(2):227–35.
56. Soar J, Pumphrey R, Cant A, et al. Emergency treatment of anaphylactic reactions: guidelines for healthcare providers. Resuscitation 2008;77(2):157–69.
57. Niedoszytko M, de Monchy J, van Doormaal JJ, et al. Mastocytosis and insect venom allergy: diagnosis, safety and efficacy of venom immunotherapy. Allergy 2009;64:1237–45.
58. Rueff F, Placzek M, Przybilla B. Mastocytosis and Hymenoptera venom allergy. Curr Opin Allergy Clin Immunol 2006;6:284–8.
59. Gonzalez de Olano D, Varez-Twose I, Esteban-Lopes MI, et al. Safety and effectiveness of immunotherapy in patients with indolent systemic mastocytosis presenting with Hymenoptera venom anaphylaxis. J Allergy Clin Immunol 2008; 121:519–26.
60. Fricker M, Helbling A, Schwartz L, et al. Hymenoptera sting anaphylaxis and urticaria pigmentosa: clinical findings and results of venom immunotherapy in ten patients. J Allergy Clin Immunol 1997;100:11–5.
61. Rueff F, Wenderoth A, Przybilla B. Patients still reacting to a sting challenge while receiving Hymenoptera venom immunotherapy are protected by increased venom doses. J Allergy Clin Immunol 2001;108:1027–32.
62. Elberink JNGO, de Monchy JGR, Kors JW, et al. Fatal anaphylaxis after yellow jacket sting, despite venom immunotherapy, in two patients with mastocytosis. J Allergy Clin Immunol 1997;99:153–4.
63. Reimers A, Müller U. Fatal outcome of a vespula sting in a patient with mastocytosis after specific immunotherapy with honey bee venom. Allergy Clin Immunol Int J WAO Org 2005;17(1):69–70.
64. Carter MC, Uzzaman A, Scott LM, et al. Pediatric mastocytosis: routine anesthetic management for a complex disease. Anesth Analg 2008;197(2):422–7.
65. Sokol KC, Ghazi A, Kelly BC, et al. Omalizumab as a desensitizing agent and treatment in mastocytosis: a review of the literature and case report. J Allergy Clin Immunol Pract 2014;2(3):266–70.
66. Wimazal F, Geissler P, Shnawa P, et al. Severe life-threatening or disabling anaphylaxis in patients with systemic mastocytosis: a single-center experience. Int Arch Allergy Immunol 2012;157(4):399–405.
67. Gotlib J, Kluin-Nelemans HC, George TI, et al. Efficacy and safety of midostaurin in advanced systemic mastocytosis. N Engl J Med 2016;374(26):2530–41.
68. Arock M, Akin C, Hermine O, et al. Current treatment options in patients with mastocytosis: status in 2015 and future perspectives. Eur J Haematol 2015;94(6): 474–90.

Cutaneous Manifestation of Drug Allergy and Hypersensitivity

Anna Zalewska-Janowska, MD, PhD[a], Radoslaw Spiewak, MD, PhD[b],
Marek L. Kowalski, MD, PhD[c],*

KEYWORDS

- Drug allergy • Drug hypersensitivity • Cutaneous manifestations
- Cutaneous adverse drug reactions (CADR) • Photoallergy

KEY POINTS

- Cutaneous eruptions are the most common manifestation of both allergic and nonallergic drug hypersensitivity.
- Different medications may cause identical skin symptoms, and hypersensitivity to a single drug may manifest with various patterns of symptoms.
- Immediate drug reactions, developing within 1 hour of the drug intake, manifest with urticaria, angioedema, and/or anaphylaxis.
- Delayed type of drug hypersensitivity may manifest with virtually all other cutaneous drug eruptions.
- Analysis of morphology of drug-induced lesions as well as timing of reaction is critical for the final diagnosis

INTRODUCTION

Adverse drug reactions (ADRs) are responsible for about 6% of all hospital admissions and around 9% of hospitalization costs. Only a fraction of these reactions (less than 10%) can be defined as type B, that is, drug hypersensitivity reactions (DHRs), which are usually not predicable and occur in susceptible individuals.[1] However, DHRs may result in potentially fatal outcomes; thus, proper diagnosis and prompt, careful

The authors have no conflict of interest to disclose.
M.L. Kowalski has been partially supported by The Healthy Aging Research Center Project (REGPOT-2012-2013-1, 7FP).
[a] Department of Psychodermatology, Medical University of Lodz, 251 Pomorska Street, Lodz 92-213, Poland; [b] Department of Experimental Dermatology and Cosmetology, Faculty of Pharmacy, Jagiellonian University Medical College, 9 Medyczna Street, Krakow 30-688, Poland; [c] Department of Immunology, Rheumatology and Allergy, Medical University of Lodz, 251 Pomorska Street, Lodz 92-213, Poland
* Corresponding author.
E-mail address: kowalsml@csk.umed.lodz.pl

management is required. The pathomechanism of DHR may be either immunologic (allergy, allergic hypersensitivity) or nonimmunologic (nonallergic hypersensitivity). Although DHRs may manifest with various symptoms (organ specific or systemic), the skin is most commonly affected. Drug-induced skin symptoms are usually mild and self-limiting but may herald the development of a severe systemic and potentially lethal reaction. Drug reactions adopt many faces and should be taken into account in the differential diagnosis of numerous skin rashes. Careful clinical evaluation of visible skin lesions could greatly help in establishing a proper diagnosis.[2–4]

Allergic and Nonallergic Drug Hypersensitivity

DHRs have been defined as objectively reproducible signs or symptoms initiated by a drug at a dose usually tolerated by normal subjects and represent type B ADRs (**Fig. 1**).[5] DHRs with clearly defined immunologic (most often immunoglobulin E [IgE] mediated or T-cell mediated) mechanisms are referred to as drug allergy, whereas nonallergic drug hypersensitivity includes reactions with other, nonimmunologic pathogenic mechanisms (eg, aspirin hypersensitivity related to cyclooxygenase inhibition).[6,7] Similar drug-induced cutaneous symptoms may be evoked by both allergic and nonallergic mechanism, and a single drug can trigger reactions involving either an immunologic (allergic) or nonimmunologic mechanism. Furthermore, allergic DHRs may represent a type I, II, III, or IV drug-specific immune responses according to the Gell and Coombs classification. Distinguishing between these types of hypersensitivity reactions is important in deciding to propose alternative drugs. In drug allergy it may be possible to replace a culprit drug with a drug belonging to the same class but having a different chemical structure (eg, penicillin may be replaced by another antibiotic), whereas in the case of nonallergic hypersensitivity, the whole class of drugs should be avoided (eg, all nonsteroidal antiinflammatory drugs [NSAIDs], which are cyclooxygenase-1 [COX-1] inhibitors, will cross-react in the case of aspirin hypersensitivity).

Hypersensitivity reactions to drugs may manifest with organ-specific or systemic symptoms, ranging in severity from mild skin symptoms (eg, rash) to life-threatening reactions involving multiple organs and systems. Timing of reactions ranges from immediate symptoms, occurring within minutes (eg, penicillin allergy), to symptoms developing within several days after drug intake. Reactions occurring within the first 24 hours are called immediate or acute, whereas delayed reactions, by definition, usually appear more than 24 hours after drug intake.

Cutaneous eruptions are the most common manifestations of drug hypersensitivity and may include exanthematous eruptions, urticaria, angioedema, contact dermatitis,

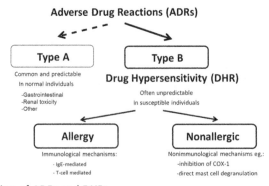

Fig. 1. Classification of ADRs and DHRs.

fixed drug eruptions (FDEs), erythema multiforme, acute generalized exanthematous pustulosis (AGEP), drug reaction with eosinophilia and systemic symptoms (DRESS), Stevens-Johnson syndrome (SJS), exfoliative dermatitis, toxic epidermal necrolysis (TEN), photosensitivity, purpura, and erythema nodosum. Different medications may cause identical skin symptoms, whereas, on the other hand, hypersensitivity to a single drug may manifest with various patterns of symptoms depending on the mechanism of the reaction. Immediate drug reactions, which develop usually within 1 hour of the intake of the culprit drug, manifest with urticaria, angioedema, and/or anaphylaxis. Delayed-type reactions may manifest with virtually all other cutaneous drug eruptions.[8] In addition to analysis of the timing of the reaction, morphology of drug-induced lesions is important for the final diagnosis. Thus, here the authors present a morphologic approach to the diagnosis of cutaneous drug eruptions. Drugs most commonly eliciting specific cutaneous lesions are summarized in **Table 1**.

Urticaria, Angioedema, and Anaphylaxis

Skin eruption
Urticaria is characterized by reddish itchy wheals. An individual wheal lasts up to 24 hours, but new wheals may continuously develop over a longer period of time. *Angioedema* presents as swelling of deep dermal and subcutaneous tissue, and drug-induced angioedema is usually unilateral and accompanied by a pain or burning sensation rather than pruritus. Generally it persists for 1 to 2 hours, but deep swelling can last even for 5 days. In an individual patient, urticaria and angioedema can develop at any location, either jointly or separately. Angiotensin-converting enzyme inhibitor (ACEI)–related angioedema is never accompanied by urticaria, and symptoms usually occur within 1 hour after drug exposure. ACEI-induced angioedema may first occur years after the beginning of treatment with an ACEI and recurs irregularly during such treatment.[9] Urticarial rash is accompanied by fever and arthralgia and, if developing after 1 to 3 weeks of the culprit drug initiation, may represent *serum sickness-like reactions*.

Anaphylaxis is a severe multisystem reaction with rapid onset and life-threatening consequences. Clinically anaphylaxis is characterized by the development of skin lesions, such as erythema, urticaria, or angioedema, followed by hypotension and/or bronchospasm. UK guidelines underline poor clinical documentation of drug allergy and subsequent patient education/information on the subject.[10]

Cutaneous histopathology
In urticaria, stratum papillare, the uppermost layer of dermis, is involved with pronounced vasodilation and moderate edema. Sparse perivascular infiltrates with neutrophils, eosinophils, monocytes, and T-lymphocytes may also be present. In angioedema, the pathologic processes are localized in the deeper layers of the dermis, stratum reticulare, and in subcutaneous or submucosal tissue, as these processes can affect both skin and mucosae. Edema dominates the picture with no or moderate vasodilation; eosinophils may be seen in allergic angioedema, but otherwise there is little or no cellular infiltrate.

Underlying mechanisms
Urticarial lesions are induced by mediators released from activated mast cells. Non-immunologic mechanisms related to COX-1 inhibition are predominant in the development of skin symptoms induced by NSAIDs.[11–13] Type I hypersensitivity reaction (involving IgE) is less frequently involved in drug-induced urticaria but seems to be frequent in anaphylactic reactions.[14] Type III hypersensitivity is responsible for serum

Table 1
Cutaneous manifestations of drug allergy and hypersensitivity in relation to the most commonly eliciting drugs

Cutaneous Manifestation	Most Commonly Eliciting Drugs
Urticaria	NSAIDs, antibiotics, narcotic analgesics
Angioedema	NSAIDs, ACE inhibitors, angiotensin antagonists
Anaphylactic reactions	NSAIDs, antimicrobials, neuromuscular blockers
Erythematous eruptions	Antibiotics, sulfonamides, antiepileptic drugs, non-nucleoside reverse transcriptase inhibitors
Acneiform eruptions	ACTH, androgens, bromides, glucocorticoids, isoniazid, iodides, lithium, phenytoin, selective serotonin reuptake inhibitors, vitamins B1, B6, B12, cyclosporine, sirolimus, isoniazid, EGF inhibitors, bevacizumab, TNF-alpha inhibitors
AGEP	Aminopenicillins, macrolides, carbamazepine, quinolones, diltiazem, antimalarials, mercury
Pseudoporphyria	NSAIDs, antibiotics
Drug-induced LABD	Vancomycin, paracetamol, amiodarone, ceftriaxone, furosemide, metronidazole, phenytoin
Drug-induced pemphigus	Penicillamine and other thiol drugs
Drug-induced pemphigoid	Psoralens, furosemide, ibuprofen, ACE inhibitors, spironolactone, ampicillin, penicillin, levofloxacin, penicillamine, metronidazole, chloroquine
Lichenoid eruptions	Beta-blockers, penicillamine, ACE inhibitors
Cutaneous pseudolymphoma reaction	Anticonvulsants
Drug-induced vasculitis	Allopurinol, penicillins, sulfonamides, phenytoin, thiazides
Drug-induced lupus	Hydralazine, isoniazid, penicillamine, minocycline
Allergic contact dermatitis to drugs	Topical: antibiotics (neomycin, gentamycin, bacitracin), glucocorticosteroids, antiseptics (chlorhexidine, quinolones, benzalkonium chloride)
Photoallergic dermatitis to drugs	NSAIDs
Phototoxic reactions	Psoralens, thiazides, chlorpropamide, nalidixic acid, phenothiazines, tetracyclines, hormonal contraceptives
FDE	Ibuprofen, sulfonamides, tetracyclines, quinolone
SJS/TEN	Allopurinol, antiretrovirals, aromatic amine anticonvulsants, NSAIDs, sulfa-antimicrobials
DRESS	Allopurinol, anticonvulsants, antiretrovirals, NSAIDs, minocycline, sulfasalazine, dapsone, fluindione, proton pump inhibitors, strontium ranelate

Abbreviations: ACE, angiotensin-converting enzyme; ACTH, adrenocorticotropic hormone; EGF, epidermal growth factor; LABD, linear IgA bullous disease; TNF, tumor necrosis factor.

sickness-like reactions presenting as urticarial rash.[15] ACEI-related angioedema is due to kinin-dependent mechanisms.[9]

Erythematous Eruptions

Skin eruptions
Erythematous eruptions (other names: maculopapular or morbilliform eruptions) are the most common clinical presentation of drug eruptions representing about 95% of

all drug-induced skin symptoms. They present as erythematous lesions without blisters or pustules (**Fig. 2**). The trunk is the most common location of the first skin lesions, which spread peripherally in a symmetric way. Almost all patients have pruritus. The first lesions usually develop within a week of the therapy introduction and resolve within 1 to 2 weeks. Typically, during the resolution phase, the eruptions fade in color from deep red into brownish hues with subsequent desquamation of variable intensity.[16]

Cutaneous histopathology
Demonstrates moderate perivascular infiltrate composed mainly of lymphocytes and eosinophils. Some vacuolization of the dermal-epidermal junction may be present.

Underlying mechanisms
It is usually a type IVc or IVb delayed-type reaction whereby T cells directly recognize the drug and activate other inflammatory cells. In some cases, viral infection is a necessary cofactor.

Pustular Eruptions

Skin eruptions
Acneiform eruptions present as scattered pustules that emerge independently of hair follicles and sebaceous glands and may, thus, localize beyond the seborrheic areas, for example, on arms, trunk, lower back, and genitals, typically with absence of comedones and cysts.[17]

Cutaneous histopathology
Inflammatory monomorphic infiltrates with intraepidermal spongiosis and pustule formation occur independent of sebaceous glands.

Underlying mechanisms
The underlying mechanisms remain mostly unknown. Delayed type IVd hypersensitivity may be responsible in some cases.

Acute Generalized Exanthematous Pustulosis

Skin eruptions
An erythematous rash with pustulosis (nonfollicular, sterile pustules <5 mm in diameter) accompanied by fever and neutrophilia develops typically within 48 hours to 3 weeks after drug ingestion. The typical localization is intertriginous areas and the face.[18,19] In most cases AGEP is a self-limited disease. The following features are

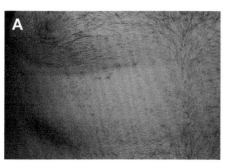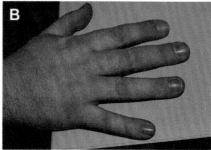

Fig. 2. Erythematous maculopapular eruption that emerged on the trunk (*A*) and on the back of the hand (*B*) after 7 days of clindamycin therapy. (*Courtesy of* Radoslaw Spiewak, MD, PhD, Krakow, Poland.)

taken into account in establishing AGEP diagnosis: pustules, erythema, distribution/ pattern, pustular desquamation, course, mucosal involvement, acute onset, resolution, fever (>38°C), neutrophils greater than 7000/mm³, and histology. The European Study of Severe Cutaneous Adverse Reactions (EuroSCAR) developed a grading system for AGEP diagnosis assigning it as possible (1–4 points), probable (5–7 points), or definite (8–12 points).[20]

Cutaneous histopathology
It typically demonstrates intraepidermal pustules with edema of the papillary dermis and perivascular infiltrates of neutrophils and eosinophils.

Underlying mechanisms
Delayed type IVd hypersensitivity related to CD4+ T cells expressing interleukin 8 initiate neutrophilic infiltration and subsequently pustule formation.[21]

Bullous Eruptions

Several types of bullous eruptions may be related to drug hypersensitivity.

Pseudoporphyria
Skin eruption Skin fragility results in formation of blisters that heal with scarring on sun exposed areas. Skin lesions can develop in the first day of the offending drug ingestion as well as after 1 year of therapy. No abnormalities in porphyrin metabolism have been found.[22]

Cutaneous histopathology It usually reveals split at the dermo-epidermal junction, absent or slight inflammation, and no damage to the epidermis.

Underlying Mechanisms The involved processes remain unknown, phototoxic mechanisms hypothesized.

Drug-Induced Linear Immunoglobulin A Bullous Diseases

Skin eruptions
Skin eruptions are quite heterogeneous and resemble erythema multiforme, bullous pemphigoid, and/or dermatitis herpetiformis. Mucosal and conjunctival lesions are less common than in the idiopathic form of linear IgA bullous diseases.

Cutaneous histopathology
Immunopathology reveals IgA deposits in the basement membrane zone.

Underlying mechanisms
Acantholysis is induced by immunologic mechanisms involving antibody production.

Drug-Induced Pemphigus

Skin eruption
Flaccid bullae and/or crusted erosions predominate. Lesions could develop up to 1 year after drug therapy.

Cutaneous histopathology
There are intraepidermal blisters with intercellular deposition of IgG within suprabasal epidermis.

Underlying mechanisms
Acantholysis is induced either by immunologic mechanisms involving antibody production or directly by drug, in the absence of antibody formation.

Drug-Induced Bullous Pemphigoid

Skin eruptions

Considerable variety is present, including a few bullous lesions; numerous, large, tense bullae on erythematous and urticarial base; and scarring plaques or nodules with bullae, with moderate involvement of the oral mucosa.

Cutaneous histopathology

There are mainly lymphocytic perivascular infiltrates with few eosinophils and neutrophils, intraepidermal vesicles, thrombi in dermal blood vessels, and lack of tissue-bound and circulating antibasal membrane zone IgG.

Underlying mechanisms

Acantholysis is induced either by immunologic mechanisms involving antibody production or directly by drug in the absence of antibody formation.

Lichenoid Eruptions

Skin eruption

There are lichenoid papules with a reddish hue, both clinically and on histopathology consistent with the idiopathic form of lichen planus. The first skin lesions typically develop on the trunk (**Fig. 3**). The mucous membranes and nails are spared. The regression of the lesions proceeds without scarring. The period from drug introduction to skin lesion development ranges between 2 months and 3 years.

Cutaneous histopathology

Cutaneous histopathology of lichenoid drug eruption demonstrates focal parakeratosis, cytoid bodies in the cornified and granular layers, focal interruption in the granular layer, and inflammatory infiltrate with eosinophils and plasma cells, also situated in the deep dermis.

Underlying mechanisms

Type IV hypersensitivity reaction is implied in the formation of lichenoid lesions.

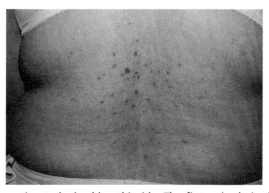

Fig. 3. Lichenoid reaction to hydrochlorothiazide. The first episode in this patient developed after 2 months of taking a combination drug including enalapril and hydrochlorothiazide. The lesions resolved within 3 weeks after stopping the medication; however, they returned in less than a week after another doctor unaware of the patient's past history prescribed her with another combination drug of hydrochlorothiazide with valsartan. (*Courtesy of* Radoslaw Spiewak, MD, PhD, Krakow, Poland.)

Cutaneous Pseudolymphoma Reaction

Skin eruptions
Skin lesions are solitary in most cases but could be fairly widespread and present as erythematous nodules, plaques, or papules. Most patients manifest fever, eosinophilia, lymphadenopathy, and hepatosplenomegaly. Skin lesions develop after at least 1 week but may even occur after up to 5 years of drug exposure.

Cutaneous histopathology
It requires specific staining for differential diagnosis with malignant lymphoma. Polymorphic infiltrates containing T or B lymphocytes are observed in the dermis and the subcutaneous tissue.

Underlying mechanisms
There is a delayed type IV reaction and disturbances in enzymatic detoxification of culprit drugs.

Drug-Induced Vasculitis

Skin eruption
Palpable purpura typically located on the lower limbs is a hallmark of cutaneous vasculitis (**Fig. 4**). Small vessel vasculitis could clinically manifest as urticarial wheals. Persistence of a single lesion in the same location for more than 24 hours is a characteristic feature of urticarial vasculitis. Hemorrhagic bullae, ulcers, nodules, and distal necrosis can develop. The vasculitic process can involve internal organs, including

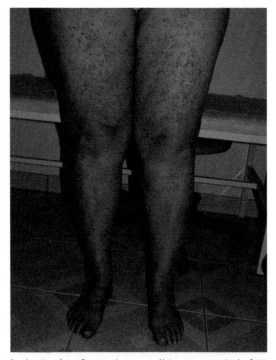

Fig. 4. This patient had episodes of recurring vasculitis over a period of 17 years. Careful diagnosis revealed that relapses were provoked by nitrofurantoin, which she took occasionally for recurring urinary tract infections. (*Courtesy of* Radoslaw Spiewak, MD, PhD, Krakow, Poland.)

the liver, gut, kidney, and central nervous system, leading to serious consequences, including life-threatening ones. Drug-induced vasculitis is frequently a diagnosis of exclusion.[23,24]

Cutaneous histopathology
Dilatation and damage of blood vessels with lymphocytic infiltrate and mast cell degranulation are observed in the edematous dermis.

Underlying Mechanisms
Type III mechanisms mediate the process.

Drug-Induced Lupus

Skin eruption
Skin eruptions are consistent with typical lupus erythematosus lesions, that is, erythematous lesions with edema. Annular or papulosquamous eruptions resembling subacute cutaneous lupus erythematosus are also encountered. Skin lesions are frequently accompanied by systemic symptoms, such as fever, weight loss, musculoskeletal complaints, pleuropulmonary involvement, and less frequently renal, neurologic, and vascular abnormalities.

Cutaneous histopathology
Epidermal atrophy, hyperkeratosis, basal layer degeneration, dermal edema, inflammatory infiltrate, is seen with occasional vasculitis, immunoglobulins, and complement at the dermo-epidermal junction.

Underlying mechanisms
Hapten/prohapten theory, direct cytotoxicity, lymphocytes activation, disturbances in immunologic tolerance.

Allergic Contact Dermatitis to Drugs
Allergic contact dermatitis (ACD; synonym: allergic contact eczema) is an inflammatory skin disease that develops in a person hypersensitive to a low-molecular-weight chemical (hapten), following reexposure to this hapten. There are 4 major clinical variants: localized ACD restricted to the area of contact with the culprit drug, localized ACD with satellites due to redistribution via lymphatic vessels of the absorbed hapten, generalized hematogenous ACD due to blood-borne redistribution of hapten absorbed through the skin, and finally the systemic reactivation of ACD (SRACD) after extracutaneous exposure to hapten (injection, ingestion, inhalation).[25] The last form frequently manifests flexural or fold involvement. Drug-related SRACD is frequently referred to as symmetric drug-related intertriginous and flexural exanthema or baboon syndrome.[26,27] The diagnosis of ACD is confirmed by patch tests that should be carried out in line with expert guidelines.[28]

Skin eruptions
There are eczematous skin lesions with exudation in the acute phase and hyperkeratosis and lichenification in the chronic phase (**Figs. 5** and **6**).

Cutaneous histopathology
Epidermal edema, dermal vessels dilatation, epidermal, dermal, and perivascular inflammatory infiltrate, keratinocyte apoptosis leading to spongiosis with formation of vesicles.

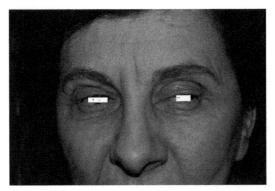

Fig. 5. ACD of eyelids in a patient with contact allergy to antibiotics gentamicin, neomycin, and preservative benzalkonium, all of which were present in ophthalmic drugs that she has used for more than 20 year for recurring sties. (*Courtesy of* Radoslaw Spiewak, MD, PhD, Krakow, Poland.)

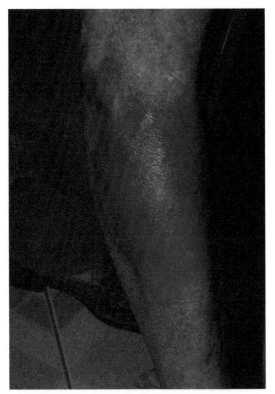

Fig. 6. ACD to a glucocorticosteroid (budesonide) on the right leg secondary to prolonged treatment of venous insufficiency and stasis dermatitis. (*Courtesy of* Radoslaw Spiewak, MD, PhD, Krakow, Poland.)

Underlying mechanisms
Delayed-type hypersensitivity, overlapping subtypes IVa, and IVc (cytotoxic lymphocytes).

Photoallergic Dermatitis to Drugs
Photoallergic dermatitis is a variant of ACD in which additional energy in the form of photons is required to initiate a photochemical reaction between hapten and carrier protein, which subsequently induces the same delayed-type hypersensitivity mechanisms as in ACD.[29] Photopatch tests are required to confirm photoallergy to a suspected drug and the ultimate diagnosis of photoallergic dermatitis.[30]

Skin eruptions
The morphology and clinical course of the disease is identical with ACD, except that irradiation (typically UVA from sunlight) is necessary for the development of the disease; thus, areas exposed to both the drug and light are involved (**Fig. 7**), regardless of the route of drug exposure (topical or systemic).[31–33]

Underlying Mechanism
There is a delayed type IV reaction.

Phototoxic Reactions

Skin eruption
There are cutaneous lesions of variable morphology (erythema, eczema, lichenoid, petechiae, bullae, hyperpigmentation) localized on sun-exposed areas. There are usually sharp borders between areas exposed to light and those covered by clothing, jewelry, watches, and so forth.[34]

Cutaneous histopathology
It is variable depending on the morphology of skin lesions.

Underlying mechanisms
There is damage to lipid membranes, proteins, and DNA by free oxygen or nitrogen radicals produced in photochemical reactions facilitated by the presence of a phototoxic drug in the skin.[35]

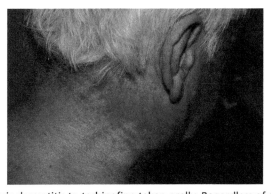

Fig. 7. Photoallergic dermatitis to terbinafine taken orally. Regardless of systemic exposure to the drug, areas covered by clothing were spared; dermatitis is also visibly milder in areas less exposed to direct sunlight, that is, under the hair, behind the ears, under the chin, in the orbital fossae. (*Courtesy of* Radoslaw Spiewak, MD, PhD, Krakow, Poland.)

Severe cutaneous adverse reactions, although often involving bullous eruptions, are presented in a separate section later.

Fixed Drug Eruption

Skin eruptions

They are characterized by solitary (or less frequently multiple) oval reddish plaques that resolve with residual grayish hyperpigmentation (**Fig. 8**). Blisters may develop within the lesions. Lesions develop at the same location each time the culprit drug is taken and are most frequently found within the genital and perianal region; however, they can occur anywhere on the skin. The lesions can develop 30 minutes to 16 hours after culprit drug ingestion. When the culprit drug is reintroduced, not only the lesion reappears in the same locations but also totally new lesions frequently develop. In the acute phase, patients can complain of a burning or stinging sensation. Sometimes fever, malaise, and abdominal symptoms even develop.

Cutaneous histopathology

Cutaneous histopathology shows erythema multiforme features with quite pronounced interface dermatitis together with signs of epithelial degeneration with

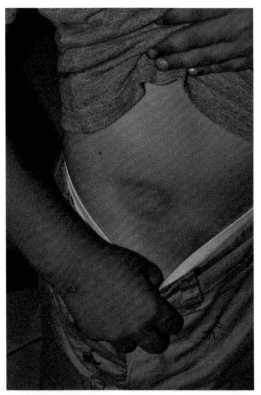

Fig. 8. Fixed drug reaction to paracetamol (acetaminophen) in an 8-year-old boy. He experienced 5 recurrences over the last 5 years because of easy access and widespread presence of paracetamol in various combination drugs for children. (*Courtesy of* Radoslaw Spiewak, MD, PhD, Krakow, Poland.)

dyskeratosis and lymphocyte infiltrates at the dermoepidermal junction. Within FDE lesions, chronic changes, including acanthosis, hypergranulosis, hyperkeratosis eosinophils, and neutrophils, could also be visible.

Underlying mechanisms
T helper and suppressor lymphocytes are increased in the lesional skin. They are thought to contribute to recurrence of the lesions in the same locations after the culprit drug ingestion.

Stevens-Johnson Syndrome/Toxic Epidermal Necrolysis
SJS and TEN are the most severe type of DHR with an estimated mortality rate of 1% to 10% and 20% to 35%, for TEN and SJS, respectively. A severity-of-illness score for TEN is the most frequently used scoring system to predict the course of SJS/TEN.[36]

In about 50% of patients with SJS/TEN, the disease begins with nonspecific prodrome symptoms, such as fever, malaise, headaches, cough, rhinitis, sore through, chest pain, arthralgias, myalgias, diarrhea, and vomiting. Those symptoms could precede skin lesion development by 1 to 14 days.

Skin eruption and organ involvement
SJS/TEN is characterized by acute-onset blistering skin lesions. SJS is diagnosed when epidermal detachment is observed on less than 10% of total body surface area (BSA). TEN requires more than 30% of the BSA epidermal detachment, whereas SJS/TEN overlap is defined as epidermal detachment of 10% to 30% BSA.

SJS/TEN presents with the following skin lesions: macular, often morbilliform rash (first on the face, neck, and central trunk areas and then spreading to the rest of the body); erosions of the mucous membranes; target lesions (with dusky center); and epidermal necrosis. Skin lesions heal with transient hypopigmentation and/or hyperpigmentation. Scarring of mucosal membranes is quite frequent, and there are late complications in about 30% of patients with TEN. The most serious consequences of scarring are observed in the eyes.

The most severely affected parts are the mucous membranes of the mouth (mainly buccal mucosa, palate, and vermilion border) and the eyes (mainly bulbar conjunctiva and anogenital region). Mucous membrane lesions occur either in parallel with or preceding the rash. All 3 sites are involved in about 40% of cases.

Patients report sore and burning sensations of the buccal mucosa, conjunctivae, and lips. Edema and erythema of the skin and mucous membranes follow with blister formation. They subsequently rupture leaving extensive, hemorrhagic erosions covered by white-grayish pseudomembranes composed of fibrin and necrotic epithelium. Numerous hemorrhagic crusts cover the lips. Oral lesions are very painful and lead to eating and breathing inconvenience and excessive saliva production.

Conjunctival involvement demonstrates mainly as inflammation, vesiculation, erosions, and lacrimation. Photophobia, pseudomembranous purulent conjunctivitis, anterior uveitis, corneal ulceration, and panophthalmitis are less frequently observed.

Genital mucous membrane involvement mainly manifests as sore hemorrhagic bullous-erosive or purulent lesions of fossa navicularis, glans penis, vulva, and vagina. Those abnormalities could lead to phimosis in males and/or urinary retention in both sexes.

Pathologic processes of the upper respiratory tract can involve the nasal cavity, gingival, tongue, pharynx, larynx, esophagus, and respiratory tree. In the course of SJS/TEN, otitis media as well as internal organ involvement may develop.

Respiratory and gastrointestinal tract symptoms are most commonly noted. However, development of the following abnormalities could be observed: cytopenias (mostly anemia and lymphocytopenia), gastritis, hepatitis, myocarditis, nephritis, and pneumonitis.

Cutaneous histopathology
It reveals massive necrosis of keratinocytes and epidermis shedding, with minimal or absent dermal inflammatory infiltrate.

Underlying mechanisms
There is a cytotoxic reaction aimed at destruction of keratinocytes expressing foreign (ie, drug-related) antigens. The drug may specifically activate CD8+ T cells, natural killer (NK) cells, and NKT cells to secrete granulysin, leading to upregulation of Fas-Ligand by keratinocytes and to activation of a death receptor–mediated apoptotic pathway. Alternatively, the drug may interact with major histocompatibility complex (MHC) I–expressing cells, causing drug-specific CD8+ cytotoxic T cells to accumulate within epidermal blisters, releasing perforin and granzyme B, which induce keratinocytes death without the need for cell contact. Recent pharmacogenomics studies documented a strong association with MHC.[37–39]

Drug Reaction with Eosinophilia and Systemic Symptoms

DRESS, also known as drug-induced hypersensitivity syndrome (DIHS) or hypersensitivity syndrome (HSS), is a potentially life-threatening condition characterized by both skin and internal organ involvement. The mortality rate in DRESS/DIHS/HSS is estimated at 10% of the affected cases, mainly due to hepatic and renal involvement. In patients with DRESS, leukocytosis at presentation could be regarded as a prognostic marker for prolonged hospitalization.[40,41]

Skin eruption and organ involvement
Clinical presentation of DRESS typically starts with such prodromal symptoms as skin itch and fever followed by cutaneous eruption of erythematous morbilliform rash and then lymphadenopathy development with pharyngitis, oral ulcers, and subsequently systemic symptoms.

Systemic abnormalities encountered in DRESS are as follows: hepatic, hematologic, gastrointestinal, renal, neurologic, cardiac, and endocrine. Liver seems to be the organ most frequently involved in DRESS. Until now, no formal diagnostic criteria for DRESS have been accepted; but in clinical practice both Japanese and RegiSCAR criteria are used.[42,43] Maculopapular rash is usually developing 3 weeks after drug administration, and clinical symptoms persist for 2 or more weeks after drug withdrawal.

Cutaneous histopathology
Coexistence of 3 patterns (ie, eczematous, interface dermatitis, and vascular) seems to be most frequently encountered and suggestive of higher trend of hematological abnormalities and human herpes virus 6 reactivation.[44]

Underlying mechanisms
DRESS has been associated with specific HLA antigens in some ethnic groups with certain culprit drugs. HLA-B*58:01 is associated with allopurinol-induced disease, whereas HLA-B*57:01 with abacavir-induced disease. HLA-B*51:01 was significantly associated with phenytoin-related DRESS.[38] DRESS seems to be more common in Asia than in other parts of the world.

SUMMARY

Cutaneous eruptions are the most common manifestation of both allergic and nonallergic drug hypersensitivity. Different medications may cause identical skin symptoms, and hypersensitivity to a single drug may manifest with various patterns of symptoms depending on the pathogenetic mechanism involved. Immediate drug reactions, developing within 1 hour of drug intake, manifest with urticaria and/or angioedema and may herald development of a severe anaphylactic reaction. A delayed type of drug hypersensitivity may manifest with various cutaneous symptoms, including exanthematous eruptions, FDEs, erythema multiforme, and purpura or erythema nodosum. The most severe reactions, SJS and TEN and some cases of DRESS, may be fatal. Analysis of morphology of drug-induced lesions as well as timing of reaction is critical for the final diagnosis. Further studies will lead to better understanding of the pathogenic mechanism (genetic, immunologic, and nonimmunologic) underlying the skin manifestation of drug hypersensitivity allowing for earlier identification of the culprit drug and more effective management and prevention.

REFERENCES

1. Demoly P, Adkinson F, Brockow K, et al. International consensus on drug allergy. Allergy 2014;69:420–37.
2. Limsuwan T, Demoly P. Acute symptoms of drug hypersensitivity (urticarial, angioedema, anaphylaxis, anaphylactic shock). Med Clin North Am 2010;94:691–710.
3. Gomes ER, Brockow K, Kuyucu S, et al. Drug hypersensitivity in children: report from the pediatric task force of the EAACI drug allergy interest group. Allergy 2016;71:149–61.
4. Tuchinda P, Chularojanamontri L, Sukakul T, et al. Cutaneous adverse drug reactions in the elderly: a retrospective analysis in Thailand. Drugs Aging 2014;31:815–24.
5. Johansson SG, Hourihane JO, Bousquet J, et al, EAACI (the European Academy of Allergology and Clinical Immunology) nomenclature task force. A revised nomenclature for allergy. An EAACI position statement from the EAACI nomenclature task force. Allergy 2001;56:813–24.
6. Naldi L, Crotti S. Epidemiology of cutaneous drug-induced reactions. G Ital Dermatol Venereol 2014;149:207–18.
7. Ardern-Jones MR, Friedmann P. Skin manifestations of drug allergy. Br J Clin Pharmacol 2011;71:672–83.
8. Schrijvers R, Gilissen L, Chiriac AM, et al. Pathogenesis and diagnosis of delayed-type drug hypersensitivity reactions, from bedside to bench and back. Clin Transl Allergy 2015;5:31.
9. Inomata N. Recent advances in drug-induced angioedema. Allergol Int 2012;61:545–57.
10. National Clinical Guideline centre (UK). Drug allergy: diagnosis and management of drug allergy in adults, children and young people. London: National Institute for Health and Care Excellence (UK); 2014.
11. Kowalski ML, Asero R, Bavbek S, et al. Classification and practical approach to the diagnosis and management of hypersensitivity to nonsteroidal anti-inflammatory drugs. Allergy 2013;68:1219–32.
12. Kowalski ML, Woessner K, Sanak M. Approaches to the diagnosis and management of patients with a history of nonsteroidal anti-inflammatory drug-related urticaria and angioedema. J Allergy Clin Immunol 2015;136:245–51.

13. Sanchez-Borges M, Caballero-Fonseca F, Capriles-Hulett A. Aspirin-exacerbated cutaneous disease. Immunol Allergy Clin N Am 2013;33:251–62.

14. Patel TK, Patel PB, Barvaliya MJ, et al. Drug-induced anaphylactic reactions in Indian population: a systematic review. Indian J Crit Care Med 2014;18:796–806.

15. Shear NH, Knowles SR, Sullivan JR, et al. Cutaneous reactions to drugs. In: Freedberg IM, Eisen AZ, Wolff K, et al, editors. Fitzpatrick's dermatology in general practice. New York: McGraw-Hill; 2003. p. 1330–7.

16. Koelblinger P, Dabade TS, Gustafson CJ, et al. Skin manifestations of outpatient adverse drug events in the United States: a national analysis. J Cutan Med Surg 2013;17:269–75.

17. Du-Thanh A, Kluger N, Bensalleh H, et al. Drug-induced acneiform eruption. Am J Clin Dermatol 2011;12:233–45.

18. Sidoroff A, Halevy S, Bavinck JNB, et al. Acute generalized exanthematous pustulosis (AGEP) – a clinical reaction pattern. J Cutan Pathol 2001;28:113–9.

19. Szatkowski J, Schwartz RA. Acute generalized exanthematous pustulosis (AGEP): a review and update. J Am Acad Dermatol 2015;73:843–8.

20. Thienvibul C, Vachiramon V, Chanprapaph K. Five-year retrospective review of acute generalized exanthematous pustulosis. Dermatol Res Pract 2015;2015: 260928.

21. Sukasem C, Puangpetch A, Medhasi S, et al. Pharmacogenomics of drug-induced hypersensitivity reactions: challenges, opportunities and clinical implementation. Asian Pac J Allergy Immunol 2014;32:111–23.

22. LaDuca JR, Bouman PH, Gaspari AA. Nonsteroidal antiinflammatory drug-induced pseudoporphyria: a case series. J Cutan Med Surg 2002;6:320–6.

23. Calvo-Rio V, Loricera J, Ortiz-Sanjuan F, et al. Revisiting clinical differences between hypersensitivity vasculitis and Henoch-Schönlein purpura in adults from a defined population. Clin Exp Rheumatol 2014;32(3 Suppl 82):S34–40.

24. Ortiz-Sanjuan F, Blanco R, Hernandez JL, et al. Drug-associated cutaneous vasculitis: study of 239 patients from a single referral center. J Rheumatol 2014;41:2201–7.

25. Spiewak R. Alergia kontaktowa i alergiczny wyprysk kontaktowy. Alergol Pol Pol J Allergol 2014;1:150–7.

26. Spiewak R. Contact dermatitis in atopic individuals. Curr Opin Allergy Clin Immunol 2012;12:491–7.

27. Jacob SE, Goldenberg A, Nedorost S, et al. Flexural eczema versus atopic dermatitis. Dermatitis 2015;26:109–15.

28. Johansen JD, Aalto-Korte K, Agner T, et al. European Society of Contact Dermatitis guideline for diagnostic patch testing - recommendations on best practice. Contact Dermatitis 2015;73:195–221.

29. Spiewak R. Patch testing for contact allergy and allergic contact dermatitis. Open Allergy J 2008;1:42–51.

30. Goncalo M, Ferguson J, Bonevalle A, et al. Photopatch testing: recommendations for a European photopatch test baseline series. Contact Dermatitis 2013;68: 239–43.

31. Spiewak R. Systemic photoallergy to terbinafine. Allergy 2010;65:1071–2.

32. European Multicentre Photopatch Test Study (EMCPPTS) Taskforce. A European multicentre photopatch test study. Br J Dermatol 2012;166:1002–9.

33. Spiewak R. The frequency and causes of photoallergic contact dermatitis among dermatology outpatients. Acta Dermatovenerol Croat 2013;21:230–5.

34. Zuba EB, Koronowska S, Osmola-Mańkowska A, et al. Drug-induced photosensitivity. Acta Dermatovenerol Croat 2016;24:55–64.

35. Spiewak R. Pathomechanisms of phototoxic dermatitis. In: Spiewak R, editor. Photoallergy and photopatch testing. DIASeries: dermato-immuno-allergo series, vol. 1. Krakow (Poland): Institute of Dermatology; 2009. p. 20–2.
36. Bastuji-Garin S, Fouchard N, Bertocchi M, et al. SCORTEN: a severity-of-illness score for toxic epidermal necrolysis. J Invest Dermatol 2000;115:149–53.
37. Gunathilake KM, Wettasinghe KT, Dissanayake VH. A study of HLA-B*15:02 in Sri Lankan population: implications for pharmacogenomic testing. Hum Immunol 2016;77:429–31.
38. Tassaneeyakul W, Prabmeechai N, Sukasem C, et al. Associations between HLA class I and cytochrome P450 2C0 genetic polymorphisms and phenytoin-related severe cutaneous adverse reaction in a Thai population. Pharmacogenet Genomics 2016;26:225–34.
39. Ghattaoraya GS, Dundar Y, Gonzalez-Galarza FF, et al. A web resource for mining HLA associations with adverse drug reactions: HLA-ADR. Database 2016;2016: 1–10.
40. Wei CH, Chung-Yee Hui R, Chang CJ, et al. Identifying prognostic factors for drug rash with eosinophilia and systemic symptoms (DRESS). Eur J Dermatol 2011;21:930–7.
41. Yang MS, Kang MG, Jung JW, et al. Clinical features and prognostic factors in severe cutaneous drug reactions. Int Arch Allergy Immunol 2013;162:346–54.
42. Kardaun SH, Sidoroff A, Valeyrie-Allanore L, et al. Variability in the clinical pattern of cutaneous side-effects of drugs with systemic symptoms: does a DRESS syndrome really exist? Br J Dermatol 2007;156:609–11.
43. Shiohara T, Iijima M, Ikezawa Z, et al. The diagnosis of a DRESS syndrome has been sufficiently established on the basis of typical clinical features and viral reactivations. Br J Dermatol 2007;156:1083–4.
44. Cho YT, Liau JY, Chang CY, et al. Co-existence of histopathological features is characteristic in drug reaction with eosinophilia and systemic symptoms and correlates with high grades of cutaneous abnormalities. J Eur Acad Dermatol Venereol 2016. [Epub ahead of print].

The Angiotensin-Converting-Enzyme-Induced Angioedema

Murat Bas, MD

KEYWORDS

• ACE inhibitor • Angioedema • Bradykinin • Bradykinin receptors

KEY POINTS

- The bradykinin B2 receptor antagonist icatibant is effective in angiotensin-converting-enzyme inhibitor-induced angioedema.
- Icatibant is not approved officially for this indication and has to be administered in an emergency situation off-label.
- Corticosteroids or antihistamines do not seem to work in this condition.

ETIOLOGY AND PATHOPHYSIOLOGY OF ANGIOEDEMA

Angioedema is an edematous swelling of deeper tissue layers, which impacts both the skin and the mucosa (**Fig. 1**). When angioedema manifests in the airways, it can cause breathing difficulties and can even, in rare cases, lead to death.[1] One can divide angioedema into allergic (urticaria) and nonallergic angioedema.[2] Typically, nonallergic angioedema, when juxtaposed to allergic urticaria, is the lack of pruritus or erythema. Central to allergic urticaria pathophysiology is histamine, whereas the main mediator of nonallergic angioedema is bradykinin (**Fig. 2**).

This difference is important in determining the appropriate treatment for the disease. Especially problematic is chronic urticaria. Angioedema, which may appear during the course of this disease, only shows in 10% of cases an allergic cause.[3,4] It is for this reason that this type of angioedema rarely reacts to standard antiallergy therapy, such as antihistamines and corticosteroids. Without the pruritus or erythema, the angioedema from chronic urticaria cannot easily be differentiated from nonallergic angioedema. These are differential diagnosis problems that lead to early treatment failures. Bradykinin-induced angioedema is owing to either an increased production of bradykinin or an arrested breakdown thereof. Bradykinin is a Nonapeptide, which is physiologically made in the kallikrein–kinin system. This system was discovered more than 100 years ago when Abelous and Bardier were investigating the blood dropping effect of urine.[5] Kinins are pharmacologically active

Clinic of Otorhinolaryngology, Klinikum rechts der Isar, Technische Universität München, Ismaninger St 22, 81675 Munich, Germany
E-mail address: m.bas.hno@gmail.com

Immunol Allergy Clin N Am 37 (2017) 183–200
http://dx.doi.org/10.1016/j.iac.2016.08.011   immunology.theclinics.com
0889-8561/17/© 2016 Elsevier Inc. All rights reserved.

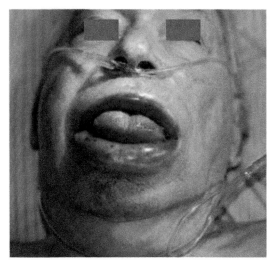

Fig. 1. Angiotensin-converting-enzyme-induced angioedema of the tongue and epiglottis.

peptides produced by the enzymatic degradation of kininogens by kallikrein. Kinins are then released into body fluids and tissue. In comparison, the C1-esterase inhibitor (C1-INH) functions as an endogenous kallikrein inhibitor, thereby slowing kinin synthesis. The family of kinins includes bradykinin, kallidin, and methionyl-iyssyl-bradykinin, which is found in blood plasma and in urine, and can quickly be converted to bradykinin.[6]

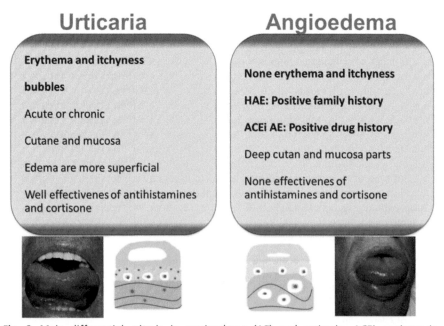

Fig. 2. Main differential criteria in angioedema (AE) and urticaria. ACEi angiotensin-converting-enzyme inhibitor; HAE, hereditary angioedema.

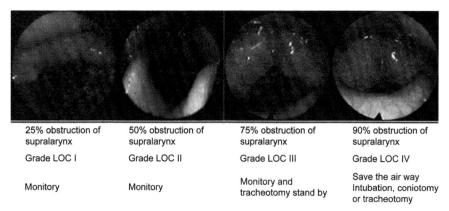

25% obstruction of supralarynx	50% obstruction of supralarynx	75% obstruction of supralarynx	90% obstruction of supralarynx
Grade LOC I	Grade LOC II	Grade LOC III	Grade LOC IV
Monitory	Monitory	Monitory and tracheotomy stand by	Save the air way Intubation, coniotomy or tracheotomy

Fig. 3. Laryngeal edema classification.

The kallikrein–kinin system is closely connected with the renin–angiotensin–aldosterone system, and to some degree even antagonizes its effects. The functional coupling between these 2 systems is owing to the unspecificity of the angiotensin-converting enzyme (ACE), which builds angiotensin II, but also degrades kinins such as bradykinin or substance P to inactive metabolites.[7,8] Other proteases besides ACE (aminopeptidase P, dipeptidylpeptidase IV, carboxpeptidase N) also partake in bradykinin degradation. If they are inhibited in addition to ACE, then one may see an extra increase in plasma and tissue bradykinin concentrations.[9–11]

BRADYKININ RECEPTORS

Bradykinin receptors are G-protein–coupled receptors that are present ubiquitously on cell membranes. As of yet, 2 types of receptor subtypes have been identified: the bradykinin-receptor types 1 (BKR-1) and 2 (BKR-2). Each seems to have different pharmacologic properties.[12–18] The human gene for BKR-2 has been localized to chromosome 14q32,[19] whereas BKR-1 was found to be on chromosome 14q32.1-q32.2.[20] The amino acid sequences from BKR-1 and BKR-2 have been shown to be 32% homologous.[18] BKR-1 is created de novo by many different organs as a reaction from tissue injury, whereas BKR-2 is usually expressed constitutively.[20–22]

BRADYKININ EFFECTS

The discovery of various selective antagonists of BKR-1 and BKR-2 in the 1980s were fundamental to the discovery of the function role of kinins.[15] Recently, the development of C1-INH and BKR-2-transgene mice has produced important information concerning the role of kinins.[23,24] This revealed the effects of bradykinin on vessel permeability through inhibition of C1-INH.[24] The anticonstrictive effects of bradykinin on peripheral and coronary arteries have been shown to lower blood pressure in normotensive animals. Additionally, it has antithrombotic, antiproliferative, and antifibrinogenic perperties.[22,25–29]

The cardiovascular effects of bradykinin are according to contemporary knowledge, mostly triggered through the BKR-2 activation on endothelial cells, which causes a release of nitrous monoxide, prostaglandin PGI2 and tissue plasminogen activator.[30,31] It has also been shown that bradykinin has a cardioprotective effect, and is involved in the "preconditioning" during myocardial ischemia and by reperfusion injury.[32] Bradykinin can decrease the size of an infarct[33,34] and can also retard the growth of cardiomyocytes.[35,36] Additionally, kinins can cause a bronchoconstriction,[37] which may be associated with the ACE inhibitor-induced dry cough, which is mediated by bradykinins and substance P.[38,39] Furthermore, the local accumulation of bradykinin can lead to an activation of locally released histamine, which may be 1 reason for the local susceptibility for the cough reflex.[40] Finally, it shown that bradykinin stimulates insulin secretion from the B-cells of the pancreas. This effect is caused by the increase in intracellular calcium as a result of a hyperglycemia.[41,42] Braydkinin also increases the insulin-dependent glucose transport.[43] Further investigations have shown that the effects of locally secreted bradykinin, namely, the intake of glucose in cells, is independent of the insulin secretion.[44,45] These results imply that the lesser degradation of bradykinin in patients with cardiovascular disease is associated with the beneficial effects of ACE inhibitors (ACEi). This includes, for example, the lower rate of long-term injuries associated with type 2 diabetes mellitus.[46]

BRADYKININ-INDUCED ANGIOEDEMA
Hereditary Angioedema

In 1882, Heinrich Irenaus Quincke described an acute and clearly circumscribed edema. Even though such an edema was described in earlier cases, it was Quincke who accurately described the illness and who clearly delineated it from urticaria.[47] Currently, the terms Quincke edema and angioedema are interchangeably used. Quincke edema is also used as an umbrella term to describe an edema without urticaria and/or pruritus.

Our contemporary understanding is that an insufficiency of the serine protease C1-INH, which is caused by a genetic defect, may play a role in the development of hereditary angioedema (HAE).[48] As a result, a series of changes within the complement system are initiated, which can be used for diagnostic purposes. Important is that the lack of C1-INH plays a physiologic role in decreased bradykinin production. This is because C1-INH are endogenous inhibitors of kallikrein. The reduced activity of C1-INH lead to a increased bradykinin production. Human C1-INH gene is located on chromosome 11 (11q12-q13.1).[49] Two variants of HAE have been described: HAE type 1 with a lowered C1-INH level and deficient function (in 85% of cases), and HAE type 2 with a normal protein concentration but a functional deficit (in 15% of cases). This is a case of a heterozygote, autosomal-dominant inheritance with an incidence of 1 in 50,000, independent of ethnicity or gender.[49] Additional causes of autosomal dominance inheritance of angioedema were discovered in 2006 as mutations in exon 9 of the F-12 gene. Amino acid position 309 of the coagulation factor XII was shown to have lysine or arginine instead of threonine.[50] A cause of the activating mutation is, as with the classical HAE types 1 and 2, an increased kinin production as a result of an increased enzymatic activity of coagulation factor XII. Activating factors XIIa change prekallikrein into kallikrein, which leads to a faster conversion of "high-molecular-weight kininogen" to bradykinin. This disease impacts mostly women, because estrogen intake is a precipitating factor. This can be explained by the fact that coagulation factor XII is synthesized in an estrogen-dependent manner. As a result, women who take medications such as oral contraceptives or who are pregnant are especially susceptible. The medication causes increased factor XII serum concentrations. Rarely are men impacted by this disease and when they are the disease is usually less pronounced. The most common symptoms of patients with HAE type 3 are swelling of the face (93%) and tongue (54%), as well as abdominal pain (50%). Larynx (25%) and uvula edema (21%) are also seen.[51] The quantitative and function of C1-INH is normal in contrast with types 1 and 2. However, only some patients have been shown to have a mutation in exon 9 of the F-12 gene. Therefore, one must assume that further unknown genetic causes for this subtype must exist. The first case of homozygote C1-INH-deficiency was discovered recently with a mutation of c.1576T>G.[51] In mice, an interruption of the C1-INH impact led to increased vessel permeability, which was shown to be reversible with human plasma pool C1-INH.[24] Other results, which were taken from transgene mice, produced further results supporting the role of BKR-2 in the pathogenesis of angioedema. In this way was one able to dramatically reduce increased vessel permeability with the BKR-2 antagonist icatibant (see the discussion in the Icatibant section).

Trigger Factors

Patients with HAE describe a large number of factors that induce angioedema, including cold exposure, mechanical trauma (eg, cold compresses, sitting or standing for long periods of time), food (eg, eggs or alcohol), infection, pesticide contact or other chemicals, stress or anxiety, and certain pharmaceuticals such as ACE inhibitors and estrogen.[48] These mostly anecdotal accounts are rarely investigated and often seem to be associated with individual patient characteristics. One exception is the intake of estrogen as seen in hormone replacement therapy. It has been shown in multiple HAE patients that women with higher estrogen levels, as seen during the menstrual cycle as well as during pregnancy or with hormone replacement therapy, all have an higher incidence rate.[51,52] Other researchers have found similar cases in men and women who used antiandrogenous medication in the form of Cyproteron.[53] Indeed, also pharmaceuticals that inhibit bradykinin *degradation* can lead to increased incidence, this is why ACE inhibitors are contraindicated in HAE patients.[54,55]

IATROGENIC INDUCED BRADYKININ ANGIOEDEMA

The most common reason for bradykinin-induced angioedema is the intake of pharmaceuticals that lead to an inhibition of the breakdown of bradykinin. This includes ACE inhibitors like enalapril as well as angiotensin-1 blockers like losartan and the renin inhibitor aliskiren. The arrested breakdown of bradykinin by this group of medications, which are often used to treat cardiovascular disease, is not a desired effect. However, it is believed that the ACE inhibitors have a stronger inhibiting effect on bradykinin breakdown than the other agents in this category.

ANGIOTENSIN-CONVERTING ENZYME INHIBITOR–INDUCED ANGIOEDEMA

A characteristic of ACE inhibitor–induced angioedema is its constant manifestation in the airways. Swelling in the head and neck areas, especially in the pharynx and larynx, make multiple-day ward stays for patients necessary.

The incidence of ACE inhibitor–induced angioedema varies in different investigations, which is most likely owing to ethnic differences. In Caucasians, an incidence of ACE inhibitor–induced angioedema of 0.1% to 0.7%[1,48,49,56,57] was found, whereas the incidence in African Americans was much higher.[58] A recent metaanalysis of the side effects of pharmaceuticals for treating cardiovascular disease found a 3 times greater relative risk for the manifestation of an ACE inhibitor–induced angioedema in African Americans as compared with Causasians.[5] With the approximately 7 million patients taking ACE inhibitors in Germany and an assumed angioedema incidence of 0.3% to 0.5%, one can extrapolate that to about 20,000 to 35,000 cases present every year. The incidence itself is calculated to be 1 in 4000. This means that ACE inhibitor–induced angioedema is more common than HAE.[59] If additional enzymes, besides ACE, that arrest bradykinin breakdown, are inhibited, then the one can assume an even higher plasma bradykinin concentration.[9–11] This effect is seen especially well with omapatrilat, which inhibits both ACE and the neutral endopeptidase. During clinical examinations a 3 times greater rate of angioedema was found in comparison with the ACE inhibitor enalapril (2.17% vs 0.68%), which is why this particular drug was not approved.

ANGIOTENSIN-1 BLOCKER–INDUCED ANGIOEDEMA

Angiotensin-1 blockers rarely cause angioedema in comparison with ACE inhibitors.[57,59] In the VALIANT Study (Valsartan in Acute Myocardial Infarction Trial), 4900 patients were treated with valsartan, captopril, or the combination of both. In the valsartan group, 0.2% of patients incurred an angioedema; in the other groups, 0.5% of the patients had this side effect. It seems surprising that angioedema can occur, when looking at the drugs method of action, through the effects of bradykinin. The fact that the combined intake of valsartan and captopril did not cause more angioedema than captopril alone suggests that it may not be associated. However, a recent clinical study showed that angiotensin-1 blockers increase bradykinin levels in hypertensive patients.[60,61] Blood levels of angiotensin II increase when patients are treated with angiotensin-1 blockers, possibly because these interrupt the physiologic negative feedback mechanism, which regulates angiotensin-II production through the secretion of renin.[62] Concurrently, all the angiotensin type 1 receptors are blocked, which allows angiotensin type 2 receptors to be activated by angiotensin II. In this context it is important to note that the activation of angiotensin type 2 receptors is regulated through an as-of-yet unknown mechanism, which also leads to an inhibition of ACE activity.[63–65] As a result, the angiotensin-1 inhibition, as seen in Campbell and colleagues' study,[61] and increased bradykinin concentration in plasma, could be owing to the inhibition of bradykinin breakdown. However, this theory needs to still be shown valid through animal experiments. Hypothetically, patients who experience an angiotensin-1 blocker–induced angioedema should not continue to receive angiotensin-1 blockers. Potential alternatives are calcium blockers. In cases with severe heart failure and renal dysfunction, the use of angiotensin-1 blockers is possible. The patients must be informed regarding side effects like angioedema. The risk to develop an angioedema with angiotensin-1 blockers are limited.

RENIN INHIBITOR–INDUCED ANGIOEDEMA

A further pharmacologic alternative to influence the renin–angiotensin–aldosterone system is through the relatively new renin inhibitor, aliskiren, which is also approved for the treatment of hypertension by the US Food and Drug Administration (FDA) and the European Medicine Agency (EMA). The inhibition of renin leads neither to a direct inhibition of ACE nor to an increased activity of angiotensin type 2 receptors, and therefore probably not to an increased plasma bradykinin concentration. However, aliskiren has not been shown to be any better than ACE inhibitor or sartans.[66–69] In the initial approval studies, all patients with mild or moderate hypertension were excluded. In contrast with other antihypertensive medications, no reduced cardiovascular morbidity or mortality has been shown with aliskiren.[66–69] Additionally, aliskiren is not indicated for patients who suffered an angioedema with ACE inhibitor or with a sartan, because this has been judged a therapeutic contraindication (Decision of the Federal Committee of initiation of an opinion process to amending the official drug guideline).

ACQUIRED ANGIOEDEMA

Acquired angioedema develops owing to a nongenetic deficiency of C1-INH, and usually impacts adults.[68] It can develop as a result of a severe disease, for example, a malignant lymphoma. Patients with lymphoproliferative diseases can develop an angioedema, which is associated with low C1-INH plasma concentrations.[70–72] In comparison with HAE with lowered C1-INH synthesis and/or activity, acquired angioedema is characterized by a greater number of idiotype anti-idiotype immune complexes (autoantibodies), which breakdown C1-INH and C1q-molecules. Other diseases, for example, liver cell carcinoma and liver cirrhosis, are also characterized by lower C1-INH concentration, although in these cases angioedema is not a known problem. To note is that some lymphoma-associated angioedema cases are known to have normal C1-INH plasma levels.[73] A recent study found that a newly discovered C1-INH mutation was associated with monocyte-inhibited C1-INH secretion.[73]

THERAPY OF THE ACUTE ANGIOTENSIN-CONVERTING ENZYME INHIBITOR–INDUCED ANGIOEDEMA

Angioedema in the head and neck region is especially dangerous owing to the danger of airway closure, and thereby asphyxiation. As a result, it is always important to inform patients about where the angioedema is found and its severity. Patients need to be informed about the possibility of asphyxiation and any need for intervention. One can differentiate different general therapeutic options of angioedema of the head and neck region; these include:

- Mechanical protection of the airways,
- Supportive therapeutic measures,
- Symptomatic (nonspecific) pharmacologic measures, and
- Causal (specific) pharmacotherapy.

Mechanical Protection of the Airways

Mechanical protection of the airways must be considered if asphyxiation is threatening if there is:

- Inability to swallow,
- Inspiratory stridor, and/or
- Cyanosis.

If these symptoms are present, one should immediately begin mechanical safeguarding of the airways.

Forms of Mechanical Safeguarding

The methods can depend on the localization of the angioedema (**Table 1**). Besides these symptoms, the severity and degree of angioedema are important in the decision. The degree of laryngeal (**Fig 3**) and tongue angioedema (**Fig. 4**) should be ascertained. Additionally, the mechanical intervention can lead to further tissue damage and inflammation, which can last for days.

Supportive Procedures in the Therapy

The use of ice cubes in cases with angioedema in the mouth cavity and oropharynx is potentially helpful. Patients with hypotension should be treated with a sodium chloride infusion. An upright position of the upper part of the body is favored.

Table 1
Forms of mechanical safeguarding of the airways

Location	Method
Lip, Face (Cheeks, Periorbital)	None Necessary
Tongue, mouth	• Nasal fiberoptic intubation ○ Wendl-Tubue
Oropharynx (soft palate, uvula, oropharyngeal back-wall, tonsillar region)	• Wendl-Tubus • Nasal fiberoptic intubation • Tracheotomy
Tongue base, hypopharynx, larynx (supralarynx)	• Nasal fiberoptic intubation • Oral intubation • Tracheotomy

Symptomatic Pharmacotherapy

Vasoconstricting agents can be helpful in the therapy of renin–angiotensin–aldosterone system blocker-induced angioedema (RAE). Epinephrine (inhalation or spray) can be (off-label) used (dosage up to 8 mg/application). Unfortunately, there are no studies demonstrating treatment efficacy of epinephrine. Treatment with epinephrine is therefore not evidence based. Treatment with all classes of analgesics is possible if required.

Nonspecific Pharmacotherapy

Corticosteroids

At the time of this writing, here is no EMA or FDA approved treatment for RAE. Despite a lack of approval, RAE has been treated in the past with glucocorticosteroids (methylprednisolone 250–500 mg) and H2 antihistamines (clemastine 2 mg). There are no studies supporting this therapeutic scheme. A retrospective case series could not show a faster remission of symptoms with glucocorticosteroids versus placebo.[74] Three of 47 patients treated with cortisone had to be tracheotomized, 2 had to be intubated, and 12 received a second dose of cortisone. The time of complete symptom remission was 33 hours and did not differ statistically from placebo. A recent

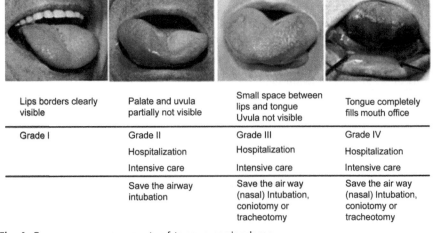

Lips borders clearly visible	Palate and uvula partially not visible	Small space between lips and tongue Uvula not visible	Tongue completely fills mouth office
Grade I	Grade II	Grade III	Grade IV
	Hospitalization	Hospitalization	Hospitalization
	Intensive care	Intensive care	Intensive care
	Save the airway intubation	Save the air way (nasal) Intubation, coniotomy or tracheotomy	Save the air way (nasal) Intubation, coniotomy or tracheotomy

Fig. 4. Emergency managements of tongue angioedema.

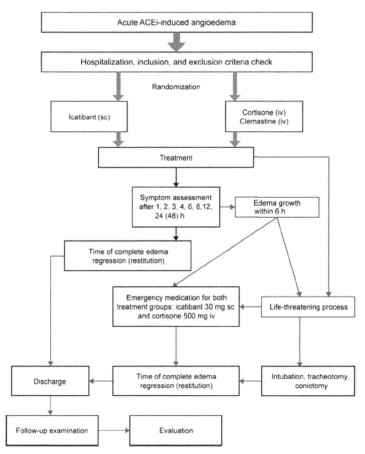

Fig. 5. Study design of AMACE (AMelioration of Angiotensin Converting Enzyme Inhibitor Induced Angioedema Study). ACEi, angiotensin-converting enzyme inhibitor; IV, intravenous; SC, subcutaneous.

randomized controlled study could show a mean time to complete symptom remission of 27 hours after treatment with cortisone and H2 antihistamines and therefore confirmed a lack of efficacy of this therapeutic concept.[74] It can be concluded that there is no evidence for the effectiveness of glucocorticosteroid or H2 antihistamines in the therapy of RAE.

SPECIFIC PHARMACOTHERAPY

Because it can be safely assumed that RAE belong to the group of ACE inhibitor–induced angioedema in which a potential effectiveness of pharmacotherapeutic agents reducing the production of bradykinin or blocking the bradykinin 2 receptor can be expected. The aim of this therapy is to prevent the angioedema from spreading to the upper airways and to reduce an existing edema.

Icatibant

Because most of the nonallergic angioedema are related to a pathologic increase in bradykinin concentration an effectiveness of the synthetic B2 receptor antagonist icatibant (Firazyr) can be assumed. Icatibant is a competitive receptor antagonist. Icatibant is approved by the FDA an EMA for the treatment of acute type 1 and 2 HAE attacks. Standard therapy is applied subcutaneously in the belly region. Standard dosage is 30 mg. A first symptom improvement can be expected in average after 45 minutes. Systemic side effects have not been reported up until now. A local erythema at the injection site appears regularly.

Since market approval, dozens of ACE inhibitor patients have been successfully off-label treated with icatibant. There are 4 original papers on the subject. Three of these are case series showing successful treatment in a total of 33 patients. Parts of the patients had previously received glucocorticosteroids or had been intubated. Complete remission of symptoms had been approximately reached after 4 to 5 hours.

The fourth publication is a randomized, double blind controlled 2-armed multicenter trial. Thirty-two patients were screened and 30 patients were included in the study. The patients received icatibant plus placebo versus prednisolone plus clemastine plus placebo in a randomized fashion.[74]

Eligible patients were randomly assigned, in a 1:1 ratio, to receive, within 10 hours after symptom onset, subcutaneous icatibant at a dose of 30 mg injected into the abdominal wall or standard therapy consisting of intravenous prednisolone (Solu-Decortin H, Merck, Kenilworth, NJ) at a dose of 500 mg plus clemastine (Tavegil, Novartis, Basel, Switzerland) at a dose of 2 mg. Randomization was performed online with the use of variable block sizes to ensure that the number of study participants in the treatment groups was balanced. Normal saline (0.9%, B. Braun, Melsungen, Germany) was administered as an intravenous placebo in patients who were receiving icatibant and as a subcutaneous placebo in those who were receiving standard therapy. The patients and the investigators who were responsible for the assessment of efficacy outcomes were unaware of the study assignments; the investigators who were responsible for randomization, study drug administration, and assessment of injection site reactions were aware of the study assignments.

Patients assessed the intensity of 6 symptoms (pain, shortness of breath, dysphagia, change in voice, sensation of a foreign body, and feeling of pressure) before treatment and at 1, 2, 3, 4, 6, 8, 12, 24, and 48 hours after treatment with the use of a visual analog scale that ranged from 0 to 10, with higher scores indicating more severe symptoms. A composite score on the visual analog scale was calculated as the average of the measurements for the 6 symptoms. Investigators who were unaware of the treatment assignments also assessed the severity of the same 6 symptoms at the same time points, using a scale from 0 (no symptoms) to 3 (severe symptoms); a composite symptom score was calculated from the average of the 6 symptom scores. In addition, investigators assessed the severity of angioedema at 4 locations (lips and cheeks, tongue, oropharynx, and hypopharynx or larynx), using a scale from 0 (no angioedema) to 4 (very severe angioedema). Angioedema of the oropharynx and hypopharynx was assessed by an ear, nose, and throat specialist, who performed endoscopy when necessary. A composite angioedema score was calculated as the average of the 4 symptom scores (**Fig. 5**).

If no reduction in symptoms had occurred by 6 hours after treatment, the investigator could administer rescue medication (30 mg of icatibant with 500 mg of prednisolone), regardless of the group to which the patient had been randomly assigned. In life-threatening situations, appropriate rescue procedures (including intubation or tracheotomy) could be implemented. A final follow-up visit was scheduled 14 days after hospital admission.

The primary endpoint was the time to the complete resolution of edema after administration of the study treatment, as evaluated on the basis of investigator-assessed and patient-assessed symptom scores, as well as the investigator's assessment of the severity of angioedema on the basis of the physical examination. Secondary end-points included the proportion of patients who did not have a response to treatment (ie, patients who required rescue therapy); the proportion of patients with complete resolution of edema at 4 hours after treatment; the time to the onset of symptom relief, which was defined as the time to the first improvement (ie, decrease) of at least 1 point in the composite score of the investigator-assessed symptom score, the angioedema score, or the score on the patient-assessed visual analog scale; and the composite and individual investigator-assessed symptom scores, angioedema scores, and scores on the patient-assessed visual analog scale, as well as the change in the composite scores from the pretreatment scores, at each protocol-specified time point. Safety was evaluated by assessment of the incidence of and time to rescue intervention, adverse event reporting, documentation of local (injection site) reactions, measurement of vital signs, and clinical laboratory testing.

All patients in the per protocol population had complete resolution of edema; however, 3 patients in the standard therapy group required rescue therapy (icatibant and prednisolone) and were classified as having had treatment failure. One of these patients also required a tracheotomy for dyspnea that was classified as a serious adverse event (see below; **Fig. 6**). The maximum recorded time to the complete resolution of edema (61.2 hours) was used to replace the data for these 3 patients in the primary efficacy analysis.

The median time to the complete resolution of edema was 8.0 hours (interquartile range, 3.0–16.0) with icatibant as compared with 27.1 hours (interquartile range, 20.3–48.0) with standard therapy ($P = .002$; **Table 2**). The respective mean ± standard deviation times to complete resolution of edema were 15.4 ± 18.8 hours and 33.2 ± 18.0 hours. Kaplan–Meier sensitivity analyses in which the data for the 3 patients

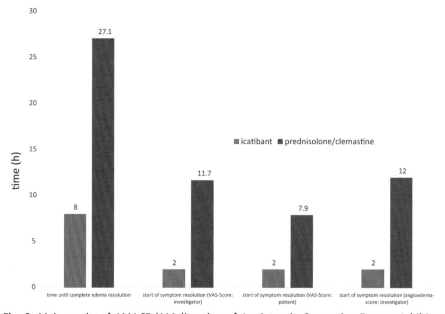

Fig. 6. Main results of AMACE (AMelioration of Angiotensin Converting Enzyme Inhibitor Induced Angioedema Study) icatibant (*blue*) and prednisolone/clemastin (*red*). VAS, visual analog scale.

Table 2
Results of AMACE

Outcome	Icatibant (n = 13)	Standard Therapy (n = 14)	P Value
Median (IQR) time to complete edema resolution (primary end point), h	8.0 (3.0–16.0)	27.1 (20.3–48.0)	.002
Proportion of patients with complete edema resolution at 4 h after treatment, n (%)	5 (39)	0 (0)	.02
Median (95% CI) time to onset of symptom relief (composite investigator-assessed symptom score), h	2.0 (1.0–8.1)	11.7 (8.0–18.0)	.03
Median (95% CI) time to onset of symptom relief (composite patient VAS score), h	2.0 (2.0–6.3)	7.9 (1.2–11.8)	.36
Median (95% CI) time to onset of symptom relief (composite investigator-assessed angioedema score), h	2.0 (2.0–12.0)	12.0 (11.3 to NE)	.003

Abbreviations: AMACE, AMelioration of Angiotensin Converting Enzyme Inhibitor Induced Angioedema Study; CI, confidence interval; IQR, interquartile range; VAS, visual analog scale.

who received rescue intervention were censored at the time of the first rescue event resulted in similar estimates of the median time to complete resolution of edema— 8.0 hours (95% confidence interval [CI], 3.0–16.0) with icatibant versus 23.7 hours (95% CI, 17.8–35.9) with standard therapy (P = .008). Five patients (38%) who received icatibant, as compared with none who received standard therapy, had complete resolution of edema within 4 hours after treatment (P = .02). On the basis of Kaplan–Meier analyses, the median time to the onset of symptom relief was shorter with icatibant than with standard therapy—2.0 hours (95% CI, 1.0–8.1) versus 11.7 hours (95% CI, 8.0–18.0; P = .03). In conclusion, the AMACE (AMelioration of Angiotensin Converting Enzyme Inhibitor Induced Angioedema Study) study demonstrated the effectiveness of icatibant, a bradykinin B2 receptor blocker in ACE inhibitor induced angioedema.

C1 INHIBITOR

Two human C1-INH concentrates (Berinert and Cinryze) are available for the treatment of HAE attacks. A third C1-INH concentrate, obtained from transgenic rabbits milk, is approved for the treatment of acute HAE. It has been hypothesized that C1-INH concentrates, which inhibits the synthesis of bradykinin, would also be an effective therapy for ACE inhibitor-induced angioedema.[75–77] However, data on clinical effectiveness are lacking. In **Table 3**, published cases are listed. Recently, a case series was published with first data about C1-INH in ACE inhibitor–induced angioedema. A small group of patients suffering from ACE inhibitor–induced angioedema was treated with C1-INH, and we compared the outcomes to those of a historical control group that had been treated conventionally with corticosteroids and antihistamines.[75,78]

The mean time ± standard deviation interval to first improvement of symptoms after pasteurized C1-INH administration (1000 IE) was 88 ± 39 minutes, and the mean ± standard deviation time to complete resolution of symptoms after drug administration was 10.1 ± 3.0 hours. Further interventions such as intubation, tracheotomy,

Table 3
Published data about the effectiveness of C1-esterase-inhibitor in angiotensin-converting-enzyme-induced angioedema

Author	Journal	Type	First Onset of Symptom Relief	Time to Complete Symptom Resolution	Conclusion	Notes
Gelée et al,[81] 2008	Rev Med Interne	1 Case	20 min	—	Successful treatment	1000 IE
Nielsen et al,[79] 2006	Acta Anaesthesiol Stand	1 Case	20 min	—	Successful treatment	1500 IE treatment after 8 h AE onset
Steinbach et al,[80] 2001	Anaesthesiol Reanim	1 Case	—	—	Successful treatment	—
Greve et al,[75] 2015	Laryngoscope	Case series	—	10 h	Successful	—

retreatment with pasteurized C1-INH, or additional medication such as corticosteroids were not necessary. No local side effects or systemic serious adverse events were reported directly after the injection or over a follow-up period of 3 months to 2 years. Furthermore, there were no recurrent angioedema within 6 months to 2 years after the cessation of ACE inhibitor treatment.

SUMMARY

The bradykinin B2 receptor antagonist icatibant is effective in ACE inhibitor–induced angioedema. The drug is not officially approved for this indication and has to be administered in emergency situation off-label. Corticosteroids or antihistamines do not seem to work in this condition. The effectiveness of C1 INH in ACE inhibitor–induced angioedema must be verified in a double-blind study.

REFERENCES

1. Bas M, Hoffmann TK, Kojda G. Evaluation and management of angioedema of the head and neck. Curr Opin Otolaryngol Head Neck Surg 2006;14:170–5.
2. Bas M, Adams V, Suvorava T, et al. Non-allergic angioedema. Role of bradykinin. Allergy 2007;62(8):842–56.
3. Kaplan AP, Greaves M. Pathogenesis of chronic urticaria. Clin Exp Allergy 2009; 39:777–87.
4. Maurer M, Grabbe J. Urticaria: its history-based diagnosis and etiologically oriented treatment. Dtsch Arztebl Int 2008;105:458–66.
5. McDowell SE, Coleman JJ, Ferner RE. Systematic review and meta-analysis of ethnic differences in risks of adverse reactions to drugs used in cardiovascular medicine. BMJ 2006;332:1177–81.
6. Sharma JN. Does kinin mediate the hypotensive action of angiotensin converting enzyme (ACE) inhibitors? Gen Pharmacol 1990;21:451–7.
7. Yang HY, Erdos EG, Levin Y. Characterization of a dipeptide hydrolase (kininase II: angiotensin I converting enzyme). J Pharmacol Exp Ther 1971;177:291–300.
8. Yang HY, Erdos EG, Levin Y. A dipeptidyl carboxypeptidase that converts angiotensin I and inactivates bradykinin. Biochim Biophys Acta 1970;214:374–6.
9. Nussberger J, Cugno M, Amstutz C, et al. Plasma bradykinin in angio-oedema. Lancet 1998;351:1693–7.
10. Adam A, Cugno M, Molinaro G, et al. Aminopeptidase P in individuals with a history of angio-oedema on ACE inhibitors. Lancet 2002;359:2088–9.
11. Lefebvre J, Murphey LJ, Hartert TV, et al. Dipeptidyl peptidase IV activity in patients with ACE-inhibitor-associated angioedema. Hypertension 2002;39:460–4.
12. Vavrek RJ, Stewart JM. Competitive antagonists of bradykinin. Peptides 1985;6: 161–4.
13. Roberts RA. Bradykinin receptors: characterization, distribution and mechanisms of signal transduction. Prog Growth Factor Res 1989;1:237–52.
14. Regoli D, Rhaleb NE, Drapeau G, et al. Kinin receptor subtypes. J Cardiovasc Pharmacol 1990;6(15 Suppl):S30–8.
15. Regoli D, Barabe J. Pharmacology of bradykinin and related kinins. Pharmacol Rev 1980;32:1–46.
16. Hess JF, Borkowski JA, Young GS, et al. Cloning and pharmacological characterization of a human bradykinin (BK-2) receptor. Biochem Biophys Res Commun 1992;184:260–8.
17. McEachern AE, Shelton ER, Bhakta S, et al. Expression cloning of a rat B2 bradykinin receptor. Proc Natl Acad Sci U S A 1991;88:7724–8.

18. Menke JG, Borkowski JA, Bierilo KK, et al. Expression cloning of a human B1 bradykinin receptor. J Biol Chem 1994;269:21583–6.
19. Ma JX, Wang DZ, Ward DC, et al. Structure and chromosomal localization of the gene (BDKRB2) encoding human bradykinin B2 receptor. Genomics 1994;23:362–9.
20. Chai KX, Ni A, Wang D, et al. Genomic DNA sequence, expression, and chromosomal localization of the human B1 bradykinin receptor gene BDKRB1. Genomics 1996;31:51–7.
21. Regoli DC, Marceau F, Lavigne J. Induction of beta 1- receptors for kinins in the rabbit by a bacterial lipopolysaccharide. Eur J Pharmacol 1981;71:105–15.
22. Bhoola KD, Figueroa CD, Worthy K. Bioregulation of kinins: kallikreins, kininogens, and kininases. Pharmacol Rev 1992;44:1–80.
23. Madeddu P, Emanueli C, Gaspa L, et al. Role of the bradykinin B2 receptor in the maturation of blood pressure phenotype: lesson from transgenic and knockout mice. Immunopharmacology 1999;44:9–13.
24. Han ED, MacFarlane RC, Mulligan AN, et al. Increased vascular permeability in C1 inhibitor- deficient mice mediated by the bradykinin type 2 receptor. J Clin Invest 2002;109:1057–63.
25. Groves P, Kurz S, Just H, et al. Role of endogenous bradykinin in human coronary vasomotor control. Circulation 1995;92:3424–30.
26. Hall JM. Bradykinin receptors: pharmacological properties and biological roles. Pharmacol Ther 1992;56:131–90.
27. Ellis EF, Heizer ML, Hambrecht GS, et al. Inhibition of bradykinin- and kallikrein induced cerebral arteriolar dilation by a specific bradykinin antagonist. Stroke 1987;18:792–5.
28. Marceau F, Regoli D. Bradykinin receptor ligands: therapeutic perspectives. Nat Rev Drug Discov 2004;3:845–52.
29. Duchene J, Schanstra JP, Pecher C, et al. A novel protein- protein interaction between a G protein-coupled receptor and the phosphatase SHP-2 is involved in bradykinin-induced inhibition of cell proliferation. J Biol Chem 2002;277:40375–83.
30. Busse R, Fleming I. Regulation of endothelium-derived vasoactive autacoid production by hemodynamic forces. Trends Pharmacol Sci 2003;24:24–9.
31. Smith D, Gilbert M, Owen WG. Tissue plasminogen activator release in vivo in response to vasoactive agents. Blood 1985;66:835–9.
32. Giannella E, Mochmann HC, Levi R. Ischemic preconditioning prevents the impairment of hypoxic coronary vasodilatation caused by ischemia/reperfusion: role of adenosine A1/A3 and bradykinin B2 receptor activation. Circ Res 1997;81:415–22.
33. Zhu P, Zaugg CE, Simper D, et al. Bradykinin improves postischaemic recovery in the rat heart: role of high energy phosphates, nitric oxide, and prostacyclin. Cardiovasc Res 1995;29:658–63.
34. Leesar MA, Stoddard MF, Manchikalapudi S, et al. Bradykinin-induced preconditioning in patients undergoing coronary angioplasty. J Am Coll Cardiol 1999;34(3):639–50.
35. Ritchie RH, Marsh JD, Lancaster WD, et al. Bradykinin blocks angiotensin II-induced hypertrophy in the presence of endothelial cells. Hypertension 1998;31:39–44.
36. Maestri R, Milia AF, Salis MB, et al. Cardiac hypertrophy and microvascular deficit in kinin B2 receptor knockout mice. Hypertension 2003;41:1151–5.
37. Fuller RW, Dixon CM, Cuss FM, et al. Bradykinin-induced bronchoconstriction in humans. Mode of action. Am Rev Respir Dis 1987;135:176–80.

38. Tsukagoshi H, Sun J, Kwon O, et al. Role of neutral endopeptidase in bronchial hyperresponsiveness to bradykinin induced by IL-1 beta. J Appl Physiol (1985) 1995;78:921–7.
39. Mukae S, Aoki S, Itoh S, et al. Bradykinin B(2) receptor gene polymorphism is associated with angiotensin-converting enzyme inhibitor-related cough. Hypertension 2000;36:127–31.
40. Hulsmann AR, Raatgeep HR, Saxena PR, et al. Bradykinin-induced contraction of human peripheral airways mediated by both bradykinin beta 2 and thromboxane prostanoid receptors. Am J Respir Crit Care Med 1994;150:1012–8.
41. Yang C, Hsu WH. Glucose-dependency of bradykinin-induced insulin secretion from the perfused rat pancreas. Regul Pept 1997;71:23–8.
42. Damas J, Bourdon V, Lefebvre PJ. Insulin sensitivity, clearance and release in kininogen-deficient rats. Exp Physiol 1999;84:549–57.
43. Duka I, Shenouda S, Johns C, et al. Role of the B(2) receptor of bradykinin in insulin sensitivity. Hypertension 2001;38:1355–60.
44. Rett K, Wicklmayr M, Dietze GJ. Metabolic effects of kinins: historical and recent developments. J Cardiovasc Pharmacol 1990;15(Suppl 6):S57–9.
45. Kishi K, Muromoto N, Nakaya Y, et al. Bradykinin directly triggers GLUT4 translocation via an insulin-independent pathway. Diabetes 1998;47:550–8.
46. Yusuf S, Sleight P, Pogue J, et al. Effects of an angiotensin-converting-enzyme inhibitor, ramipril, on cardiovascular events in high-risk patients. The Heart Outcomes Prevention Evaluation Study Investigators. N Engl J Med 2000;342:145–53.
47. Goring HD, Bork K, Spath PJ, et al. Hereditary angioedema in the German-speaking region. Hautarzt 1998;49:114–22 [in German].
48. Agostoni A, Ygoren-Pursun E, Binkley KE, et al. Hereditary and acquired angioedema: problems and progress: proceedings of the third C1 esterase inhibitor deficiency workshop and beyond. J Allergy Clin Immunol 2004;114:S51–131.
49. Kaplan AP, Greaves MW. Angioedema. J Am Acad Dermatol 2005;53:373–88.
50. Bork K, Fischer B, Dewald G. Recurrent episodes of skin angioedema and severe attacks of abdominal pain induced by oral contraceptives or hormone replacement therapy. Am J Med 2003;114:294–8.
51. Blanch A, Roche O, Urrutia I, et al. First case of homozygous C1 inhibitor deficiency. J Allergy Clin Immunol 2006;118:1330–5.
52. Bouillet L, Ponard D, Drouet C, et al. Angioedema and oral contraception. Dermatology 2003;206:106–9.
53. Pichler WJ, Lehner R, Spath PJ. Recurrent angioedema associated with hypogonadism or anti-androgen therapy. Ann Allergy 1989;63:301–5.
54. Agostoni A, Cicardi M, Cugno M, et al. Angioedema due to angiotensin-converting enzyme inhibitors. Immunopharmacology 1999;44:21–5.
55. Berkun Y, Shalit M. Hereditary angioedema first apparent in the ninth decade during treatment with ACE inhibitor. Ann Allergy Asthma Immunol 2001;87:138–9.
56. Messerli FH, Nussberger J. Vasopeptidase inhibition and angio-oedema. Lancet 2000;356:608–9.
57. Agostoni A, Cicardi M. Drug-induced angioedema without urticaria. Drug Saf 2001;24:599–606.
58. Gainer JV, Nadeau JH, Ryder D, et al. Increased sensitivity to bradykinin among African Americans. J Allergy Clin Immunol 1996;98:283–7.
59. Pfeffer MA, McMurray JJ, Velazquez EJ, et al. Valsartan, captopril, or both in myocardial infarction complicated by heart failure, left ventricular dysfunction, or both. N Engl J Med 2003;349:1893–906.

60. Kostis JB, Packer M, Black HR, et al. Omapatrilat and enalapril in patients with hypertension: the Omapatrilat Cardiovascular Treatment vs. Enalapril (OCTAVE) trial. Am J Hypertens 2004;17:103–11.
61. Campbell DJ, Krum H, Esler MD. Losartan increases bradykinin levels in hypertensive humans. Circulation 2005;111:315–20.
62. Goodfriend TL, Elliott ME, Catt KJ. Angiotensin receptors and their antagonists. N Engl J Med 1996;334:1649–54.
63. Hiyoshi H, Yayama K, Takano M, et al. Stimulation of cyclic GMP production via AT2 and B2 receptors in the pressure-overloaded aorta after banding. Hypertension 2004;43:1258–63.
64. Gohlke P, Pees C, Unger T. AT2 receptor stimulation increases aortic cyclic GMP in SHRSP by a kinin-dependent mechanism. Hypertension 1998;31:349–55.
65. Hellebrand MC, Kojda G, Hoffmann TK, et al. Angioedema due to ACE inhibitors and AT(1) receptor antagonists. Hautarzt 2006;57(9):808–10 [in German].
66. Oparil S, Yarows SA, Patel S, et al. Efficacy and safety of combined use of aliskiren and valsartan in patients with hypertension: a randomised, double-blind trial. Lancet 2007;370:221–9.
67. Oparil S, Yarows SA, Patel S, et al. Dual inhibition of the renin system by aliskiren and valsartan. Lancet 2007;370:1126–7.
68. Yarows SA, Oparil S, Patel S, et al. Aliskiren and valsartan in stage 2 hypertension: subgroup analysis of a randomized, double-blind study. Adv Ther 2008; 25:1288–302.
69. Solomon SD, Appelbaum E, Manning WJ, et al. Effect of the direct Renin inhibitor aliskiren, the Angiotensin receptor blocker losartan, or both on left ventricular mass in patients with hypertension and left ventricular hypertrophy. Circulation 2009;119:530–7.
70. Agostoni A, Cicardi M. Hereditary and acquired C1- inhibitor deficiency: biological and clinical characteristics in 235 patients. Medicine (Baltimore) 1992;71: 206–15.
71. Cicardi M, Zingale LC, Pappalardo E, et al. Autoantibodies and lymphoproliferative diseases in acquired C1-inhibitor deficiencies. Medicine (Baltimore) 2003;82: 274–81.
72. Markovic SN, Inwards DJ, Frigas EA, et al. Acquired C1 esterase inhibitor deficiency. Ann Intern Med 2000;132:144–50.
73. Gaur S, Cooley J, Aish L, et al. Lymphoma associated paraneoplastic angioedema with normal C1- inhibitor activity: does danazol work? Am J Hematol 2004;77:296–8.
74. Baş M, Greve J, Stelter K, et al. A randomized trial of icatibant in ACE-inhibitor-induced angioedema. N Engl J Med 2015;372(5):418–25.
75. Greve J, Bas M, Hoffmann TK, et al. Effect of C1-Esterase-inhibitor in angiotensin-converting enzyme inhibitor-induced angioedema. Laryngoscope 2015;125(6): E198–202.
76. Rasmussen ER, Bygum A. ACE-inhibitor induced angio-oedema treated with complement C1-inhibitor concentrate. BMJ Case Rep 2013.
77. Lipski SM, Casimir G, Vanlommel M, et al. Angiotensin-converting enzyme inhibitors-induced angioedema treated by C1 esterase inhibitor concentrate (Berinert®): about one case and review of the therapeutic arsenal. Clin Case Rep 2015;3(2):126–30.
78. Bas M, Greve J, Stelter K, et al. Therapeutic efficacy of icatibant in angioedema induced by angiotensin-converting enzyme inhibitors: a case series. Ann Emerg Med 2010;56(3):278–82.

79. Nielsen EW, Gramstad S. Angioedema from angiotensin-converting enzyme (ACE) inhibitor treated with complement 1 (C1) inhibitor concentrate. Acta Anaesthesiol Scand 2006;50(1):120–2.
80. Steinbach O, Schweder R, Freitag B. C1-esterase inhibitor in ACE inhibitor-induced severe angioedema of the tongue. Anaesthesiol Reanim 2001;26(5): 133–7 [in German].
81. Gelée B, Michel P, Haas R, et al. Angiotensin-converting enzyme inhibitor-related angioedema: emergency treatment with complement C1 inhibitor concentrate. Rev Med Interne 2008;29(6):516–9 [in French].

Differential Diagnosis of Chronic Urticaria and Angioedema Based on Molecular Biology, Pharmacology, and Proteomics

CrossMark

David H. Dreyfus, MD, PhD

KEYWORDS

- Autoantigen • Proteomics • Virokine • HERV • Herpes • Metagenome
- Microbiome omalizumab • Autoimmune

KEY POINTS

- Differential diagnosis and classification of chronic urticaria and angioedema should reflect advances in molecular biology, pharmacology, and proteomics.
- Advances in molecular biology and genetics illustrate the importance of the acquired immune system, autoreactive autoantibodies, pattern recognition molecules, and complement proteins.
- Chronic inflammation in chronic urticaria and angioedema may be related to complex interactions between the host immune system and the metagenome.

INTRODUCTION

Several recent practice guidelines have produced consensus differential diagnosis schemes for urticaria and angioedema with input from both US and European investigators.[1-5] The reader is referred to these comprehensive summaries for a traditional perspective on the differential diagnosis and therapy of urticaria and angioedema. Although historical classification schemes are useful, many patients with chronic urticaria do not neatly fit into current categories. Novel agents such as omalizumab (Xolair) approved for therapy of chronic urticaria, also often defy current classification schemes because some forms of chronic urticaria thought to be distinct in mechanism have similar responses to omalizumab therapy.

For the purposes of this article, urticaria and angioedema that persist for more than 6 to 8 weeks are termed "chronic urticaria," whatever the disease phenotype. However,

Conflicts of Interest: None.
Yale School of Medicine, Gesher LLC, Allergy, Asthma and Clinical Immunology, 4 Clifton Avenue, Waterbury CT 06710, USA
E-mail address: dhdreyfusmd@gmail.com

many forms of urticaria and angioedema that seem to be phenotypically similar differ in mechanisms and response to therapy.[6–9] Familial or hereditary forms of urticaria, although rare, have recently also been extensively characterized at a molecular level, and some patients even with no family history of urticaria may in the future be found to harbor some variants of these novel genes. With the decreasing costs of whole exome and whole genome sequencing and it is likely in the future that many families will have questions regarding genetic data available regarding specific gene mutations either in germ line cells or somatic tissues that were not available previously.[10–12]

For example, patients with angioedema owing to hereditary defects in the C1 inhibitor protein require different therapy than patients with angioedema owing to medications or autoreactive autoantibodies. Depending on the underlying mechanism recurrent episodes of angioedema, which can occur both with and without urticaria, some cases respond to omalizumab, some cases to discontinuation of medications such as angiotensin-converting enzyme inhibitors, whereas other cases respond to a variety of new therapies targeting the C1 inhibitor protein.[1,13] A diagnosis of hereditary angioedema, which is covered in more detail elsewhere in this issue, is currently divided into at least 3 categories (types 1, 2, and 3) based on distinct molecular mechanisms affecting the C1 inhibitor protein function or levels, but other proteins in the complement pathway may also be involved, leading to altered requirements and response to therapy.[1] The acquired form of angioedema associated with deficiency of C1 inhibitor proteins is usually associated with either malignant (type 1) or autoimmune disease (type 2) also recently characterized both by molecular mechanisms and response to therapy.[13]

Autoreactive antibodies are also present in many cases of chronic urticaria as are associations with other autoimmune syndromes such as autoimmune thyroid disease, although the mechanism underlying these associations is debated.[14–17] Improved methods of immune assays such as peptide arrays and proteomics can provide detailed molecular information about the targets of autoreactive antibodies in some forms of chronic urticaria, as will be discussed in more detail elsewhere in this review. Contributing still more complexity, increasing understanding of the microbiome and the metagenome (viruses, bacteriophage, and endogenous retroviruses) is likely to provide additional insight into urticaria and angioedema diagnosis as the prevalence of both atopy and autoimmune disease increases.[18]

In this review, the author provides a brief summary of conventional classification of urticaria and angioedema based on disease phenotype, because characterization of disease based on phenotype is a sufficient for clinicians in many cases. However, the author also proposes that new information with regard to disease mechanisms should be incorporated into future classification schemes (**Fig. 1**). The author then provides some suggestions regarding how a new understanding of disease mechanisms should ideally be incorporated and combined with new molecular information and response to therapy into any new classification schemes of urticaria and angioedema. The intention of the author is to augment the existing schemes of classification as outlined by incorporating specific molecular features of the innate immune system versus acquired immunity as well as response to conventional antihistamines, corticosteroids, and novel therapy such as cyclosporine and omalizumab into the diagnostic framework.

TRADITIONAL SCHEMES OF CLASSIFICATION OF CHRONIC URTICARIA BASED ON DISEASE PHENOTYPE AND THEIR LIMITATIONS IN DIFFERENTIAL DIAGNOSIS

As shown in **Fig. 1**, chronic urticaria and angioedema can be classified on the phenotypic presentation without any reference to underlying mechanism. In the author's own

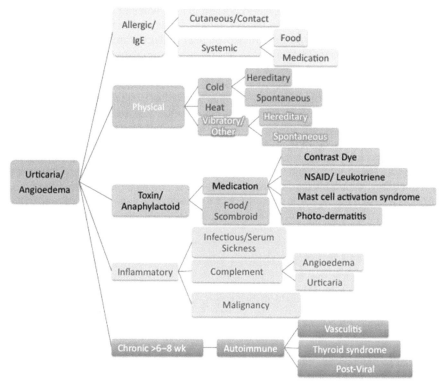

Fig. 1. Phenotypic classification of urticaria and angioedema. This figure is intended to provide a framework for clinical use based on the author's and others' experience that most presentations of urticaria and angioedema can be grouped in distinct categories that can predict prognosis and response to therapy. IgE, immunoglobulin E.

clinical experience most cases fall into 5 basic clinical presentations: (1) allergic or immunoglobulin (Ig)E mediated, (2) physical, (3) toxin mediated, (4) inflammatory, and (5) chronic. Of course, these categories are not mutually exclusive; for example, patients with an inflammatory urticaria owing to a malignancy may have exacerbations owing to allergy, cold, heat or other physical stimuli, medications, or toxins. Each of these categories may in turn be further divided, for example, with physical urticaria owing to cold versus heat, pressure, or vibration.

Often, these phenotypes show little or no overlap; for example, patients with cold urticaria very rarely or never in the author's experience present with simultaneous heat-triggered urticaria. For this reason, some classification schemes have proposed that the underlying mechanisms of, for example, cold-induced physical urticaria might be owing to a cold-sensitive immunoglobulin, whereas heat-induced urticaria (often also termed cholinergeric urticaria) might reflect cholinergic neuromediators rather than immunoglobulins. Although published literature beyond the scope of this review supports each of these mechanisms, in the authors opinion terms such as "cholinergic" are mechanistic rather than based on phenotype and should be reserved for cases in which specific neuromediators have been demonstrated. For clinical purposes, it is often sufficient to state that the patient's symptoms are triggered by reduction or elevation of local or core body temperature, or other physical causes without speculating about the mechanism or mechanisms involved.

Conversely, as shown in **Box 1**, it is important to note whether the patient's urticaria is related to a specific IgE and thus allergic in nature, because in most cases the presence of a specific IgE can be determined by skin testing or immunoassay and this finding may then be considered part of the disease phenotype. Testing for specific IgE is of great importance, for example, in establishing whether a patient who has had 6 months of daily hives has chronic urticaria or instead is suffering from living with a new partner who has pet cats. However, as noted in recent guidelines, extensive and unfocussed "screens" for environment or food triggers in patients with urticaria and angioedema are seldom productive and not useful or recommended. Similarly, if all the clients of a certain restaurant are suddenly incapacitated with urticaria and angioedema after eating a certain fish dish, the disease phenotype obtained by history is sufficient in many cases to implicate scrombroid or other food toxins without further testing for a specific IgE to fish.

Also as noted in **Fig. 1**, some phenotypes of urticaria and angioedema are extremely important in suggesting appropriate therapy, for example, angioedema without urticaria should immediately suggest a different approach to therapy, such as discontinuation of angiotensin-converting enzyme inhibitors, evaluation for an occult malignancy, or evaluation of the patient and other family members for hereditary angioedema or a related defect in complement the C1 inhibitor protein, as reviewed elsewhere in this issue. Also as noted, if a specific IgE can be associated with the urticaria angioedema phenotype, or a particular medication such as nonsteroidal antiinflammatory drugs can be implicated, then desensitization may be useful and even life saving in many cases. Urticaria and angioedema related to ingestion of a class of medications such as several different nonsteroidal antiinflammatory drugs is usually related to a metabolic imbalance in leukotriene and prostaglandin metabolism, whereas a reaction to a single nonsteroidal antiinflammatory drug may suggest an IgE-mediated pathology. Often, although not always, IgE-, physical-, or toxin-mediated urticaria and angioedema will respond to conventional antihistamines and oral corticosteroids, whereas inflammatory or chronic forms of urticaria and angioedema often will not respond to conventional therapy.

Box 1
Chronic urticaria/angioedema mechanism based terminology: an outline

1. Acute urticaria and angioedema
   a. IgE/allergy
   b. IgG/infection
   c. Complement
   d. Innate/mast cell hyperrelease syndrome

2.1. Chronic, familial
   Urticaria predominant/"gene name"
   Angioedema predominant/"gene name"[a]

2.2. Chronic, acquired
   IgG/IgE autoimmune predominant
      Autoantigen (s)
      Antibody type
      Viral or infection related[a]
   Physical predominant
   Angioedema predominant[a]

The author proposes that terms such as "idiopathic" and "spontaneous" should be eliminated and replaced by specific molecular and genetic data to the extent that these are known.
   [a] These terms are discussed in more detail in the text and figures.

Phenotypic classification schemes as shown in **Fig. 1** have been less useful, or in many cases of no use at all in the author's experience, in the case of chronic urticaria. Chronic urticaria often seems to resist any classification at all other than the fact that the urticaria and angioedema goes on for more than 6 to 8 weeks, and often for years. Although some associations with autoimmune disease have been established, it is often difficult to correlate these observations with prognosis or response to therapy, suggesting that there is some a lack of understanding of the mechanism underlying the phenotype. In frustration, many clinicians have adopted terms such as "idiopathic" and/or "spontaneous" to categorize chronic urticaria, terms that in the author's opinion add little or nothing to the diagnosis. Instead, for the remainder of this work, the author focuses on how new technology may clarify the underlying mechanisms of chronic urticaria and angioedema, and suggest that this information should be incorporated into future terminology and differential diagnosis.

DIFFERENTIAL DIAGNOSIS OF CHRONIC URTICARIA AND ANGIOEDEMA SHOULD INCORPORATE TERMS DERIVED FROM ADVANCES IN MOLECULAR BIOLOGY AND GENETICS

As noted, traditionally depending on the phenotype urticaria and angioedema were considered to have either "immunologic" or "nonimmunologic" mechanisms depending on whether immunoglobulin played a role in the disease.[13,17] More recently, this terminology has become antiquated with the discovery of the innate immune system that does not rely on immunoglobulin but rather conserved "pattern receptors."[19,20] Thus, the author proposes that the differential diagnosis of hereditary or acquired urticaria and angioedema should contain specific terms indicating whether the disease is primarily mediated by either the innate or the acquired system. Also, complement interacts with both acquired and innate immunity, and complement proteins if responsible should be identified (see **Box 1**). Terms such as "idiopathic" or "spontaneous" should be phased out whenever possible in the diagnosis of chronic urticaria, and instead components of the acquired or innate immune system including numerous specific pattern recognition molecules or by immunoglobulins or antibodies generated by the acquired immune should be specified to the extent that this information is known.

Hereditary syndromes are particularly useful and important in understanding underlying mechanisms of chronic urticaria, particularly because there are few or no animal model for chronic urticaria. Increasing numbers of single human gene mutations have been defined in the past several decades. The importance of these mutations is that they show that apparently urticarial phenotype can be generated entirely by an abnormal innate immune response.[10–12,19,21] Perhaps somatic mutations in these innate immune response genes may also play a role in acquired forms of urticaria and angioedema as well as a diverse population of immunoglobulin-independent "mast cell activation syndromes."[22,23] As the cost of genome sequencing decreases, it is likely that these innate immune gene mutations will be detected both in germ line tissues and also in somatic tissues contributing to or causing disease.

Similarly, hereditary angioedema without urticaria has historically been categorized as "type 1" resulting from a defect in the C1 inhibitor protein level, "type 2" resulting from a defect in protein function with normal or near normal C1 inhibitor protein levels, and "type 3" resulting from the disease without detected abnormal C1 inhibitor protein levels or function.[5] The term "type 3" has also sometimes been used to denote a specific form of estrogen-sensitive familial urticaria that in some ethnic groups is associated with a specific abnormality in the factor XII protein.[24–29] However, most clinicians who see significant numbers of patients with chronic angioedema encounter patients who do not fall neatly into any of these groups. A more detailed discussion of hereditary angioedema diagnosis, mechanisms and therapy is presented elsewhere in this issue.

To illustrate the limitations of phenotype-based diagnosis of angioedema, for the past decade the author has cared for a family in which females have normal C1 inhibitor protein levels and function by the most sensitive assays, and no described or detectable mutation in factor XII protein and yet have severe estrogen-sensitive angioedema with decreased complement C4 levels during attacks. Females in the family also have severe dysfunctional menstrual bleeding, suggesting that some other component of the coagulation pathway may be involved. Two of the affected females also have allergic urticaria and food-induced IgE-mediated anaphylaxis, possibly unrelated to the hereditary angioedema. Rather than adding more phenotypic subtypes, the author proposes that, like acquired urticaria and angioedema, hereditary angioedema would more accurately be described by the specific mutations in the complement or other proteins when this is known, or by the molecular phenotype such as "hereditary angioedema, estrogen dependent with decreased C4 levels and elevated IgE" in the specific family described.

DIFFERENTIAL DIAGNOSIS OF URTICARIA AND ANGIOEDEMA SHOULD INCLUDE PHARMACOLOGIC INFORMATION INDICATING RESPONSE TO THERAPY

Therapy over the past decade has been revolutionized concurrently with advances in molecular biology and genetics of chronic urticaria. Whereas a decade ago therapy for urticaria was limited largely to antihistamines and occasional oral corticosteroids, most clinicians now use monoclonal antibodies such as omalizumab and immune response–modifying agents such as cyclosporine. Although a full review of on- and off-labels uses for therapy of urticaria and angioedema is beyond the scope of this review, omalizumab may illustrate the complexity of response to these new therapies.

Omalizumab was first developed and FDA approved for asthma, and later found effective in chronic urticaria.[6] Omalizumab interferes with free IgE binding to high- and low-affinity IgE receptors on mast cells, basophils, and other hematopoietic cells; however, the effects of xolair in chronic urticaria may or may not be related to its effects on IgE receptors.[16,30,31] Almost immediately it was noted that most but not all patients with phenotypically similar chronic urticaria responded to omalizumab. In some patients, response was complete, in others partial, and in some not at all.[32] In addition, it was soon noted that there is not a simple relationship between serum IgE levels or other autoantibodies such as antithyroid antibodies and response to therapy.[33] This has led to the hypothesis that more complicated or indirect effects such as the downregulation of other cytokine receptors or endogenous viruses may contribute to the response to omalizumab.[34]

In addition, other forms of chronic urticaria such as physical urticarias triggered by cold seem in many cases to respond rapidly to omalizumab despite no apparent direct mechanistic link between these physical urticarias and IgE.[35–39] So-called mast cell activation syndromes, although relatively IgE and immunoglobulin independent, may also respond to omalizumab.[22,23] To help clarify these mysteries, some inclusion of response to therapy would be helpful; for example, it may be that chronic idiopathic or spontaneous urticaria that responds to xolair uses different molecular pathways than the same phenotype or apparent condition that does not respond to xolair. Alternatively, the same mechanism, such as alteration of inflammatory cytokines in the skin might be involved in both responsive and unresponsive forms, but with a dose-related window of efficacy.[33,40,41] Alternatively, autoantibodies might be present in some patients that neutralize omalizumab. Similarly, characterization of a response to therapy should be included in the differential diagnosis and description of "mast cell activation" syndromes.[22,23,42–45]

Hereditary and acquired angioedema had no FDA-approved treatment a decade ago and a single specific therapy, androgens; however, there has been a remarkable increase in both molecular diagnosis and therapy of these conditions as been reviewed extensively elsewhere.[5] Remarkably, in the case of hereditary angioedema, response among patients is variable with some having almost complete cessation of attack with addition of prophylactic administration of replacement C1 inhibitor protein, whereas others require a second rescue medication for treatment. Obviously, as in the case of chronic urticaria, in hereditary angioedema it would also be helpful to have a diagnostic schema including previous response to therapy to facilitate care among multiple providers and to develop more effective prophylactic therapy.

In the acquired form of angioedema, there is normal to increased synthesis of normal C1 inhibitor protein and either an excessive consumption of C1 inhibitor protein or a formation of circulating anti–C1 inhibitor protein antibodies that cleaves or otherwise transforms C1 inhibitor protein into a nonfunctional form.[13] In theory, acquired angioedema should not respond well to additional replacement C1 inhibitor proteins because the circulating abnormal proteins or immunoglobulins should inactivate the replacement protein rapidly; however, this has not been studied systematically.[5] The acquired form of C1 inhibitor protein has been divided into types 1 and 2, a distinction that may influence therapy.[13]

Type 1 acquired angioedema is associated with lymphoproliferative disorders and thus require chemotherapy of the underlying malignant or premalignant condition and responds to therapy directed at the underlying disease, whereas type 2 has been associated with autoimmune syndromes. In patients with acquired angioedema related to autoimmune disease, a wide variety of therapies have been attempted including therapy with androgens also useful in hereditary angioedema, unsuccessful depletion of autoreactive antibodies through plasmapheresis, replacement of C1 INH, eternacept blocking inflammatory tumor necrosis factor, as well as agents that interfere with generation of bradykinin. Remarkably, patients with both types of acquired angioedema seem to respond to depletion of B-lymphocytes with chimeric antibodies such as rituximab.[13] Rituximab, which depletes memory B-lymphocytes has been used successfully (and sometimes unsuccessfully) in both chronic urticaria and other autoimmune diseases such as rheumatoid arthritis, idiopathic thrombocytopenic purpura, idiopathic urticaria, autoimmune hemolytic anemia, systemic lupus erythematosis, multiple sclerosis, and acquired hemophilia.[46]

DIFFERENTIAL DIAGNOSIS OF URTICARIA AND ANGIOEDEMA SHOULD INCLUDE INFORMATION FROM NOVEL PROTEOMIC TECHNOLOGY

In many cases, chronic urticaria is a disease primarily of the acquired immune system associated with generation of abnormal or pathologic immunoglobulins in conditions previously termed "idiopathic" or "spontaneous."[14,15,47–49] These autoreactive antibodies have been proposed to trigger mast cells and basophils by binding and cross-linking surface IgE leading to release of mediators responsible for urticaria and angioedema. An advance has been the clinical availability of assays for basophil activation using donor basophils exposed to serum from patients with chronic urticaria.[49] Basophil activation tests or autologous skin tests that suggest the presence of serum-mediated activation of mast cells may prove useful particularly if positive, for example, to differentiate between angioedema mediated by complement pathways versus autoreactive antibodies as a guide for therapy.

However, basophil activation assays provide only a qualitative rather than quantitative answer and often are negative in the authors experience despite other evidence suggesting a component of an autoreactive immunoglobulin component, such as a comorbid autoimmune condition. Similarly, although in some cases of acquired angioedema a specific mechanism of complement depletion such as a premalignant lymphoma or complement autoreactive antibody can be detected, often these methods lack sensitivity, specificity and are not clinically available, except at a few specialized laboratories.[13] As shown in **Fig. 2**, it is likely that the next clinical advance will include proteomic methods in development for autoimmune diseases that could also radically alter classification of urticaria and angioedema.[50]

For example, the author has used proteomic technology for identification of novel sperm autoantigens in chronic urticaria after vasectomy (unpublished observations). After more than a year of daily urticaria after a vasectomy, a patient's serum was used to probe a sperm-specific protein library generated by gel electrophoresis. Using proteomic analysis of sperm proteins, 2 proteins were identified that could serve as triggering sperm antigens in this putative syndrome: (1) testis-specific protein 1 (NCBI accession # NP_003287) and (2) similar to the alpha subunit, or the macropapain iota subunit of the proteosome multicatalytic endopeptidase complex (NCBI accession # CAA43964 and # AAH5552). Evidence of IgE autoantibodies to both proteins were present in addition to autoreactive IgG. Antithyroid microsomal and peroxidase antibodies and a positive basophil activation test were also present. A full discussion of this patient will be recounted elsewhere; however, the power of

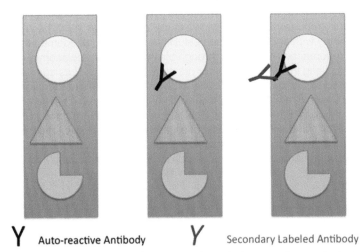

Y Auto-reactive Antibody   Y Secondary Labeled Antibody

Fig. 2. Replacement of labor-intensive proteomic techniques such as gel electrophoresis with more advanced technology to identify autoantibodies is predicted to occur through arrays of antigen printed microchips. As shown, individual proteins or peptides (shown as 3 different shapes), are bound to a chip and incubated with patient and control serum. After washing, bound autoantibodies are detected with secondary antibody binding only to 1 of the 3 proteins (*top circle*). With miniaturization of this new technology, thousand of autoantigens and corresponding autoantibodies can be bound chronic urticaria to serum immunoglobulin, washed, and labeled to detect and characterize bound autoantibodies in mass production.

proteomics has recently been established independently in published peer-reviewed studies.[15,33] For example, in chronic urticaria associated with thyroid autoimmunity, organ-specific IgE as well as IgG can be demonstrated. Whatever the mechanisms responsible for the generation of these abnormal disease-associated antibodies, it will be of great interest to see to what extent specific autoimmune IgE and IgG are correlated with disease prognosis and response to therapy.

DIFFERENTIAL DIAGNOSIS OF CHRONIC URTICARIA AND ANGIOEDEMA SHOULD INCLUDE MECHANISMS IDENTIFIED IN OTHER SYSTEMIC AUTOIMMUNE AND INFLAMMATORY DISEASES AND SYNDROMES

Viral proteins, like sperm proteins, frequently contain enzymatic activities such as proteases and nucleases. Also like sperm, viral proteins are foreign to the immune system developed in infancy through the acquired immune system. Thus, like sperm proteins that come in contact with the immune system after vasectomy, viral proteins from acute viral infection or reactivation may trigger some forms of chronic urticaria.[34,46] Although some patients with chronic urticaria respond to antiviral therapy such as acyclovir, most do not, suggesting that once autoantibodies and autoreactive inflammatory processes are present, they may trigger pathology independent of active infection.

Extensive observations suggest that systemic lupus erythematosis and other systemic syndromes such as scleroderma causing epithelial disease are associated with abnormal response to chronic infection with some herpesviridae, specifically human herpes virus (HHV)-4 and HHV-6.[46,51] In other autoimmune syndromes affecting the neuroepithelium such as multiple sclerosis, serology to HHV-4 antigens is

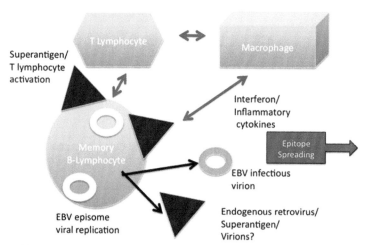

Fig. 3. Possible role of human endogenous retrovirus (HERV) in autoimmune disease. Both gamma herpes viruses such as human herpes virus (HHV)-4 (Epstein-Barr virus [EBV]) latent in memory B lymphocytes and HHV-6 in infected CD4 T-lymphocytes transactivate HERV superantigens that can both activate and suppress immune responses during viral reactivation as discussed in more detail in the text. Herpes reactivation may also reflect altered T helper cell type 2 cytokine balance in the host owing to hygiene, other illness, or factors; chronic urticaria thus could provide a useful means to study human autoimmune disease in situ in humans because a skin biopsy can be obtained much more readily than a brain biopsy in multiple sclerosis or other systemic autoimmune syndromes.

detected years or decades before presentation of clinical disease and may correlate with disease exacerbations.[46] Possibly, a common mechanism or mechanism may underlie autoimmune pathogenesis because beta and gamma herpesviruses are capable of triggering both systemic and localized inflammation through a variety of mechanisms including viral encoded cytokines (virokines), and viral encoded microRNA.[18]

As shown in **Fig. 3**, an intriguing possibility is that HHV-6 and HHV-4 viruses are particularly associated with autoimmune syndromes because they replicate in lymphocytes and activate endogenous superantigens expressed on lymphocytes encoded by extinct retroviruses or human endogenous retroviruses.[46] Herpes virus replication and gene expression are not independent of the host, but instead influenced by host T helper cell type 2 cytokine and other inflammatory cytokine expression, and viral gene expression in turn interacts with host T helper cell type 2 cytokine expression in epithelial tissues.[41] As the prevalence of both T helper cell type 2–mediated atopic disease and also autoimmune disease increase in modern societies, it is

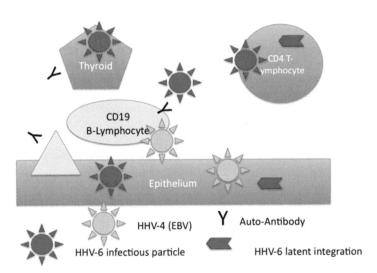

Fig. 4. The chronic viral urticaria (CVU) paradigm. In the CVU model, the initial triggering event in chronic urticaria (CU) is localized cutaneous inflammation owing to reactivation of beta and gamma herpes viruses that subsequently activate superantigens from endogenous human endogenous retroviruses (HERV). Perhaps many years after primary human herpes virus (HHV)-6 infection, reactivation of gene expression from HHV-6–infected CD4 lymphocytes and epithelial cells could trigger a chronic inflammatory state associated with HERV reactivation and clinically observed autoimmune pathology as well as depletion of mast cells in the skin and basophils in the serum. This inflammatory state would be sufficient to trigger urticaria analogous to the exanthem of primary herpes infection. Long-term cutaneous inflammation would also stimulate proliferation in situ of local autoreactive HHV-4 positive B lymphocyte clones. Many questions remain unresolved, for example, whether use of omalizumab is correlated with decreased viral reactivation of herpes and herpes and HERV gene expression in the skin. Related questions include whether level of elevation of initial HHV-6 and HHV-4 titers predict a clinical response to omalizumab and a response to anti-viral therapy, and to what extent mechanisms of chronic urticaria are shared with severe drug allergy syndromes such as drug reaction with eosinophilia and systemic symptoms and/or delayed hypersensitivity with systemic symptoms (see text).

probable that increased T helper cell type 2 bias in the skin would also predict an increased prevalence of chronic urticaria.[18]

Based on analysis of a response to antiviral therapy in some patients with chronic urticaria, the author recently presented a working model of urticaria pathogenesis in some cases as a syndrome termed chronic viral urticaria related to partial or complete reactivation of a beta or gamma herpes virus or viruses in both endocrine and cutaneous tissues[34,46] (**Fig. 4**). An important and long-standing observation in chronic urticaria is an association with autoimmune thyroid disease that may also have HHV-6 as a cofactor.[52] HHV-4 and HHV-6 reactivation also is implicated in severe cutaneous drug allergy syndromes termed drug reaction with eosinophilia and systemic symptoms and/or delayed hypersensitivity with systemic symptoms driven by increased gene expression of a chronic viral pathogen.[34] A common underlying etiology for the underlying inflammation in thyroid disease, drug reaction with eosinophilia and systemic symptoms and chronic urticaria could open a new window into definitive or curative therapies both in all of these autoimmune conditions.

Long-standing clinical observations have suggested that patients who report multiple drug and antibiotics allergy often have underlying chronic urticaria, supporting a common mechanism that might be a target for new therapy. A related and unresolved clinical question concerns whether all forms of chronic urticaria and angioedema, including physical urticaria syndromes, share some common inflammatory pathway because physical urticaria, although phenotypically diverse, also often responds to omalizumab. If in some forms of chronic urticaria the underlying defect is related to abnormal gene expression of reactivated herpes viruses and human endogenous retroviruses in cutaneous tissues, then monitoring of herpes and human endogenous retroviruses serology or related markers for viral infection could be useful in predicting response to both conventional and antiviral therapy. Similarly, proteomics, and messenger RNA or other gene profiling methods might be helpful in discriminating between patients with active cutaneous viral gene expression and replication and those with inflammation not related to active viral replication to predict response to therapy.

SUMMARY

New molecular and pharmacologic techniques and therapies have blurred many of the traditional categories of differential diagnosis and therapy particularly for chronic urticaria and angioedema. Rather than the impossible task of attempting to review all of these developments, instead the author has used selective examples from his own literature review and clinical experience to illustrate the limitations of phenotype based diagnosis and corresponding complexity of urticaria and angioedema diagnosis by molecular mechanism and response to therapy. Apparently, new genomic methods such as whole exome and whole genome sequencing both of germ line and somatic tissues, proteomics, and new targeted therapies will permit very detailed characterization of chronic urticaria and angioedema and this information must somehow be incorporated into new classification schemes.

The author has focused also on the role of inflammation in triggering chronic urticaria, and the author suggests there may be significant overlap between chronic urticaria and other autoimmune conditions detected by proteomic technology in the future. Chronic urticaria may also yield insights into acute urticaria, either IgE mediated or postviral, physical urticaria and mast cell activation syndromes, as well as severe drug allergy such as drug reaction with eosinophilia and systemic symptoms and/or delayed hypersensitivity with systemic symptoms, which may also share innate and acquired immune response owing to chronic viral reactivation.[34,46] Importantly, many or even most phenotypically distinct cases of familial urticaria and angioedema can now be characterized as the results of specific gene mutations, often in the innate and complement components of the immune system rather than resulting from defects in the acquired immune system (see **Box 1**). Because of these advances in molecular biology and pharmacology, the author suggests that poorly defined terms such as "idiopathic" and "spontaneous" do not provide any additional information and should be eliminated from future terminology.

Classification of response to therapy is also useful in differential diagnosis of urticaria although often surprisingly unpredictable (**Box 2**). With respect to the role of the acquired immune system, autoreactive antibodies are certainly present in many acquired chronic urticaria and angioedema phenotypes, but a causal role for these antibodies is more difficult to establish and may benefit in the future from more advanced combinations of proteomic and immunologic technologies (see **Fig. 2**). As shown in **Fig. 2**, the proteomic methods outlined also can be combined with immunologic methods into very powerful screens to detect hundreds or thousands of autoreactive antigens and antibodies.

As increasing data regarding specific autoantibody specificity emerges from novel technology, it will be interesting to what extent these observations can be integrated into diagnostic algorithms (see **Box 1**) and correlated with response to therapy (see **Box 2**). It is likely that correlations with other cutaneous autoimmune and inflammatory syndromes will also emerge from this data. In summary, many different phenotypic forms of chronic urticaria, particularly nonhereditary forms, may result from complex and chaotic interactions between the genome, pharmacologic therapy, and the microbiome and metagenome (see **Figs. 3** and **4**). Clinicians seeking accurate differential diagnosis of chronic urticaria and angioedema should continue to use phenotypic classification schemes as outlined in **Fig. 1** of this work, but also bear in mind Jonathan Swift (1667–1745) who wrote in his poem for children "Syphonaptera" more than 300 years ago shortly after the first microscopes revealed unexpected complexity of microscopic organisms:

> *Big fleas have little fleas,*
> *Upon their backs to bite 'em,*
> *And little fleas have lesser fleas,*
> *and so, ad infinitum.*

Box 2
Classification of chronic urticaria subtypes by response to therapy: an outline

Antihistamine responsive, unresponsive

Antiviral/antibiotic responsive, unresponsive

Corticosteroid responsive, unresponsive

Cyclosporine responsive, unresponsive

Omalizumab responsive, unresponsive

Other responsive, unresponsive

The author proposes that terms such as "idiopathic" and "spontaneous" should be eliminated and replaced by specific pharmacologic response data to the extent that this is known. This box is not intended to provide an exhaustive list of all possible reported therapy for chronic urticaria, but instead to provide a framework for more definitive future nomenclature.

ACKNOWLEDGMENTS

The author acknowledges Marcus Maurer, MD, Charite Hospital, Berlin, Germany, and Alessandra Farina, Boston University Medical School, Boston, Massachusetts, for helpful discussions. The author also acknowledges his urticaria and angioedema patients over the years who have often provided their own insights into diagnosis and therapy.

REFERENCES

1. Bernstein JA, Lang DM, Khan DA, et al. The diagnosis and management of acute and chronic urticaria: 2014 update. J Allergy Clin Immunol 2014;133:1270–7.
2. Kaplan AP. Therapy of chronic urticaria: a simple, modern approach. Ann Allergy Asthma Immunol 2014;112:419–25.
3. Weller K, Zuberbier T, Maurer M. Chronic urticaria: tools to aid the diagnosis and assessment of disease status in daily practice. J Eur Acad Dermatol Venereol 2015;29(Suppl 3):38–44.
4. Zuberbier T, Aberer W, Asero R, et al, European Academy of Allergy and Clinical Immunology, Global Allergy and Asthma European Network, European Dermatology Forum, World Allergy Organization. The EAACI/GA(2) LEN/EDF/WAO Guideline for the definition, classification, diagnosis, and management of urticaria: the 2013 revision and update. Allergy 2014;69:868–87.
5. Zuraw BL, Bernstein JA, Lang DM, et al, American Academy of Allergy, Asthma and Immunology, American College of Allergy, Asthma and Immunology. A focused parameter update: hereditary angioedema, acquired C1 inhibitor deficiency, and angiotensin-converting enzyme inhibitor-associated angioedema. J Allergy Clin Immunol 2013;131:1491–3.
6. Kaplan AP, Joseph K, Saini SS. How omalizumab came to be studied as a therapy for chronic spontaneous/idiopathic urticaria. J Allergy Clin Immunol Pract 2015;3:648.
7. Magerl M, Staubach P, Altrichter S, et al. Effective treatment of therapy-resistant chronic spontaneous urticaria with omalizumab. J Allergy Clin Immunol 2010;126: 665–6.
8. Vieira Dos Santos R, Locks Bidese B, Rabello de Souza J, et al. Effects of omalizumab in a patient with three types of chronic urticaria. Br J Dermatol 2014;170: 469–71.
9. Zuberbier T, Maurer M. Omalizumab for the treatment of chronic urticaria. Expert Rev Clin Immunol 2015;11:171–80.
10. Boyden SE, Desai A, Cruse G, et al. Vibratory urticaria associated with a missense variant in ADGRE2. N Engl J Med 2016;374:656–63.
11. Milner JD. PLAID: a syndrome of complex patterns of disease and unique phenotypes. J Clin Immunol 2015;35:527–30.
12. Ombrello MJ, Remmers EF, Sun G, et al. Cold urticaria, immunodeficiency, and autoimmunity related to PLCG2 deletions. N Engl J Med 2012;366:330–8.
13. Dreyfus DH, Na CR, Randolph CC, et al. Successful rituximab B lymphocyte depletion therapy for angioedema due to acquired C1 inhibitor protein deficiency: association with reduced C1 inhibitor protein autoantibody titers. Isr Med Assoc J 2014;16:315–6.
14. Altrichter S, Peter HJ, Pisarevskaja D, et al. IgE mediated autoallergy against thyroid peroxidase–a novel pathomechanism of chronic spontaneous urticaria? PLoS One 2011;6:e14794.

15. Chang TW, Chen C, Lin CJ, et al. The potential pharmacologic mechanisms of omalizumab in patients with chronic spontaneous urticaria. J Allergy Clin Immunol 2015;135:337–42.

16. Dreyfus DH. Observations on the mechanism of omalizumab as a steroid-sparing agent in autoimmune or chronic idiopathic urticaria and angioedema. Ann Allergy Asthma Immunol 2008;100:624–5.

17. Greaves M. Autoimmune urticaria. Clin Rev Allergy Immunol 2002;23:171–83.

18. Dreyfus DH. Herpesviruses and the microbiome. J Allergy Clin Immunol 2013; 132:1278–86.

19. McDermott MF, Aksentijevich I. The autoinflammatory syndromes. Curr Opin Allergy Clin Immunol 2002;2:511–6.

20. Philpott DJ, Sorbara MT, Robertson SJ, et al. NOD proteins: regulators of inflammation in health and disease. Nat Rev Immunol 2014;14:9–23.

21. Fritz JH, Ferrero RL, Philpott DJ, et al. Nod-like proteins in immunity, inflammation and disease. Nat Immunol 2006;7:1250–7.

22. Frieri M. Mast cell activation syndrome. Clin Rev Allergy Immunol 2016. [Epub ahead of print].

23. Jagdis A, Vadas P. Omalizumab effectively prevents recurrent refractory anaphylaxis in a patient with monoclonal mast cell activation syndrome. Ann Allergy Asthma Immunol 2014;113:115–6.

24. Gompel A, Fain O, Bouillet L. Progestins are efficient agents in estrogen-sensitive nonhistaminic angioedema. Am J Med 2014;127:e7.

25. Binkley KE. Factor XII mutations, estrogen-dependent inherited angioedema, and related conditions. Allergy Asthma Clin Immunol 2010;6:16.

26. Duan QL, Binkley K, Rouleau GA. Genetic analysis of Factor XII and bradykinin catabolic enzymes in a family with estrogen-dependent inherited angioedema. J Allergy Clin Immunol 2009;123:906–10.

27. Hentges F, Hilger C, Kohnen M, et al. Angioedema and estrogen-dependent angioedema with activation of the contact system. J Allergy Clin Immunol 2009;123:262–4.

28. McGlinchey PG, McCluskey DR. Hereditary angioedema precipitated by estrogen replacement therapy in a menopausal woman. Am J Med Sci 2000;320:212–3.

29. Binkley KE, Davis A 3rd. Clinical, biochemical, and genetic characterization of a novel estrogen-dependent inherited form of angioedema. J Allergy Clin Immunol 2000;106:546–50.

30. Gericke J, Ohanyan T, Church MK, et al. Omalizumab may not inhibit mast cell and basophil activation in vitro. J Eur Acad Dermatol Venereol 2015;29:1832–6.

31. Staubach P, Metz M, Chapman-Rothe N, et al. Effect of omalizumab on angioedema in H1 -antihistamine resistant chronic spontaneous urticaria patients: results from X-ACT, a randomised controlled trial. Allergy 2016;71:1135–44.

32. Kaplan A, Ledford D, Ashby M, et al. Omalizumab in patients with symptomatic chronic idiopathic/spontaneous urticaria despite standard combination therapy. J Allergy Clin Immunol 2013;132:101–9.

33. Altrichter S, Hawro T, Hanel K, et al. Successful omalizumab treatment in chronic spontaneous urticaria is associated with lowering of serum IL-31 levels. J Eur Acad Dermatol Venereol 2016;30:454–5.

34. Dreyfus DH. Serological evidence that activation of ubiquitous human herpesvirus-6 (HHV-6) plays a role in chronic idiopathic/spontaneous urticaria (CIU). Clin Exp Immunol 2016;183:230–8.

35. Kaplan A, Ferrer M, Bernstein JA, et al. Timing and duration of omalizumab response in patients with chronic idiopathic/spontaneous urticaria. J Allergy Clin Immunol 2016;137:474–81.

36. Kaplan AP, Popov TA. Biologic agents and the therapy of chronic spontaneous urticaria. Curr Opin Allergy Clin Immunol 2014;14:347–53.
37. Metz M, Ohanyan T, Church MK, et al. Omalizumab is an effective and rapidly acting therapy in difficult-to-treat chronic urticaria: a retrospective clinical analysis. J Dermatol Sci 2014;73:57–62.
38. Netchiporouk E, Nguyen CH, Thuraisingham T, et al. Management of pediatric chronic spontaneous and physical urticaria patients with omalizumab: case series. Pediatr Allergy Immunol 2015;26:585–8.
39. Zhao ZT, Ji CM, Yu WJ, et al. Omalizumab for the treatment of chronic spontaneous urticaria: A meta-analysis of randomized clinical trials. J Allergy Clin Immunol 2016;137:1742–50.e4.
40. de Koning HD, van Vlijmen-Willems IM, Rodijk-Olthuis D, et al. Mast-cell interleukin-1beta, neutrophil interleukin-17 and epidermal antimicrobial proteins in the neutrophilic urticarial dermatosis in Schnitzler's syndrome. Br J Dermatol 2015;173:448–56.
41. Kay AB, Clark P, Maurer M, et al. Elevations in T-helper-2-initiating cytokines (interleukin-33, interleukin-25 and thymic stromal lymphopoietin) in lesional skin from chronic spontaneous ('idiopathic') urticaria. Br J Dermatol 2015;172:1294–302.
42. Afrin LB, Cichocki FM, Patel K, et al. Successful treatment of mast cell activation syndrome with sunitinib. Eur J Haematol 2015;95:595–7.
43. Asawa A, Simpson KH, Bonds RS. Ketotifen use in a patient with fire ant hypersensitivity and mast cell activation syndrome. Ann Allergy Asthma Immunol 2015;114:443–6.
44. Kounis NG, Kounis GN, Soufras GD, et al. Therapeutic hypothermia, stent thrombosis and the Kounis mast cell activation-associated syndrome. Int J Cardiol 2015;179:504–6.
45. Sabato V, Van De Vijver E, Hagendorens M, et al. Familial hypertryptasemia with associated mast cell activation syndrome. J Allergy Clin Immunol 2014;134:1448–50.e3.
46. Dreyfus DH. Autoimmune disease: a role for new anti-viral therapies? Autoimmun Rev 2011;11:88–97.
47. Kolkhir P, Pogorelov D, Olisova O, et al. Comorbidity and pathogenic links of chronic spontaneous urticaria and systemic lupus erythematosus - a systematic review. Clin Exp Allergy 2016;6:275–87.
48. Maurer M, Altrichter S, Bieber T, et al. Efficacy and safety of omalizumab in patients with chronic urticaria who exhibit IgE against thyroperoxidase. J Allergy Clin Immunol 2011;128:202–9.e5.
49. Yasnowsky KM, Dreskin SC, Efaw B, et al. Chronic urticaria sera increase basophil CD203c expression. J Allergy Clin Immunol 2006;117:1430–4.
50. Putterman C, Wu A, Reiner-Benaim A, et al. SLE-key((R)) rule-out serologic test for excluding the diagnosis of systemic lupus erythematosus: developing the ImmunArray iCHIP((R)). J Immunol Methods 2016;429:1–6.
51. Farina A, Cirone M, York M, et al. Epstein-Barr virus infection induces aberrant TLR activation pathway and fibroblast-myofibroblast conversion in scleroderma. J Invest Dermatol 2014;134:954–64.
52. Caselli E, Zatelli MC, Rizzo R, et al. Virologic and immunologic evidence supporting an association between HHV-6 and Hashimoto's thyroiditis. Plos Pathog 2012;8:e1002951.

Cutaneous Manifestation of Food Allergy

Jonathan S. Tam, MD

KEYWORDS

• Food allergy • Atopic dermatitis • Urticaria • Contact dermatitis • Contact urticaria

KEY POINTS

- Urticaria is the most common symptom in patients experiencing food-induced anaphylaxis, but the prevalence across all IgE-mediated food reactions is unknown.
- Contact urticaria can be immunologic or nonimmunologic. Immunologic contact urticaria may be associated with development of a protein contact dermatitis.
- Atopic dermatitis commonly occurs with food sensitization and is a significant risk factor for the development of IgE-mediated food allergy.
- The prevalence of food-induced exacerbations of atopic dermatitis is unclear; food is likely more important in young children with atopic dermatitis.
- Food elimination should be done with caution in correctly selected patients.

Food allergy is defined by the National Institute of Allergy and Infectious Diseases expert panel "as an adverse health effect arising from a specific immune response that occurs reproducibly on exposure to a given food".[1] As defined, food allergy encompasses a wide array of clinical and immunologic adverse reactions to food. Manifestations of food allergy are diverse and reflect the complex interactions of the food protein, gastrointestinal system, immune system, and target organs. Although food initially contacts the gastrointestinal mucosa, allergic manifestations commonly occur outside the gastrointestinal tract, affecting distant target sites. The skin is not only the largest organ of the human body but also one of the most frequently targeted organs for food hypersensitivity reactions. As such, clinical manifestations for food reactions range from IgE-mediated reactions (urticaria, angioedema, flushing, pruritus, and erythematous morbilliform rash), cell-mediated reactions (contact dermatitis and dermatitis herpetiformis), and mixed IgE-mediated and cell-mediated (atopic dermatitis [AD]) reactions (**Table 1**).

Given the apparent increase of IgE-mediated food allergy in developed countries[2,3] and the emergence as a potential health threat in countries with rapid industrialization,[4]

Disclosure Statement: The author listed below has identified no professional or financial affiliation for themselves or their spouse/partner: J.S. Tam.
Division of Clinical Immunology and Allergy, Department of Pediatrics, Children's Hospital Los Angeles, 4650 Sunset Boulevard MS#75, Los Angeles, CA 90027, USA
E-mail address: jstam@chla.usc.edu

Immunol Allergy Clin N Am 37 (2017) 217–231
http://dx.doi.org/10.1016/j.iac.2016.08.013
0889-8561/17/© 2016 Elsevier Inc. All rights reserved.

Table 1
Cutaneous food reactions

Reaction Type	Timing	Diagnostic Evaluation
Urticaria	Immediate	Skin prick testing, food-specific IgE testing, oral food challenge
Contact urticaria		
IgE-mediated	Immediate	Skin prick testing
Non–immune mediated	Immediate	Skin prick testing, repeat open application testing
Oral allergy syndrome	Immediate	Fresh fruit/vegetable prick-by-prick testing + aeroallergen testing (skin prick or specific IgE), oral food challenge
Contact dermatitis		
ACD	Delayed	Patch testing
ICD	Immediate	Empiric avoidance
PCD	Immediate, chronic/recurrent	Patch testing
Phototoxic contact dermatitis	Delayed	Photo-patch testing
Photoallergic contact dermatitis	Delayed	Photo-patch testing
Systemic contact dermatitis	Immediate or delayed	Patch testing
AD	Immediate or delayed	Skin prick testing, food-specific IgE testing may be used to guide food challenge ± specific elimination diets

it is important to recognize adverse food reactions and their possible cutaneous manifestations. For most of these skin manifestations provoked by food, pruritus is a hallmark of the disease. Itch may help differentiate mimickers of food allergy such as auriculotemporal syndrome (Frey syndrome).[5,6] These cutaneous manifestations provide an opportunity to better understand the diversity of adverse immunologic responses to food and the interconnected pathways that produce them.

URTICARIA

Urticaria is characterized by the appearance of pruritic, erythematous papules or plaques, with superficial swelling of the dermis. Urticaria affects approximately 20% of the population at some point.[7] Urticaria is categorized by its chronicity; urticaria lasting less than 6 weeks is considered acute, whereas urticaria recurring frequently for longer than 6 weeks is considered chronic.[8,9] The distinction is somewhat arbitrary, except that acute urticaria is more often associated with an identifiable cause than in chronic urticaria.[10] Acute urticaria tends to be more common in younger patients,[11] occurs more often in atopic patients, and is much more likely to be caused by food allergy than is chronic urticaria. In contrast, chronic urticaria is rarely caused by IgE-mediated reactions to foods, but food is frequently perceived by patients as a potential cause; yet, virtually no reported food reactions in chronic urticaria patients are confirmed by double-blind, placebo-controlled food challenge (DBPCFC). At most, studies suggest that foods provoke chronic urticaria in 1% to 2% of all patients.[10,12,13]

Conversely, IgE-mediated allergic reactions to food are known to play a role in acute urticaria. Urticaria and angioedema are thought to be some of the most common presentations of food allergy. Although urticaria is the most common symptom in patients experiencing food-induced anaphylaxis,[14–16] the prevalence across all IgE-mediated food reactions is unknown, and estimates vary greatly.[17,18] Several studies using food challenges found that most positive food reactions have some cutaneous manifestations.[19–21] These studies found that cutaneous reactions occurred in 75% of the positive challenges, generally consisting of pruritic, morbilliform, or macular eruptions. Looking at food challenges over 16 years of DBPCFCs, cutaneous reactions were the most frequent symptoms for all foods tested[22]; cutaneous symptoms were present in 62% of all reactions. Looking at the presentation of food-allergic and anaphylactic events from 34 participating emergency departments in the National Electronic Injury Surveillance System in the United States, Ross and colleagues[23] found skin symptoms were the most common complaint presenting for care. Urticaria and angioedema were the most common with urticaria accounting for 38%. In contrast, a German study of adults found only 8.7% reporting skin reactions,[24] whereas a population-based study in France reported 57% of those affected reporting urticaria and 26% reporting angioedema.[25]

In children, the most frequently reported foods causing urticaria are egg, milk, peanuts, and tree nuts. In adults, fish, shellfish, tree nuts and peanuts are reported as the most common.[1] However, the prevalence of any particular food allergy may vary by location. For example, in a French population study, the most frequently reported foods were rosaceae fruits, vegetables, milk, crustaceans, fruit cross-reacting with latex, egg, tree nuts, and peanut.[25] Similarly, in a Mediterranean adult population from Turkey, vegetables, egg, and fruits were the most frequent foods to cause urticaria and angioedema.[26]

After consumption of the offending food, urticaria or angioedema may appear rapidly within minutes or take up to 2 hours to appear. Flushing, pruritus, and morbilliform rash may precede the development of urticaria or angioedema. The shape and size of wheals vary from millimeters to a few centimeters; some may coalesce to form giant lesions with raised borders. The wheals may appear in one location and fade in another within minutes or hours, but an individual wheal should not persist for greater than 24 hours.

Histologic examination of these urticarial lesions find that skin mast cells have degranulated in the dermis.[27] Mast cells express high-affinity IgE receptors that bind to the constant region domain of IgE. Food allergens interact with IgE bound to the patient's tissue mast cells and trigger the reaction upon re-exposure to the antigen. This event elicits mast cell degranulation and the subsequent release of vasoactive mediators. Histamine, which is critical to the formation of the urticarial lesions,[27] is released by preformed granules in the mast cells and is noted to be elevated in biopsied skin.[28,29]

Histamine causes vasodilation and vascular permeability. The peripheral release of neurotransmitters like substance P from type C cutaneous fibers and resulting end-organ effect is known as an *axon reflex*, which helps perpetuate and further the allergic inflammation.[30] Substance P, in particular, also further stimulates mast cells to increase their histamine release. Other membrane-derived mediators such as prostaglandins and leukotrienes are subsequently released, contributing to vasodilation and an increase in microvascular permeability, all of which allow fluid leakage into the superficial tissues.

Lymphocytes, neutrophils, eosinophils and basophils can be found migrating into the perivascular space of the skin lesion.[27] Like mast cells, basophils release histamine and other inflammatory mediators (prostaglandins, leukotrienes, cytokines) on activation and are capable of causing local vasodilation, itch, and swelling in the skin. Roles for eosinophils, lymphocytes, and neutrophils have not fully been elucidated.

CONTACT URTICARIA

Acute urticaria may be the result of ingestion and processing of antigens through the gastrointestinal tract or a local reaction from topical exposure to a food. The food can directly contact the skin or contact in the form of dust, steam, and aerosolized proteins (produced during cooking or boiling).[31,32] The reaction may begin locally, but disseminate with systemic symptoms.[33]

These contact reactions can be categorized as immunologic or nonimmunologic. Immunologic (allergic) contact urticaria is caused by immediate-type hypersensitivity (IgE mediated), whereas nonallergic contact dermatitis is caused by direct stimulation and the release of vasoactive substances like histamine from mast cells.[34] Both forms present similarly with a rapid onset of wheal-and-flare reaction on an erythematous base. Because symptoms occur so rapidly after exposure, the etiology is usually obvious.

Both forms of these reactions are most commonly reported because of occupational exposures. For example, bakers and preparers of processed food were found to rank among the most commonly affected by occupational contact urticaria in Finland.[35] Any job that entails food handling is a potential cause of contact urticaria. Raw meats, seafood, raw vegetables, and fruits are among the foods that have been most commonly implicated.[36–38]

Nonimmunologic contact urticaria is most commonly reported with foods high in histamine/histamine-related compounds (sauerkraut, pickled herring, tuna), foods that cause direct release of histamine (strawberry), or with other food additives found in soft drinks, chewing gum, or baked goods (benzoic acid, sorbic acid, cinnamic acid, cinnamic aldehyde, and balsam of Peru).[34,39,40]

A common form of immediate contact allergy is oral allergy syndrome, also known as *pollen-food allergy syndrome*, which occurs in people who have pollen allergy[1,41]; patients often report itching or mild swelling of the mouth and throat immediately after ingestion of certain uncooked fruits, vegetables, or nuts. Usually, symptoms are mild, self-limited, and localized to the oral mucosa, although they may sometimes become generalized and life threatening. Symptoms improve rapidly after the food is swallowed because of proteolytic denaturation by the gastrointestinal enzymes of these type 2 allergens. Heating of the food helps prevent symptoms for most allergens.[42,43]

CONTACT DERMATITIS

In addition to urticaria, contact reactions to food include irritant contact dermatitis, allergic contact dermatitis, protein contact dermatitis, photo contact dermatitis (phototoxic and photoallergic), and systemic contact dermatitis.

Irritant contact dermatitis (ICD) is the most common and is the result of direct toxic effect of an agent on the epidermis without a need for prior sensitization. The pathophysiologic mechanism involves activation of the innate immune system and skin barrier disruption leading to proinflammatory mediators (eg, tumor necrosis factor-α, interleukin-1) that directly recruit and activate T lymphocytes.[44] Even though the mechanism of ICD does not require immunologic memory, atopy does seem to increase susceptibility to irritant contact dermatitis. Specifically, patients with AD are at increased risk, possibly because of changes in skin barrier function.[45] Case-control studies looking at patients with ICD in Germany identified that loss-of- function polymorphisms in the filaggrin gene have been associated with an increased susceptibility to chronic ICD.[46] Foods that commonly induce ICD include garlic, onion, spices, citrus fruits, potatoes, pineapple, corn, radish, carrots, and mustard.[34,47,48] Spices and their essential oils are also known irritants.

Allergic contact dermatitis (ACD) can be difficult to distinguish from ICD. ACD may be more acute in presentation with significant pruritus and possible vesicle formation, frank blistering, and swelling. Unlike in ICD, the borders of lesions in ACD are often poorly defined. Additionally, ACD may undergo a phenomenon known as *secondary spread*, in which additional lesions can appear on other parts of the body that have not come into contact with the allergen.[34]

ACD is a classic delayed hypersensitivity reaction (type IV) in the skin occurring in a sensitized individual on contact. ACD is initiated by allergen bypassing the outer layers of skin and finding its way to major histocompatibility complex class II on antigen-presenting cells below. Although ACD overall may be common, ACD caused by food is thought to be rare.[34] These antigens tend to be low-molecular-weight substances requiring haptenization. The classic example of ACD related to food is mango dermatitis. The plant family Anacardiaceae (poison ivy and poison oak) contains other species such as mango, cashew, and ginkgo, which all contain the identical oleoresin urushiol that cross-react with poison ivy. Mango dermatitis most commonly develops around the mouth and on the hands from exposure to the peel, leaves, or stem of the mango and not the juice.[47,49]

Protein contact dermatitis (PCD) is a combination of immediate (type I) and delayed (type IV) hypersensitivity. The causative allergens are high-molecular-weight proteins in foods that can only penetrate the skin and cause sensitization if the epidermis is damage such as in AD. Not surprisingly, given the mixed pathophysiology of PCD, immunologic contact urticaria may be associated with development of a PCD.[50,51] Patients with PCD report a history of immediate reactions such as urticaria, erythema, and itching 30 minutes after exposure to the food, followed by chronic relapsing eczematous dermatitis. The most frequently reported foods to cause PCD are raw seafood, eggs, and flour.[47,48]

Photo contact dermatitis results when substances or food are converted into an irritant (phototoxic) or an allergen (photoallergic) as a result of sun exposure. This conversion usually requires a specific wavelength for specific substance, principally in the ultraviolet A range (wavelength, 320–400 nm).[34] Phototoxicity is more common, as many plants can cause a phototoxic response. The classic example is skin exposure to lime juice; citrus fruits (Rutaceae), as well as many other plant families, contain psoralens (furocoumarins). After sun exposure, these substances can lead to angulated, streaky erythema on the areas of exposure and hyperpigmentation, which can last months.[47]

Photoallergic contact dermatitis resembles allergic contact dermatitis on sun-exposed areas; however, as in ACD, borders may be poorly defined and extend into covered areas. The most commonly reported cases are caused by diallyl disulfide in garlic.[52]

Systemic contact dermatitis may occur when a sensitized individual is exposed to allergens from routes other than skin exposure, such as orally, parenterally, or by inhalation. Several foods have been described as responsible for systemic contact dermatitis including garlic, onion, herbs, fish, cashew nuts, various spices, and food additives.[34,47,53]

ATOPIC DERMATITIS

AD is a chronic relapsing inflammatory skin disease, which is characterized by extreme pruritus and a distinctive skin distribution.[54] Patients with AD have higher rates of allergic diseases than the general population, with up to 80% of children with AD having asthma or allergic rhinitis later in childhood.[55] The relationship between

AD and food allergy is complicated and somewhat controversial. Although it is undeniable that the 2 diseases commonly present concurrently, their relationship influencing one another is an area of active investigation.

Food allergy has been strongly correlated with the persistence of AD, especially during infancy and early childhood.[56,57] High levels of food-specific IgE have been associated with earlier age of onset for AD and increased disease severity.[58–60] Moreover, patients with AD are at risk for the development of immediate food hypersensitivity reactions. Based on DBPCFCs, up to 40% of children with moderate-to-severe AD have a concomitant IgE-mediated food allergy.[61] An even higher proportion of children with AD were found to produce IgE to common food allergens.[58,62] In a multicenter, international study of 2184 children with active eczema, 64% of infants with severe AD that developed before 3 months of age had high levels of food-specific IgE, indicating an association between early-onset severe AD and significant sensitization to these food allergens.[58]

This close relationship with food allergy and AD seems strongest in infant and young children, and is thought to be less important in adults. Food-exacerbated AD is thought to be rare in adults, based on a poor response to elimination diets in unselected cases.[63] However, a study from Japan found that 44% of the 195 adults with AD had positive challenges to foods; interestingly, the causative foods listed in this study were uncommon allergens, including chocolate, coffee, and rice.[64] Another German study found that certain adult subjects who were sensitized to pollen allergens were consequently also sensitized to pollen-associated food allergens.[65]

Food-specific IgE in Atopic Dermatitis

Unfortunately, food-specific IgE was found in AD to poorly correlate with clinically relevant food allergy.[66] In a retrospective chart review, 125 children with AD and positive food-specific IgE were evaluated by oral food challenge; only a small proportion of these children had clinical reactions on exposure to these foods. In this study, there was poor correlation between food sensitization and both immediate and delayed eczematous reactions in childhood AD.[21] In general, patients with AD have a high rate of sensitization to foods ranging from 30% to 80%, but the actual rate of confirmed food allergy is much lower.[67–70] In a birth cohort from Denmark, 52% of children who had AD during the first 6 years of life were sensitized to at least 1 food allergen, but only 15% had challenge-proven food allergy.[69]

This limitation in the utility of food specific IgE in AD has led some clinicians to conclude that food allergy is not a factor in AD, whereas others think that food triggers play a significant role in exacerbating AD in young children. Nevertheless, clinicians have all experienced parents who report a history of foods worsening their child's eczema. This finding may be tied to the parent's desire to have an explanation for their child's condition but does not explain symptom improvement for some select children with elimination diets. So although it is clear patients with AD are at increased risk of development of IgE-mediated food allergy, the reverse relationship of food-exacerbated AD has been more controversial.

Evaluations of Food Exacerbating Atopic Dermatitis

Part of the difficulty in evaluating food as an exacerbating factor for AD centers around the timing of reactions and difficulty excluding other confounding factors. Also, reactions to food in patients with AD may take one of 3 forms[71]:

- Immediate urticaria but no flare in AD
- Pruritus with subsequent excoriation leading to exacerbation of AD
- Isolated exacerbations of AD after 6 to 48 hours, termed *late reactions*

Studies using food challenge testing have not been as consistent in reporting these late reactions. A study from Germany looking retrospectively at 106 DBPCFCs to cow's milk, hen's egg, wheat, and soy in 64 children with AD found isolated late eczematous reactions in 12% of all positive challenges.[72] Similarly, Niggemann and colleagues[73] found that late eczematous reactions (after 2 hours) occurred in 18.9% of positive reactions. In a recent study looking at outcomes of 1186 DBPCFCs performed for suspicion of food allergy, 54.9% of those challenges had a current history of AD and on challenge, late eczematous reactions were unlikely to occur without other immediate symptoms preceding.[74] In this study, late eczematous reactions alone were uncommon, but unlike the prior studies, late reactions were only ascertained by semistructured telephone interview 48 hours after challenge rather than direct observation.

Immunopathology of Food and Atopic Dermatitis

The focus on IgE may distract from other parts of the immune system, which could be playing a significant role in food-sensitive AD. Patients with AD have high systemic immune activation with increased T helper 2 (Th2) polar differentiation of effector and memory T cells, particularly in those T cells homing to the skin.[75,76] Several studies helped clarify the role of food allergen–specific T cells in the underlying inflammatory process in AD. Food-specific T cells have been isolated and cloned from active AD lesions.[77–80] These food-specific T cells have also been identified in peripheral blood in subjects with food allergy–associated AD.[77–80] Further evidence of T-lymphocyte involvement in the development of AD in food-allergic patients relates to the homing of allergen-specific T cells to the skin.[77] The extravasation of T cells at sites of inflammation critically depends on the activity of homing receptors that are involved in endothelial cell recognition and binding. Studies in patients with peanut allergy found T cells with high expression of skin-homing receptor CLA in the serum.[81] Additionally, peanut component Ara h1-reactive T cells in the serum of peanut-allergic individuals expressed high levels of CCR4, another skin homing receptor.[82]

Genetic mutations resulting in primary immune deficiency have also helped elucidate this tight genetic relationship between AD and food allergy. IPEX (immune dysregulation, polyendocrinopathy, enteropathy, X-linked) is caused by a gene mutation that affects the FOXP3 protein and generation of regulatory T cells.[83,84] Food allergies and eczema develop in these patients, demonstrating a failure of tolerance.[84] Patients with Netherton syndrome, caused by mutations in serine protease inhibitor Karzal type 5 (SPINK5), also have a severe AD-like rash, Th2 polarization, increased IgE levels, and food allergy.[85,86] Japanese investigators found an association of SPINK5 mutations in children with AD.[87,88] Furthermore, a SPINK5 polymorphism was significantly associated with increased disease severity among Japanese children younger than 10 years with AD and food allergy.[86]

Important genetic mutations in the epidermal structural protein filaggrin (FLG) have been identified as key defects resulting in epidermal barrier dysfunction.[89] As discussed earlier, FLG is a risk factor for the development of ICD. Loss-of-function genetic mutations result in decreased epidermal defense mechanisms against allergens and microbes. FLG gene mutations and resultant epidermal barrier dysfunction have been linked to the development, progression, and severity of AD and increased susceptibility to skin infections.[54]

Epidermal barrier dysfunction may result in increased penetration of allergens through the skin, thereby making the skin a potentially important route by which individuals are sensitized to food and airborne allergens. The importance of FLG deficiency in allergic sensitization was found in several murine studies using the FLG loss-of-function mutation in the flaky tail (ft/ft) mouse. In a study of these flaky tail mice, ovalbumin was applied to the skin to elicit inflammatory infiltrates and enhance allergen priming.[90] Although the normal mice did not develop any specific IgE response, the flaky tail mice showed elevated ovalbumin-specific IgE without any additional adjuvant or abrasion of the skin. However, transmembrane protein 79 (Tmeme79/matt) gene, rather than *FLG*, was later proven to be responsible for the spontaneous development of dermatitis in the flaky tail mouse model.[91,92] *Tmem79/matt* gene encodes for lamella granular proteins, which are responsible for processing filaggrin, lipids, proteases, and antimicrobial peptides.

Filaggrin has been associated with increased food allergy and several diseases with known barrier defects such as ichthyosis vulgaris and AD.[93] Depending on the study, *FLG* has been found in high percentages of up to 56% in these conditions.[94] In food allergy, the impaired skin barrier resulting from defects in filaggrin expression has been hypothesized as a gateway for food allergens and as a way to avoid the oral tolerance pathways of the gut mucosa.[95] *FLG* loss of function has been variably associated with human food allergy. An analysis of 71 peanut-allergic patients from Europe compared with 1000 nonallergic patients showed a strong and statistically significant connection between the occurrence of the allergy and *FLG*. This risk was further replicated in analysis of the results from 390 Canadian patients.[96] Brough and colleagues[97] found that in patients from the United Kingdom, the probability of peanut allergen sensitization correlated linearly with environmental peanut exposure in children with AD and loss-of-function *FLG* mutations. However, the same group did not find the same association with peanut exposure in children with AD and loss-of-function FLG mutations in the United States.[98] They did show that severe AD (associated with immune-mediated skin barrier dysfunction) was associated with environmental peanut exposure. Interestingly, a recent study in adults found that filaggrin gene mutations, without concomitant AD, were not associated with food and aeroallergen sensitization.[99] This finding that the key mechanism is the skin barrier dysfunction rather than the filaggrin gene mutation itself leading to risk of food allergy.

Disruptions of skin barrier function other than filaggrin deficiency are generally required for experimental epicutaneous sensitization. In most mouse models of epicutaneous sensitization, the stratum corneum needs to be mechanically impaired by tape stripping, patch dressing, or treatment with adjuvant.[100,101] The one notable exception to the requirement of barrier disruption seems to be peanut. In mice, peanut skin exposure alone without any skin stripping promotes a Th2-dependent sensitization to peanut allergens.[102] This special adjuvant activity of peanut not only shows the unique nature of peanut allergy, but also underscores the skin as a key site of sensitization.

AD more commonly precedes the development of food allergy; however, a prospective birth cohort of 552 infants in Australia with a family history of atopic disease noted that in some infants, sensitization precedes and predicts the development of AD, whereas in others, AD precedes and predicts the development of sensitization.[103] This finding may reflect how AD and food allergy arise from complex pathologic interaction between several factors, including a genetic predisposition, dysregulated immune response, and environmental triggers that include allergens, irritants, and microbes.

How gene–environment interactions influence clinical outcomes is a significant gap in understanding. *Staphylococcus aureus* can cause significant skin barrier dysfunction and might thereby promote food allergy in patients with AD through epicutaneous entry of antigen. IgE sensitization to egg white has been significantly associated with IgE sensitization to staphylococcal superantigens in older children.[59] Further, food allergy is associated with *S aureus* colonization in children with AD.[104]

Elimination Diets in Atopic Dermatitis

AD and food allergy seem to be epidemiologically and mechanistically linked, but the most significant controversy lies in the role of food elimination diets for AD. There is a question of efficacy and of risk. There is a risk of a more severe reaction, including anaphylaxis, when foods are reintroduced.[105] In a retrospective study of 298 patients, 19% of patients with food-triggered AD and no previous history of immediate reactions had new immediate food reactions after initiation of an elimination diet.[106]

Although several studies attempted to address the therapeutic effect of food elimination diets in AD, many of these trials had significant limitations. A meta-analysis showed lack of benefit for exclusion diets in patients with AD[107]; however, 9 of 10 of the randomized trials in this meta-analysis enrolled patients with AD who were not selected for a suspicion of food allergy based on clinical history or test results. The one trial that did select for patients with suspected egg allergy (positive specific IgE to egg) found that an egg elimination diet led to improvements in the extent and severity of AD in half of infants.[108] A study of children between the ages of 2 and 8 years with AD showed marked improvement in two-thirds of subjects during a double-blind crossover trial of milk and egg exclusion.[109] Unfortunately, this study was complicated by high dropout and exclusion rates and lack of control of environmental factors and other triggers of AD. Taken in aggregate, the studies support the role of food elimination diets in properly selected children but may be limited in adults.

Children with AD should not have food introductions delayed in hopes of preventing allergy. Recent evidence strongly argues that early oral exposure helps build oral tolerance.[110,111] Evidence supporting the role of early exposure in decreasing food allergy has been well demonstrated with egg and peanut allergy.[112,113] This early exposure was particularly dramatic in high-risk children including those with AD; the Learning Early about Peanut Allergy study found a dramatic difference in peanut allergy prevalence in the peanut avoidance group (17.2%) compared with the peanut consumption group (3.2%),[114] which was durable after a period of avoidance.[115]

SUMMARY

Cutaneous manifestations represent some of the most common presentations of food allergy and provide a framework to evaluate the mutual and divergent immunologic mechanisms of the diseases. Diagnosis for some may be simpler than others, but all involve identification of the causative food through history and testing followed by confirmation of clinical allergy.[116,117] Most importantly, clinicians should maintain a high index of suspicion for the potential role of food allergy to best manage their patients with cutaneous symptoms. The diagnosis may be complicated, requiring a combination of history, laboratory assessment, and dietary manipulation with oral food challenge. Patient selection and re-evaluation are critical in difficult cases. Food challenges should be performed in these cases to confirm clinical reactivity to the food and prevent inappropriate food avoidance.[118]

REFERENCES

1. Boyce JA, Assa'ad A, Burks AW, et al. Guidelines for the diagnosis and management of food allergy in the United States: report of the NIAID-sponsored expert panel. J Allergy Clin Immunol 2010;126(6):S1–58.
2. Sicherer SH, Muñoz-Furlong A, Sampson HA. Prevalence of peanut and tree nut allergy in the United States determined by means of a random digit dial

telephone survey: a 5-year follow-up study. J Allergy Clin Immunol 2003;112(6): 1203–7.

3. Liew WK, Williamson E, Tang MLK. Anaphylaxis fatalities and admissions in Australia. J Allergy Clin Immunol 2009;123(2):434–42.

4. Chen J, Hu Y, Allen KJ, et al. The prevalence of food allergy in infants in Chongqing, China. Pediatr Allergy Immunol 2011;22(4):356–60.

5. Beck SA, Burks WA, Woody RC. Auriculotemporal syndrome seen clinically as food allergy. Pediatrics 1989;83(4):601–3.

6. Sicherer SH, Sampson HA. Auriculotemporal syndrome: a masquerader of food allergy. J Allergy Clin Immunol 1996;97(3):851–2.

7. Greaves MW. Chronic Urticaria. N Engl J Med 1995;332(26):1767–72.

8. Bailey E, Shaker M. An update on childhood urticaria and angioedema. Curr Opin Pediatr 2008;20(4):425–30.

9. Bernstein JA, Lang DM, Khan DA, et al. The diagnosis and management of acute and chronic urticaria: 2014 update. J Allergy Clin Immunol 2014;133(5): 1270–7.

10. Sehgal VN, Rege VL. An interrogative study of 158 urticaria patients. Ann Allergy 1973;31(6):279–83.

11. Monroe EW, Jones HE. Urticaria: an updated review. Arch Dermatol 1977; 113(1):80–90.

12. Champion RH, Roberts SOB, Carpenter RG, et al. Uritcaria and Angio-oedema. Br J Dermatol 1969;81(8):588–97.

13. Nizami RM, Baboo MT. Office management of patients with urticaria: an analysis of 215 patients. Ann Allergy 1974;33(2):78–85.

14. Sampson HA, Muñoz-Furlong A, Bock SA, et al. Symposium on the definition and management of anaphylaxis: summary report. J Allergy Clin Immunol 2005;115(3):584–91.

15. Simons FER. Anaphylaxis. J Allergy Clin Immunol 2010;125(2 Suppl 2):S161–81.

16. Järvinen KM. Food-induced anaphylaxis. Curr Opin Allergy Clin Immunol 2011; 11(3):255–61.

17. Bahna SL. Clinical expressions of food allergy. Ann Allergy Asthma Immunol 2003;90(6 Suppl 3):41–4.

18. Burks W. Skin manifestations of food allergy. Pediatrics 2003;111(Suppl 3): 1617–24.

19. Fleischer DM, Conover-Walker MK, Christie L, et al. The natural progression of peanut allergy: resolution and the possibility of recurrence. J Allergy Clin Immunol 2003;112(1):183–9.

20. Mankad VS, Williams LW, Lee LA, et al. Safety of open food challenges in the office setting. Ann Allergy Asthma Immunol 2008;100(5):469–74.

21. Fleischer DM, Bock SA, Spears GC, et al. Oral food challenges in children with a diagnosis of food allergy. J Pediatr 2011;158(4):578–83.e1.

22. Bock SA, Atkins FM. Patterns of food hypersensitivity during sixteen years of double-blind, placebo-controlled food challenges. J Pediatr 1990;117(4):561–7.

23. Ross MP, Ferguson M, Street D, et al. Analysis of food-allergic and anaphylactic events in the National electronic injury surveillance system. J Allergy Clin Immunol 2008;121(1):166–71.

24. Schäfer T, Böhler E, Ruhdorfer S, et al. Epidemiology of food allergy/food intolerance in adults: associations with other manifestations of atopy. Allergy 2001; 56(12):1172–9.

25. Kanny G, Moneret-Vautrin D-A, Flabbee J, et al. Population study of food allergy in France. J Allergy Clin Immunol 2001;108(1):133–40.

26. Gelincik A, Büyüköztürk S, Gül H, et al. Confirmed prevalence of food allergy and non-allergic food hypersensitivity in a Mediterranean population. Clin Exp Allergy 2008;38(8):1333–41.
27. Ying S, Kikuchi Y, Meng Q, et al. TH1/TH2 cytokines and inflammatory cells in skin biopsy specimens from patients with chronic idiopathic urticaria: comparison with the allergen-induced late-phase cutaneous reaction. J Allergy Clin Immunol 2002;109(4):694–700.
28. Claveau J, Lavoie A, Brunet C, et al. Chronic idiopathic urticaria: possible contribution of histamine-releasing factor to pathogenesis. J Allergy Clin Immunol 1993;92(1):132–7.
29. Kaplan AP, Horáková Z, Katz SI. Assessment of tissue fluid histamine levels in patients with urticaria. J Allergy Clin Immunol 1978;61(6):350–4.
30. McDonald DM, Bowden JJ, Baluk P, et al. Neurogenic inflammation. A model for studying efferent actions of sensory nerves. Adv Exp Med Biol 1996;410: 453–62.
31. Crespo JF, Pascual C, Dominguez C, et al. Allergic reactions associated with airborne fish particles in IgE-mediated fish hypersensitive patients. Allergy 1995;50(3):257–61.
32. Martínez Alonso JC, Callejo Melgosa A, Fuentes Gonzalo MJ, et al. Angioedema induced by inhalation of vapours from cooked white bean in a child. Allergol Immunopathol (Madr) 2005;33(04):228–30.
33. Bourrain JL. Occupational contact urticaria. Clin Rev Allergy Immunol 2006; 30(1):39–46.
34. Killig C, Werfel T. Contact reactions to food. Curr Allergy Asthma Rep 2008;8(3): 209–14.
35. Kanerva L, Toikkanen J, Jolanki R, et al. Statistical data on occupational contact urticaria. Contact Derm 1996;35(4):229–33.
36. Fisher AA. Contact urticaria from handling meats and fowl. Cutis 1982;30(6): 726.
37. Jovanovic M, Oliwifcki S, Beck MH. Occupational contact urticaria from beef associated with hand eczema. Contact Derm 1992;27(3):188–9.
38. Delgado J, Castillo R, Quiralte J, et al. Contact urticaria in a child from raw potato. Contact Derm 1996;35(3):179–80.
39. Yamaguchi J, Inomata N, Hirokado M, et al. A case of occupational contact urticaria and oral allergy syndrome due to seafood. Arerugi 2007;56(1):49–53.
40. Fasano MB. Dermatologic food allergy. Pediatr Ann 2006;35(10):727–31.
41. Konstantinou GN, Grattan CEH. Food contact hypersensitivity syndrome: the mucosal contact urticaria paradigm. Clin Exp Dermatol 2008;33(4):383–9.
42. Breiteneder H, Ebner C. Molecular and biochemical classification of plant-derived food allergens. J Allergy Clin Immunol 2000;106(1 Pt 1):27–36.
43. Bohle B, Zwölfer B, Heratizadeh A, et al. Cooking birch pollen–related food: divergent consequences for IgE- and T cell–mediated reactivity in vitro and in vivo. J Allergy Clin Immunol 2006;118(1):242–9.
44. Ale IS, Maibach HI. Irritant contact dermatitis. Rev Environ Health 2014;29(3): 195–206.
45. Slodownik D, Lee A, Nixon R. Irritant contact dermatitis: a review. Australas J Dermatol 2008;49(1):1–11.
46. De Jongh CM, Khrenova L, Verberk MM, et al. Loss-of-function polymorphisms in the filaggrin gene are associated with an increased susceptibility to chronic irritant contact dermatitis: a case–control study. Br J Dermatol 2008;159(3): 621–7.

47. Amado A, Jacob SE. Contact dermatitis caused by foods. Actas Dermosifiliogr 2007;98(7):452–8.
48. Warshaw EM, Belsito DV, DeLeo VA, et al. North American Contact Dermatitis Group Patch-Test Results, 2003-2004 study period. Dermatitis 2008;19(3):129–36.
49. Hershko K, Weinberg I, Ingber A. Exploring the mango – poison ivy connection: the riddle of discriminative plant dermatitis. Contact Derm 2005;52(1):3–5.
50. Hjorth N, Roed-Petersen J. Occupational protein contact dermatitis in food handlers. Contact Derm 1976;2(1):28–42.
51. Wakelin SH. Contact urticaria. Clin Exp Dermatol 2001;26(2):132–6.
52. Borrelli F, Capasso R, Izzo AA. Garlic (Allium sativum L.): adverse effects and drug interactions in humans. Mol Nutr Food Res 2007;51(11):1386–97.
53. Erdmann SM, Werfel T. Hematogenous contact eczema induced by foods. Hautarzt 2006;57(2):116–20.
54. Leung DYM. Clinical implications of new mechanistic insights into atopic dermatitis. Curr Opin Pediatr 2016;28(4):456–62.
55. Eichenfield LF, Hanifin JM, Beck LA, et al. Atopic dermatitis and asthma: parallels in the evolution of treatment. Pediatrics 2003;111(3):608–16.
56. Sampson HA, Scanlon SM. Natural history of food hypersensitivity in children with atopic dermatitis. J Pediatr 1989;115(1):23–7.
57. Burks AW, Mallory SB, Williams LW, et al. Atopic dermatitis: clinical relevance of food hypersensitivity reactions. J Pediatr 1988;113(3):447–51.
58. Hill DJ, Hosking CS, De Benedictis FM, et al. Confirmation of the association between high levels of immunoglobulin E food sensitization and eczema in infancy: an international study. Clin Exp Allergy 2008;38(1):161–8.
59. Ong PY. Association between egg and staphylococcal superantigen IgE sensitizations in atopic dermatitis. Allergy Asthma Proc 2014;35(4):346–8.
60. Guillet G, Guillet M. Natural history of sensitizations in atopic dermatitis: a 3-year follow-up in 250 children: food allergy and high risk of respiratory symptoms. Arch Dermatol 1992;128(2):187–92.
61. Eigenmann PA, Sicherer SH, Borkowski TA, et al. Prevalence of IgE-mediated food allergy among children with atopic dermatitis. Pediatrics 1998;101(3):e8.
62. Sampson HA. Update on food allergy. J Allergy Clin Immunol 2004;113(5):805–19.
63. Bath-Hextall F, Delamere FM, Williams HC. Dietary exclusions for improving established atopic eczema in adults and children: systematic review. Allergy 2009;64(2):258–64.
64. Uenishi T, Sugiura H, Uehara M. Role of foods in irregular aggravation of atopic dermatitis. J Dermatol 2003;30(2):91–7.
65. Worm M, Forschner K, Lee H-H, et al. Frequency of atopic dermatitis and relevance of food allergy in adults in Germany. Acta Derm Venereol 2006;86(2):119–22.
66. Spergel JM, Boguniewicz M, Schneider L, et al. Food allergy in infants with atopic dermatitis: limitations of food-specific IgE measurements. Pediatrics 2015;136(6):e1530–8.
67. Sampson HA. Food allergy. Part 2: diagnosis and management. J Allergy Clin Immunol 1999;103(6):981–9.
68. Hill DJ, Heine RG, Hosking CS. The diagnostic value of skin prick testing in children with food allergy. Pediatr Allergy Immunol 2004;15(5):435–41.
69. Eller E, Kjaer HF, Høst A, et al. Food allergy and food sensitization in early childhood: results from the DARC cohort. Allergy 2009;64(7):1023–9.

70. Kvenshagen B, Jacobsen M, Halvorsen R. Atopic dermatitis in premature and term children. Arch Dis Child 2009;94(3):202–5.
71. Werfel T, Breuer K. Role of food allergy in atopic dermatitis. Curr Opin Allergy Clin Immunol 2004;4(5):379–85.
72. Breuer K, Heratizadeh A, Wulf A, et al. Late eczematous reactions to food in children with atopic dermatitis. Clin Exp Allergy 2004;34(5):817–24.
73. Niggemann B, Sielaff B, Beyer K, et al. Outcome of double-blind, placebo-controlled food challenge tests in 107 children with atopic dermatitis. Clin Exp Allergy 1999;29(1):91–6.
74. Roerdink EM, Flokstra-de Blok BMJ, Blok JL, et al. Association of food allergy and atopic dermatitis exacerbations. Ann Allergy Asthma Immunol 2016; 116(4):334–8.
75. Czarnowicki T, Malajian D, Shemer A, et al. Skin-homing and systemic T-cell subsets show higher activation in atopic dermatitis versus psoriasis. J Allergy Clin Immunol 2015;136(1):208–11.
76. Tatsuno K, Fujiyama T, Yamaguchi H, et al. TSLP directly interacts with skin-homing Th2 cells highly expressing its receptor to enhance IL-4 production in atopic dermatitis. J Invest Dermatol 2015;135(12):3017–24.
77. Abernathy-Carver KJ, Sampson HA, Picker LJ, et al. Milk-induced eczema is associated with the expansion of T cells expressing cutaneous lymphocyte antigen. J Clin Invest 1995;95(2):913–8.
78. Reekers R, Beyer K, Niggemann B, et al. The role of circulating food antigen-specific lymphocytes in food allergic children with atopic dermatitis. Br J Dermatol 1996;135(6):935–41.
79. Werfel T, Ahlers G, Schmidt P, et al. Detection of a κ-casein-specific lymphocyte response in milk-responsive atopic dermatitis. Clin Exp Allergy 1996;26(12): 1380–6.
80. van Reijsen F, Felius A, Wauters EAK, et al. T-cell reactivity for a peanut-derived epitope in the skin of a young infant with atopic dermatitis. J Allergy Clin Immunol 1998;101(2):207–9.
81. Chan S, Turcanu V, Stephens A, et al. Cutaneous lymphocyte antigen and α4β7 T-lymphocyte responses are associated with peanut allergy and tolerance in children. Allergy 2012;67(3):336–42.
82. DeLong JH, Simpson KH, Wambre E, et al. Ara h 1–reactive T cells in individuals with peanut allergy. J Allergy Clin Immunol 2011;127(5):1211–8.e3.
83. Chatila TA, Blaeser F, Ho N, et al. JM2, encoding a fork head–related protein, is mutated in X-linked autoimmunity–allergic disregulation syndrome. J Clin Invest 2000;106(12):R75.
84. Torgerson TR, Linane A, Moes N, et al. Severe food allergy as a variant of IPEX syndrome caused by a deletion in a noncoding region of the FOXP3 gene. Gastroenterology 2007;132(5):1705–17.
85. Renner ED, Hartl D, Rylaarsdam S, et al. Comèl-Netherton syndrome defined as primary immunodeficiency. J Allergy Clin Immunol 2009;124(3):536–43.
86. Kusunoki T, Okafuji I, Yoshioka T, et al. SPINK5 polymorphism is associated with disease severity and food allergy in children with atopic dermatitis. J Allergy Clin Immunol 2005;115(3):636–8.
87. Kato A, Fukai K, Oiso N, et al. Association of SPINK5 gene polymorphisms with atopic dermatitis in the Japanese population. Br J Dermatol 2003;148(4):665–9.
88. Nishio Y, Noguchi E, Shibasaki M, et al. Association between polymorphisms in the SPINK5 gene and atopic dermatitis in the Japanese. Genes Immun 2003; 4(7):515–7.

89. Leung DYM. New insights into atopic dermatitis: role of skin barrier and immune dysregulation. Allergol Int 2013;62(2):151–61.

90. Fallon PG, Sasaki T, Sandilands A, et al. A homozygous frameshift mutation in the mouse FLG gene facilitates enhanced percutaneous allergen priming. Nat Genet 2009;41(5):602–8.

91. Sasaki T, Shiohama A, Kubo A, et al. A homozygous nonsense mutation in the gene for Tmem79, a component for the lamellar granule secretory system, produces spontaneous eczema in an experimental model of atopic dermatitis. J Allergy Clin Immunol 2013;132(5):1111–20.e4.

92. Saunders SP, Goh CS, Brown SJ, et al. Tmem79/Matt is the matted mouse gene and is a predisposing gene for atopic dermatitis in human subjects. J Allergy Clin Immunol 2013;132(5):1121–9.

93. Irvine AD, McLean WI, Leung DY. Filaggrin mutations associated with skin and allergic diseases. N Engl J Med 2011;365(14):1315–27.

94. Brown SJ, Irvine AD. Atopic eczema and the filaggrin story. Semin Cutan Med Surg 2008;27(2):128–37.

95. Lack G. Epidemiologic risks for food allergy. J Allergy Clin Immunol 2008; 121(6):1331–6.

96. Brown SJ, Asai Y, Cordell HJ, et al. Loss-of-function variants in the filaggrin gene are a significant risk factor for peanut allergy. J Allergy Clin Immunol 2011; 127(3):661–7.

97. Brough HA, Simpson A, Makinson K, et al. Peanut allergy: effect of environmental peanut exposure in children with filaggrin loss-of-function mutations. J Allergy Clin Immunol 2014;134(4):867–75.e1.

98. Brough HA, Liu AH, Sicherer S, et al. Atopic dermatitis increases the effect of exposure to peanut antigen in dust on peanut sensitization and likely peanut allergy. J Allergy Clin Immunol 2015;135(1):164–70.e1.

99. Thyssen JP, Tang L, Husemoen LLN, et al. Filaggrin gene mutations are not associated with food and aeroallergen sensitization without concomitant atopic dermatitis in adults. J Allergy Clin Immunol 2015;135(5):1375–8.e1.

100. Bartnikas LM, Gurish MF, Burton OT, et al. Epicutaneous sensitization results in IgE-dependent intestinal mast cell expansion and food-induced anaphylaxis. J Allergy Clin Immunol 2013;131(2):451–60.e1-6.

101. Spergel JM, Mizoguchi E, Brewer JP, et al. Epicutaneous sensitization with protein antigen induces localized allergic dermatitis and hyperresponsiveness to methacholine after single exposure to aerosolized antigen in mice. J Clin Invest 1998;101(8):1614.

102. Tordesillas L, Goswami R, Benedé S, et al. Skin exposure promotes a Th2-dependent sensitization to peanut allergens. J Clin Invest 2014;124(11): 4965–75.

103. Lowe AJ, Abramson MJ, Hosking CS, et al. The temporal sequence of allergic sensitization and onset of infantile eczema. Clin Exp Allergy 2007;37(4):536–42.

104. Jones AL, Curran-Everett D, Leung DYM. Food allergy is associated with Staphylococcus aureus colonization in children with atopic dermatitis. J Allergy Clin Immunol 2016;137(4):1247–8.e1-3.

105. Spergel JM, Beausoleil JL, Fiedler JM, et al. Correlation of initial food reactions to observed reactions on challenges. Ann Allergy Asthma Immunol 2004;92(2): 217–24.

106. Chang A, Robison R, Cai M, et al. Natural history of food-triggered atopic dermatitis and development of immediate reactions in children. J Allergy Clin Immunol Pract 2016;4(2):229–36.e1.

107. Bath-Hextall FJ, Delamere FM, Williams HC. Dietary exclusions for established atopic eczema. Cochrane Database Syst Rev 2008;(1):CD005203.
108. Lever R, MacDonald C, Waugh P, et al. Randomised controlled trial of advice on an egg exclusion diet in young children with atopic eczema and sensitivity to eggs. Pediatr Allergy Immunol 1998;9(1):13–9.
109. Atherton DJ, Soothill JF, Sewell M, et al. A double-blind controlled crossover trial of an antigen-avoidance diet in atopic eczema. Lancet 1978;311(8061):401–3.
110. Du Toit G, Katz Y, Sasieni P, et al. Early consumption of peanuts in infancy is associated with a low prevalence of peanut allergy. J Allergy Clin Immunol 2008;122(5):984–91.
111. Lack G. Update on risk factors for food allergy. J Allergy Clin Immunol 2012; 129(5):1187–97.
112. Du Toit G, Lack G. Can food allergy be prevented? The current evidence. Pediatr Clin North Am 2011;58(2):481–509.
113. Perkin MR, Logan K, Tseng A, et al. Randomized trial of introduction of allergenic foods in breast-fed infants. N Engl J Med 2016;374(18):1733–43.
114. Du Toit G, Roberts G, Sayre PH, et al. Randomized trial of peanut consumption in infants at risk for peanut allergy. N Engl J Med 2015;372(9):803–13.
115. Du Toit G, Sayre PH, Roberts G, et al. Effect of avoidance on peanut allergy after early peanut consumption. N Engl J Med 2016;374(15):1435–43.
116. Bergmann MM, Caubet J-C, Boguniewicz M, et al. Evaluation of food allergy in patients with atopic dermatitis. J Allergy Clin Immunol Pract 2013;1(1):22–8.
117. Schneider L, Tilles S, Lio P, et al. Atopic dermatitis: a practice parameter update 2012. J Allergy Clin Immunol 2013;131(2):295–9.e1-27.
118. Rancé F. Food allergy in children suffering from atopic eczema. Pediatr Allergy Immunol 2008;19(3):279–84.

Printed and bound by CPI Group (UK) Ltd, Croydon, CR0 4YY

07/10/2024

01040504-0006